a LANGE medical book

CURRENT
Diagnosis & Treatment in Sports Medicine

Edited by

Patrick J. McMahon, MD
McMahon Orthopedics & Rehabilitation
University of Pittsburgh
Pittsburgh, Pennsylvania

Lange Medical Books/McGraw-Hill
Medical Publishing Division

New York   Chicago   San Francisco   Lisbon   London   Madrid   Mexico City   Milan
New Delhi   San Juan   Seoul   Singapore   Sydney   Toronto

The *McGraw-Hill* Companies

Current Diagnosis & Treatment in Sports Medicine

1 2 3 4 5 6 7 8 9 0   DOC/DOC   0 9 8 7 6

ISBN 13: 978-0-07-141063-2
ISBN-10 : 0-07-141063-5
ISSN: 1931-8480

Notice

Medicine is an ever-changing science. AS new research and clinical experience broaden our knowledge, changes in treatment and drug therapy are required. The authors and the publisher of this work have checked with sources believed to be reliable in their efforts to provide information that is complete and generally in accord with the standards accepted at the time of publication. However, in view of the possibility of human error or changes in medical sciences, neither the authors nor the publisher nor any other party who has been involved in the preparation or publication of this work warrants that the information contained herein is in every respect accurate or complete, and they disclaim all responsibility for any errors or omissions or for the results obtained from use of the information contained in this work. Readers are encourage to confirm the information contained herein with other sources. For example and in particular, readers are advised to check product information sheet included in the package of each drug they plan to administer to be certain that the the information contained in this work is accurate and that changes have not been made in the recommended dose or in the contraindications for administration. This recommendation is of particular importance in connection with new or infrequently used drugs.

This book was set in Adobe Garamond by International Typesetting and Composition.
The editors were Harriet Lebowitz and Patrick Carr.
The production supervisor was Phil Galea.
The index was prepared by Michael Ferreira.

Cover design by Mary McKeon.
Cover photos: SPL/Photo Researchers, Inc. (upper left); John Lund/Getty Images (lower left); Neil Borden/Photo Researchers, Inc. (right).

RR Donnelley was printer and binder.

This book is printed on acid-free paper

To my father, William J. McMahon, MD

In memory of Kevin L. Armstrong, MD, for his outstanding patient care, easy smile, and laughter

Contents

Authors

Derek Armfield, MD
Assistant Professor, Divison of Musculoskeletal
   Radiology, University of Pittsburgh Medical Center,
   Pittsburgh, Pennsylvania
armfielddr@upmc.edu
Lower Leg, Ankle, & Foot Injuries

Michael W. Collins, PhD
Assistant Professor, Department of Orthopaedic
   Surgery; Assistant Director, UPMC Sports Concussion
   Program, University of Pittsburgh Medical Center,
   Pittsburgh, Pennsylvania
collinsmw@msx.upmc.edu
Concussion

Adam C. Crowl, MD
Fellow, Spine Surgery, University of Pittsburgh Medical
   Center, Pittsburgh, Pennsylvania
acrowl@adelphia.net
Spine

Hussein Elkousy, MD
Volunteer Clinical Faculty, University of Texas Health
   Sciences Center, Houston; Fondren Orthopedic
   Group, Houston, Texas
be50@fondren.com
Hip & Pelvis Problems

Frank Fumich, MD
Fellow, Spine Surgery, University of Pittsburgh Medical
   Center, Pittsburgh, Pennsylvania
Spine

Jan S. Grudziak, MD, PhD
Assistant Professor, University Of Pittsburgh;
   Department of Orthopedics, Children's Hospital of
   Pittsburgh, Pittsburgh, Pennsylvania
grudziakjs@upmc.edu
The Youth Athlete

Ranjan Gupta, MD
Assistant Professor, Hand & Upper Extremity Surgery,
   University of California, Irvine, Orange, California
ranjang@uci.edu
Elbow, Wrist, & Hand Injuries

Tanya J. Hagen, MD
Assistant Professor, Department of Orthopedics,
   University of Pittsburgh Medical Center; Associate
   Director, UPMC Sports Medicine Fellowship; Head
   Physician, Robert Morris University Athletics; Head
   Physician, Point Park University Athletics and Dance;
   Assistant Physician, university of Pittsburgh Athletics,
   Pittsburgh, Pennsylvania
hagentj@upmc.edu
Medical Aspects of Sports Medicine

Nicholas Honkamp, MD
Resident, Orthopedic Surgery, University of Wisconsin
   Department of Orthopedics and Rehabilitation,
   Madison, Wisconsin
Knee Injuries

James J. Irrgang, PhD, PT, ATC
Assistant Professor, University of Pittsburgh School of
   Health and Rehabilitation Sciences; Director, Clinical
   Research, UPMC Center for Sports Medicine; Vice
   President, Quality Improvement and Outcomes, Centers
   for Rehabilitation Services, Pittsburgh, Pennsylvania
irrgangjj@upmc.edu
Rehabilitation Principles

James D. Kang, MD
Associate Professor of Orthopaedic and Neuroscurgery;
   Vice Chairman, Department of Orthopedic Surgery,
   University of Pittsburgh, School of Medicine, Pittsburgh,
   Pennsylvania
kangjd@upmc.edu
Spine

Lee Kaplan, MD
Assistant Professor, Department of Orthopedics &
   Rehabilitation, University of Wisconsin; Orthopedic
   Surgeon, University of Wisconsin Sports Medicine
   Clinic, Madison, Wisconsin
kaplan@orthorehab.wisc.edu
Knee Injuries

Ryan Kehoe, MD
Resident, Orthopedic Surgery, University of Wisconsin
   Department of Orthopedics and Rehabilitation,
   Madison, Wisconsin
Knee Injuries

Christian Lattermann, MD
Visiting Clinical Instructor, University of Pittsburgh; Visiting Instructor, Orthopaedic Department, University of Pittsburgh Medical Center, Pittsburgh, Pennsylvania
Clattermann@gmail.com
Lower Leg, Ankle, & Foot Injuries

Patrick J. McMahon, MD
McMahon Orthopedics & Rehabilitation, University of Pittsburgh, Pittsburgh, Pennsylvania
mcmahonp@upmc.edu
Shoulder & Knee Injuries

Volker Musahl, MD
Resident, Department of Orthopaedic Surgery, University of Pittsburgh Medical Center, Pittsburgh, Pennsylvania
vmusahl@hotmail.com
The Youth Athlete

Jamie E. Pardini, PhD
Instructor, Department of Orthopaedic Surgery, University of Pittsburgh Medical Center; Neuropsychology Fellow, University of Pittsburgh Sports Medicine Concussion Program, Pittsburgh, Pennsylvania
Concussion

Alexandre Rasouli, MD
Resident, Orthopaedic Surgery, University of California, Irvine, Orange, California
rasouli@uci.edu
Elbow, Wrist, & Hand Injuries

Tara M. Ridge, MS, PT, SCS
Senior Physical Therapist, Centers for Rehabilitation Services, University of Pittsburgh Medical Center, Pittsburgh, Pennsylvania
ridgetm@upmc.edu
Rehabilitation Principles

Shane Seroyer, MD
Resident, Orthopedic Surgery, University of Pittsburgh Medical Center, Pittsburgh, Pennsylvania
serost@upmc.edu
Injuries Specific to the Female Athlete

Gregory Stocks, MD
Fondren Orthopaedic Group, Houston, Texas
stocks@fondren.com
Hip & Pelvis Problems

Jennifer Swanson, DPT
Physical Therapist, Centers for Rehabilitation Services, University of Pittsburgh Medical Center, Pittsburgh, Pennsylvania
swansonjb@upmc.edu
Rehabilitation Principles

Jonathon Tueting, MD
Resident, Orthopedic Surgery, Department of Orthopedics and Rehabilitation, University of Wisconsin, Madison, Wisconsin
Knee Injuries

Armando F. Vidal, MD
Blue Sky Orthopedics & Sports Medicine, Brighton, Colorado
Shoulder Injuries

Leslie S. Beasley Vidal, MD
Denver Orthopedics & Sports Medicine, Denver, Colorado
lesliebvidal@hotmail.com
Shoulder Injuries

Robin West, MD
Assistant Professor, University of Pittsburgh; Head Team Physician, University of Pittsburgh Men's Basketball, Carnegie Mellon University; Assistant Team Physician, Pittsburgh Steelers, Pittsburgh, Pennsylvania
westrv@upmc.edu
Injuries Specific to the Female Athlete

Dane K. Wukich, MD
Assistant Professor of Orthopaedic Surgery; Chief, Division of Foot Ankle, University of Pittsburgh School of Medicine, Pittsburgh, Pennsylvania
wukichdk@upmc.edu
Lower Leg, Ankle, & Foot Injuries

Preface

Current Diagnosis & Treatment in Sports Medicine is an easy-to-read reference for all clinicians involved in the care of athletes—the weekend warrior as well as the elite athlete. Physicians, physical therapists, athletic trainers, and nurses will find information on, not only musculoskeletal injuries, but also important medical conditions. Knowledge in all of these areas is valuable in keeping the athlete healthy and performing best.

Each chapter is organized in a straightforward and consistent style to promote quick comprehension. A guide for pre-participation and on-the-field evaluation of the athlete is presented first. Medical and musculoskeletal conditions, which are the topics of the subsequent chapters, are organized by body part from the lower extremity to the upper extremity and spine. Specific information affecting female athletes and the latest data in treating concussions follow. The final chapter presents rehabilitation principles for preventing injury and returning the athlete to play after injury.

Outstanding Features

- An easy-to-read, complete text that can be carried to the office, training room, and field of play
- A straightforward and consistent organizational style throughout the book
- Evidence-based recommendations
- Numerous figures and tables for easy comprehension
- Complete evaluation and management of musculoskeletal injuries of the extremities and spine
- Nonoperative and operative therapies
- Specifics for the female athlete
- The latest data in treating and preventing concussions
- Rehabilitation principles to prevent injury and return the athlete to play after injury

Intended Audience

All clinicians caring for athletes, including physicians, physical therapists, athletic trainers, and nurses will find this text a useful resource. Written for those in training, it is an excellent resource for practicing clinicians as well. Numerous figures and detailed information in both tabular and text forms provide a ready reference for evaluation, selecting diagnostic procedures, and management.

Unlike larger manuals that sit on a shelf and are used only as a reference, this book is compact enough to be carried to the office, training room, and the field of play. In addition, its easy readability makes it possible to read in its entirety.

Acknowledgments

I would like to acknowledge all those, including patients, who have taught me that while medicine is a science, its practice is an art. I am also grateful to the staff at McGraw-Hill, especially Harriet Lebowitz and Hilarie Surrena, for their professionalism and dedication. Most importantly, I thank my family for educating and encouraging me and God, who is my strength.

Patrick J. McMahon, MD

Medical Aspects of Sports Medicine

Tanya J. Hagen, MD

MEDICAL BENEFITS OF EXERCISE & PARTICIPATION IN SPORTS

A continuously growing body of evidence indicates that regular physical activity is associated with dramatic reductions in cardiac events and all-cause mortality. Despite this, there are an estimated 200,000 deaths annually in the United States related to sedentary lifestyle. In addition to the well-known cardiovascular benefits, improvements in social, mental, and other aspects of physical wellness with sports participation and exercise have been documented. Some of these benefits are listed in Table 1–1.

As more and more research reveals the tremendous benefits of exercise, physicians are expected to encourage and even prescribe physical activity to their patients. With this, they must be aware not only of the potential injuries associated with sports and exercise involvement, but also of the potential medical issues pertinent to each patient and specific to particular sports. It is important to note that all medical issues are of potential concern in an active population. Therefore, the goals of this chapter are to provide an introduction to some medical issues that (1) can be associated with significant morbidity and/or mortality in an active population (eg, arrhythmias related to acute chest trauma or congenital cardiac disease), (2) are very common in general (eg, diabetes mellitus), or (3) may be unique to physically active individuals (eg, exercise-associated asthma).

PREPARTICIPATION EVALUATION

In the 2002–2003 school year in the United States there were 6.9 million high school athletes and over 375,000 National Collegiate Athletic Association (NCAA) athletes participating in school-sponsored sports programs, and these numbers are steadily increasing. The American Heart Association, the American Medical Society for Sports Medicine, the American Academy of Family Practice, the American Orthopedic Society for Sports Medicine, and other health and sports organizations have made recommendations regarding the usefulness of a preparticipation evaluation (PPE). Despite the large number of athletes, the above recommendations, and decades of history, the structure, the appropriate content, and even the overall utility of the PPE are still under debate.

The goals of the PPE come from many perspectives (athlete, school, preventive health care, safety, legal issues, etc). These goals include (1) screening for life-threatening illness or injury that would preclude participation in sports; (2) identifying medical or musculoskeletal conditions that could predispose the athlete to further problems or could limit the athlete's performance; (3) collecting baseline data such as medical history, allergies, and vital signs, and in some cases neuropsychological testing, body composition measurements, and other components that can be referred to if the need arises; (4) providing what is often the only exposure of young healthy individuals to the healthcare system with education on issues such as smoking, sexually transmitted diseases (STDs), and supplement use; and (5) meeting organizational or state/school requirements for legal and/or insurance reasons.

Although the exact structure of the evaluation varies between organizations, all are based on a good history and physical examination (Figure 1–1). It has been shown that the history is the most important component of the PPE, often providing clues to issues that require further investigation. The history should include not only the basics (past medical history, family history, medications, allergies), but also a detailed review of systems and a questionnaire regarding symptoms that could raise concern for a particular problem, for example, increased risk of concussion, disordered eating, or exercise-induced asthma. A positive screening question should then prompt a more detailed, targeted history and examination in that area of concern. Although few conditions preclude sports participation completely, the examiner must be aware of these. The conditions of most concern are those that increase the risk of sudden cardiac death. Although the cardiovascular benefits of physical activity and participation in sports are well

Preparticipation physical evaluation

History

Date of exam _____

Name _____ Sex _____ Age _____ Date of birth _____

Grade _____ School _____ Sport(s) _____

Address _____

Personal physician _____ Phone _____

In case of emergency, contact

Name _____ Relationship _____ Phone (H) _____ (W) _____

Explain "Yes" answers below.
Circle questions you don't know the answers to.

	Yes	No
1. Have you had a medical illness or injury since your last check up or sports physical?	☐	☐
Do you have an ongoing or chronic illness?	☐	☐
2. Have you ever been hospitalized overnight?	☐	☐
Have you ever had surgery?	☐	☐
3. Are you currently taking any prescription or nonprescription (over-the-counter) medications or pills or using an inhaler?	☐	☐
Have you ever taken any supplements or vitamins to help you gain or lose weight or improve your performance?	☐	☐
4. Do you have any allergies (for example, to pollen, medicine, food, or stinging insects)?	☐	☐
Have you ever had a rash or hives develop during or after exercise?	☐	☐

	Yes	No
10. Do you use any special protective or corrective equipment or devices that aren't usually used for your sport or position (for example, knee brace, special neck roll, foot orthotics, retainer on your teeth, hearing aid)?	☐	☐
11. Have you had any problems with your eyes or vision?	☐	☐
Do you wear glasses, contacts, or protective eyewear?	☐	☐
12. Have you ever had a sprain, strain, or swelling after injury?	☐	☐
Have you broken or fractured any bones or dislocated any joints?	☐	☐
Have you had any other problems with pain or swelling in muscles, tendons, bones, or joints?	☐	☐
If yes, check appropriate box and explain below		
☐ Head ☐ Elbow ☐ Hip		
☐ Neck ☐ Forearm ☐ Thigh		

Figure 1–1. **Sample preparticipation history and physical examination.** (Source: Leawood KS. American Academy of Family Physicians, American Academy of Pediatrics, American Medical Society for Sports Medicine, American Orthopaedic Society for Sports Medicine, American Osteopathic Academy of Sports Medicine, 1992, 1996.)

5. Have you ever passed out during or after exercise?
   Have you ever been dizzy during or after exercise?
   Have you ever had chest pain during or after exercise?
   Do you get tired more quickly than your friends do during exercise?
   Have you ever had racing of your heart or skipped heartbeats?
   Have you had high blood pressure or high cholesterol?
   Have you ever been told you have a heart murmur?
   Has any family member or relative died of heart problems or of sudden death before age 50?
   Have you had a severe viral infection (for example, myocarditis or mononucleosis) within the last month?
   Has a physician ever denied or restricted your participation in sports for any heart problems?
6. Do you have any current skin problems (for example, itching, rashes, acne, warts, fungus, or blisters)?
7. Have you ever had a head injury or concussion?
   Have you ever been knocked out, become unconscious, or lost your memory?
   Have you ever had a seizure?
   Do you have frequent or severe headaches?
   Have you ever had numbness or tingling in your arms, hands, legs, or feet?
   Have you ever had a stinger, burner, or pinched nerve?
8. Have you ever become ill from exercising in the heat?
9. Do you cough, wheeze, or have trouble breathing during or after activity?
   Do you have asthma?
   Do you have seasonal allergies that require medical treatment?

☐ Back ☐ Wrist ☐ Knee
☐ Chest ☐ Hand ☐ Shin/calf
☐ Shoulder ☐ Finger ☐ Ankle
☐ Upper arm ☐ Foot

13. Do you want to weigh more or less than you do now?
    Do you lose weight regularly to meet weight requirements for your sport?
14. Do you feel stressed out?
15. Record the dates of your most recent immunizations (shots) for:
    Tetanus _____ Measles _____
    Hepatitis B _____ Chickenpox _____

Females only
16. When was your first menstrual period?
    When was your most recent menstrual period?
    How much time do you usually have from the start of one period to the start of another?
    How many periods have you had in the last year?
    What was the longest time between periods in the last year?

Explain "Yes" answers here:

I hereby state that, to the best of my knowledge, my answers to the above questions are complete and correct.

_____ Signature of athlete   _____ Signature of parent/guardian   _____ Date

Figure 1–1. (Continued)

3

Preparticipation physical evaluation

Physical examination

Name _____ Date of birth _____

Height _____ Weight _____ % Body fat (optional) _____ Pulse _____ BP ____/____/ (____/____, ____/____)

Vision R 20/ _____ L 20/ _____ Corrected: Y N   Pupils: Equal _____ Unequal _____

	Normal	Abnormal findings	Initials*
Medical			
Appearance			
Eyes/ears/nose/throat			
Lymph nodes			
Heart			
Pulses			
Lungs			
Abdomen			
Genitalia (males only)			
Skin			
Musculoskeletal			
Neck			
Back			
Shoulder/arm			
Elbow/forearm			
Wrist/hand			
Hip/thigh			
Knee			
Leg/ankle			
Foot			

*Station-based examination only

Clearance

☐ Cleared
☐ Cleared after completing evaluation/rehabilitation for: _____
_____
_____
_____

☐ Not cleared for: _____ Reason: _____
Recommendations _____
_____
_____
_____

Name of physician (print/type) _____ Date _____
Address _____ Phone _____
Signature of physician _____ MD or DO

Figure 1–1. (Continued)

Table 1–1. Potential benefits of regular physical activity.

Decreased all-cause mortality
Decreased risk of coronary disease, cardiac events, and death
Improved control of blood pressure
Slowed progression of early carotid atherosclerosis and reduction in risk of stroke
Improved lipid profile and control of obesity
Improved glycemic control and prevention of type II diabetes mellitus
Improved overall function in patients with certain chronic illnesses (cardiopulmonary, rheumatologic, cancer, etc)
Improved bone mineral density and decreased long-term risk of osteoporosis and fractures
Improved immunity
Modest protection against breast and other cancers
Decreased disability, improved cognitive function, and increased autonomy in elders
Decreased "risky" behavior (in adolescent females) including drug use, smoking, and unwanted pregnancy
Improved self-image, self-esteem, and overall mental health
Decreased health-related costs

known, participation carries a small but real risk of a serious cardiovascular event. The yearly incidence of sudden cardiac death in young athletes (<35 years of age) is quite small (approximately 1/100,000) but is nevertheless devastating. In this group, the majority of deaths are not caused by coronary artery disease as in an older population, but rather by a group of congenital and acquired conditions. Many of the cardiac and non-cardiac conditions that should preclude participation in high-intensity sports are listed in Table 1–2.

The physical examination portion of the PPE should then be performed by a clinician trained and experienced in a general medical, cardiovascular, and musculoskeletal examination. This is an opportunity to expand on issues raised by the history and to identify new potential problems. The cardiovascular examination should, at minimum, include auscultation in supine and standing positions. Occasionally, an irregular murmur or other abnormality can be identified. Unfortunately, even a thorough history and a cardiac examination are limited in terms of

sensitivity for detecting risk of sudden cardiac death. Despite this, an echocardiogram and/or stress testing are not routinely recommended unless the history or physical examination dictates. Although there is still much debate among "expert panels" and health organizations, electrocardiogram (EKG) testing is not uniformly recommended as part of the PPE. Currently, the American Heart Association and the American College of Cardiology do not recommend a routine EKG for athletes less than 35 years of age. The International Olympic Committee Medical Commission recommends EKGs every other year, and the recent 36th Bethesda Conference report states the following: the EKG "may be of use in the diagnosis of cardiovascular disease in young athletes and it has been promoted as a practical and cost-effective strategic alternative to routine echo."

If there is no previous history of injury, a general musculoskeletal screening examination is usually adequate. In the case of previous injury, an expanded examination of the affected area can identify risk factors for further injury or need for further rehabilitation. A targeted examination may also be performed on sport- or position-specific areas (eg, the dominant shoulder of a baseball pitcher) to increase sensitivity. In the majority of cases the musculoskeletal examination does not result in disqualification but clearly adds to the goals of safe participation and optimization of performance.

Armsey TD, Hosey RG: Medical aspects of sports: epidemiology of injuries, preparticipation physical examination, and drugs in sports. Clinics Sports Med 2004;23(2):255.

Garrick JG: Preparticipation orthopedic screening evaluation. Clin J Sports Med 2004;14(3):123.

Maron BJ, Zipes DP: 36th Bethesda Conference: eligibility recommendations for competitive athletes with cardiovascular abnormalities. J Am Coll Cardiol 2005;45(8):1313.

Wingfield K et al: Preparticipation evaluation, an evidence based review. Clin J Sports Med 2004;14(3):109.

THE ATHLETE "DOWN"

Acute Medical Issues & Injuries

Sideline physicians must have a "disaster plan" in place for the possibility of a catastrophic injury or event. Knowledge of the potential hazards of the competition can be very helpful. Ideally, the sideline physician is familiar with the players and their individual risks, the athletic trainers and coaches, as well as any emergency medical service (EMS) personnel covering the event. A disaster plan should include who to call, which hospital to use, and who would be in charge. Disaster protocol begins with an immediate on-field evaluation to determine the extent of injury and the urgency of the event. In the case of a persistently unconscious or otherwise unstable athlete, initiation of basic life support should begin and EMS should be activated early.

Table 1–2. Contraindications to participation in sports.

Symptomatic hypertrophic cardiomyopathy
Modest to severe aortic stenosis (and other significant valvular disease)
Modest to severe coarctation of the aorta
Symptomatic mitral valve prolapse
Long-QT syndrome, Wolff—Parkinson—White syndrome
Ventricular dysrhythmias
Symptomatic atrioventricular block
Infective carditis
Uncontrolled hypertension
Marfan's disease (with cardiac and valvular involvement)
Sickle cell disease
Uncontrolled asthma
Active tuberculosis
Pulmonary insufficiency with exercise-induced deoxygenation
Recurrent pneumothorax
Uncontrolled seizure disorder
Continued symptoms and/or cognitive deficits postconcussion

Adapted from the 36th Bethesda Conference, 2005, American Heart Association and American Academy of Pediatrics guidelines.

Collapsed or Unconscious Athlete

Loss of consciousness in the athlete is most commonly the result of trauma, but heat illness, neurologic conditions, metabolic disorders, and hypoxia can also cause a severe change in mental status. Initial evaluation begins with the "ABCs" familiar to all clinicians: *A*irway, *B*reathing, and *C*irculation. The possibility of a cervical spine injury should be assumed and appropriate precautions must be taken in every case. In a helmeted and padded athlete (eg, football player), the helmet should be left in place to avoid neck hyperextension. All medical personnel should know the on-field location of screwdrivers or clippers used to remove the facemask.

Injuries that pose an immediate threat to life require emergent treatment followed by transport to a hospital. These include respiratory and cardiac arrest. Other injuries that require urgent care include seizures, severe head, neck, and back injuries, uncontrolled hemorrhage, facial injuries, burns, heat stroke, hypothermia, near drowning, and severe

musculoskeletal trauma. Recognition and initial treatment for some of these conditions are discussed below. Also discussed are some injuries that although not particularly "life threatening," require relatively urgent treatment for optimal outcome (eg, dental injury).

Acute Pulmonary Issues

A. Respiratory Arrest

Airway obstruction can occur with aspiration of a foreign body (tooth, mouthpiece), direct neck trauma and deformation (eg, laryngeal fracture), or, more commonly, secondary to swelling and edema; or it may simply be due to relaxed oropharyngeal muscles in the supine, unconscious athlete. Maintenance of the airway is the primary concern for the physician and must be addressed immediately, preferably with a jaw thrust maneuver to avoid exacerbation of possible associated cervical spine injury. If this maneuver is unsuccessful, an emergency tracheostomy is indicated with emergent transfer to the nearest hospital. Respiratory arrest can also be the result of an acute asthma attack or anaphylaxis. Athletes with asthma and known severe allergies should be identified during the preparticipation physical. Treatment of both includes inhaled albuterol, 0.3–0.5 mL of 1:1000 epinephrine injected subcutaneously (Epi-pen), support with 100% oxygen (and intubation depending on the patient's condition), and immediate transport. Intravenous fluids should be initiated in the person with anaphylaxis because of the risk of cardiovascular collapse. Acute pulmonary edema in an athlete at high altitude can rapidly progress to respiratory arrest and is discussed later in this chapter.

B. Thoracic Trauma

Pulmonary contusions occur from compression of the air-filled lung, producing increasing pressure and tearing of the parenchyma. Often examination is unrevealing (although occasionally rales will be present), and because of this, a minor injury can go undetected. An athlete who presents with hemoptysis and pain, however, must be evaluated further and closely monitored, as rapid progression to acute respiratory distress syndrome (ARDS) and respiratory collapse may occur. Chest radiographs may reveal consolidation or nodular densities, but can take hours to develop and often underestimate the severity of the lesion. Computed tomography (CT) of the chest is more sensitive and should be used for diagnosis.

Pneumothorax may occur spontaneously or secondary to chest trauma. The athlete typically presents with unilateral chest pain, tachypnea, and dyspnea. Physical examination reveals hyperresonance and diminished or absent breath sounds on the affected side. Often symptoms can initially be mild and physical examination not be obvious. Because of this, all athletes with chest trauma must be monitored closely for increasing problems. Tension pneumothorax, presenting with cyanosis and tracheal deviation, is a potential complication and may result in vascular compromise and hypotension. If this occurs, insertion of a large-bore needle into the second intercostal space of the anterior thorax may be life saving.

Acute Cardiovascular Issues

A. CARDIAC INJURY

Myocardial contusion is a serious complication of severe blunt trauma to the chest, presenting most often with nonspecific chest pain and sinus tachycardia. Other arrhythmias, an S3 gallop, a pericardial friction rub, and pulmonary rales may be present. An echocardiogram is the diagnostic test of choice to evaluate for wall motion abnormality and pericardial effusion. An EKG may reveal conduction abnormalities, ST changes, and/or T wave inversions. Serial enzymes (CK-MB and troponin I) can also help with the diagnosis. Most athletes with myocardial contusion have complete recovery, but occasionally, ventricular dysfunction, thrombus, or other complications can result. A normal EKG and enzymes have a reliable negative predictive value for further complications. The athlete should not return to activity for several months until the echocardiogram has normalized; chest protection is then recommended.

B. SUDDEN CARDIAC DEATH

Commotio cordis is a very rare, but dramatic event defined as sudden collapse and cardiac arrest following blunt chest trauma. Up to two-thirds of the cases are seen in baseball and are the result of precordial ball impact. Adolescents and children are believed to be at higher risk because of increased chest wall compliance. Prevention is aimed at improved protection, particularly in high-risk positions such as a baseball catcher and a hockey goalie. The etiology of sudden cardiac death in this setting is likely ventricular fibrillation or acute bradycardia; thus, although no intervention to date has shown benefit, prompt recognition, cardiopulmonary resuscitation (CPR), and electroshock with an on-field automatic cardiac defibrillator could prove valuable. Causes of sudden cardiac death are listed in Table 1–3.

Sudden death in the athlete is in general a very rare yet devastating occurrence. Cardiovascular causes predominate (85% of 158 athlete deaths in the United States from 1985 to 1995). The most common cause is hypertrophic cardiomyopathy (HCM), which accounts for approximately 36% of the total sudden cardiac deaths in athletes. HCM is an inherited disease of the sarcomere that causes a hypertrophied, nondilated left ventricle. The clinical course is highly variable, with some patients remaining asymptomatic throughout their lives and others developing severe symptoms of heart failure or premature death. The clinical presentation may include dyspnea, angina, arrhythmia, or syncope, but sudden death during vigorous exercise, without antecedent

Table 1–3. Causes of sudden cardiac death in athletes.

Cardiomyopathies: hypertrophic cardiomyopathy, dilated cardiomyopathy, myocarditis, arrhythmogenic right ventricular dysplasia
Congenital malformation of coronary arteries
Coronary artery disease
Aortic rupture: Marfan's disease, coarctation of the aorta
Valvular heart disease: aortic stenosis, mitral valve prolapse
Arrhythmias: Wolff—Parkinson—White syndrome, long-QT syndrome, idiopathic ventricular tachycardia
Commotio cordis
Drugs and "supplements": anabolic steroids, amphetamines, cocaine, Ma Huang, Ephedra

symptoms, is often seen in children and young adults. Routine cardiac screening is unreliable in detecting HCM and risk of sudden cardiac death. On physical examination, a harsh, mid-systolic crescendo–decrescendo murmur that increases with decreased preload (eg, valsalva) may indicate HCM, but this is not present in many cases. An EKG may indicate left ventricular hypertrophy (LVH), left atrial enlargement (LAE), and/or conduction abnormalities, but is often normal. Diagnosis is made by echocardiogram, usually revealing asymmetric LVH >15 mm. It is important to note that persons under 15 years of age with HCM may not yet manifest significant hypertrophy and therefore the diagnosis can be missed. Also, echocardiogram alone does not reliably predict risk of sudden death. Eligibility for participation in sports may be judged on a case-by-case basis keeping in mind the risk factors listed in Table 1–4. In most athletes with HCM, competitive sports should be prohibited.

Congenital coronary artery anomalies are the second most common cause of sudden cardiac death in young athletes (<30 years). Athletes with congenital coronary artery anomalies are often asymptomatic, but may experience syncope or chest discomfort. Evaluation for exercise-induced myocardial ischemia is indicated for athletes suspected of having such an anomaly. If ischemia is found, athletic participation must be restricted and surgery should be considered. Return to competition can be considered in athletes who have had successful surgical repair and a documented absence of exercise-induced ischemia.

Myocardial ischemia secondary to atherosclerotic coronary artery disease is the most common cause of

Table 1–4. Risk factors for sudden death in patients with hypertrophic cardiomyopathy.

Ventricular tachycardia
Family history of sudden cardiac death due to hypertrophic cardiomyopathy
Syncope
Severe hemodynamic abnormalities (dynamic left ventricular outflow tract gradient >50 mm Hg, exercise-induced hypotension, moderate-to-severe mitral regurgitation)
Enlarged left atrium (>50 mm)
Paroxysmal atrial fibrillation
Abnormal myocardial perfusion

exercise-related sudden death in persons over 30 years of age. Most of these athletes have abnormal risk profiles (hypercholesterolemia, diabetes mellitus, a family history of cardiac disease, tobacco use) and often have prodromal chest pain. In any collapsed "masters" athlete, myocardial infarct should be suspected. Symptoms are similar to those presenting in nonathletes and include chest pain or tightness, diaphoresis, nausea, dyspnea, and a feeling of impending doom. Acute management includes O_2, Aspirin, nitroglycerin, Emergency Medical Services (EMS) activation, and transport to decrease morbidity and mortality. Immediate EKG monitoring and treatment of arrhythmia in the field with CPR and an automatic cardiac defibrillator can be life saving. Clinicians should be prepared for this scenario when possible. It is important to note that absence of symptoms in highly fit individuals does not guarantee that they are coronary artery disease free. Because of this, testing is recommended in patients with risk factors. Participation in high-intensity competitive sports is not recommended for athletes with documented ischemic disease, regardless of whether the patient has symptoms, has a history of myocardial infarction, or has undergone complete revascularization. Lower intensity activities may be permitted, but each athlete requires individual evaluation and assessment of risk.

Seizure

Seizure in the athlete is often the result of a closed head injury (ie, concussion), but can be primary or related to other illness. Secondary causes include heat illness, dehydration, and hyponatremia. Metabolic disorders, structural disease, and previous trauma with development of a subacute bleed should also be considered. Airway and cervical spine management is of utmost importance. Transport to stabilize the patient-athlete and to ensure

that no significant brain injury has occurred should follow. There will be further discussion on seizure in the athlete later in this chapter.

Head & Neck Injuries

Concussion, discussed in Chapter 8, is a common cause of change in mental status in the athlete. The most serious and most common complications include intracranial hemorrhage and associated spinal injury. Any concern for acute bleed as suggested by persistent altered mental status, focal neurologic findings, or severe headache and other signs of increased intracranial pressure should prompt immediate transport for further evaluation and imaging. A CT scan is a more rapid test in the potentially unstable patient, but magnetic resonance imaging (MRI) has been shown to have better sensitivity and specificity and should be considered after negative CT in the athlete who continues to have findings that are of concern. MRI is also appropriate when an athlete has subacute complaints or physical findings. Once severe associated injury is ruled out, the traumatic brain injury itself must be monitored closely.

Spinal injury should always be assumed in the "down athlete." The annual incidence of traumatic spinal cord injury is estimated to be between 30 and 45 cases/1,000,000. The majority result from motor vehicle accidents, but 5–14% occur during sports and recreational activities. Unsupervised diving accounts for 75% of these injuries, but in the United States the risk is highest in supervised sports, such as football, gymnastics, and hockey, in descending order. Once the adequate ABCs have been established, and the cervical spine is immobilized in neutral (eg, with the helmet and pads in place in football players), a thorough history and a neck and neurologic examination are necessary. Radiologic imaging (anteroposterior, lateral, and odontoid views or CT scan) is necessary when the history and physical examination are either inconclusive or of concern. Indications are listed in Table 1–5.

Table 1–5. Indications for radiologic evaluation in the athlete with possible neck injury.

High-risk mechanism of injury
Multiple trauma and/or distracting injures that do not allow for appropriate evaluation of the spine
Altered mental status and/or poor cooperation with the examination
Pain on the top of the head
Neck pain, tenderness, or deformity
Limitation of neck movement
Acute neurologic deficit

After acute musculoskeletal neck injury, contraindications to return to play include permanent dysfunction, permanent and significant peripheral nerve root dysfunction, and spinal fusion above the C5 level. In addition, stability, as assessed with dynamic radiographs, helps to dictate whether return to play is appropriate in cases of fracture and ligamentous injury. It is generally believed that athletes with cervical burners (transient brachial plexus injury) may return to play when completely asymptomatic. Return to play for athletes who have cervical cord neuropraxia (transient quadriplegia) remains controversial.

Facial Injuries

A. ORBITAL TRAUMA

The most common sports-related eye injuries are "black eye" (edema/ecchymosis), corneal abrasions, foreign bodies, and lacerations in and around the eyelid. More severe injuries that require urgent specialized evaluation and treatment include lacerations to the globe, commotio retinae (edema of the retina) and retinal hemorrhage, hyphema, and orbital blow-out fractures. Danger signs are listed in Table 1–6. Sports with a very high risk for eye injury include boxing, wrestling, and full-contact martial arts, but hockey, basketball, baseball, softball, racquet sports, and others also carry a relatively high risk. The functionally one-eyed athlete should not participate in very high-risk sports, but may participate in most other sports with the appropriate (3-mm thick polycarbonate lenses), well-fitted, protective eyewear.

B. DENTAL TRAUMA

Dental injuries such as tooth avulsions, fractures, and impactions are not uncommon from sports-related trauma. Tooth avulsion is considered a dental emergency as time

Table 1–6. Signs and symptoms of potential serious eye injury.

Acutely decreased vision or loss of field of vision (complete or partial)
Pain with eye movement
Photophobia
Diplopia
"Lightning flashes"
Halos around lights
Eye protrusion or "sunken" eye
Irregularly shaped pupil
Blood in the anterior chamber or a "red eye"

is of the essence to preserve function. The contaminated tooth should be gently rinsed and reinserted (assuming the athlete is conscious), with immediate referral to a dentist for splinting and antibiotic prophylaxis. Chances of retaining the tooth after avulsion diminish rapidly with delays in reinserting the tooth. If immediate on-scene reimplantation is not possible, the tooth should be transported in the patient's buccal sulcus, in milk, or in a specialized tooth solution. Fractures limited to the enamel may not require immediate treatment, but dental follow-up is necessary and complete diagnosis for a dental injury should include radiographs at some point. In many cases of facial injury, the airway can be rapidly compromised and needs to be constantly reassessed. Additionally, concussion frequently accompanies significant facial and dental injury and should be considered in all such cases.

Acute Gastrointestinal & Genitourinary Problems

A. ABDOMINAL & PELVIC TRAUMA

Abdominal and pelvic injuries, although not extremely common in sports participation, can be serious, can cause severe blood loss, and can lead to hypovolemic shock. The liver and spleen are the most commonly injured organs, followed by the pancreas, bowel, kidney, bladder, and blood vessels. Signs of significant injury include abdominal tenderness, rigidity and rebound, hematuria, and hypotension. When any of these signs are present, urgent transport for further imaging and patient-athlete stabilization and treatment are warranted.

B. HEMATURIA

Major renal trauma will often cause acute pain, but may present with delayed bleeding. Evaluation by ultrasound, CT scan, and/or intravenous pyelogram (IVP) is necessary as this often requires surgical intervention. Minor renal trauma usually presents with hematuria alone. If bleeding is mild, history, physical examination, and urinalysis are usually adequate, with return to play after 2–3 weeks of relative rest. Renal calculi cause painful hematuria and occur in 12% of men and 5% of women, making kidney stones a relatively common issue in both athletes and the general population. Dehydration can increase the risk of calculi, but in general, athletes are not considered to be at increased risk overall.

A common cause of painless hematuria in athletes who run is believed to be secondary to mild bladder wall trauma. The incidence of this "runners hematuria" is between 17% and 69%, with the highest incidence in ultramarathon runners. Hematuria may also arise from the perineal trauma experienced in bicycle, motocross, and recreational cyclists. Athletic pseudonephritis is a combination of hematuria, proteinuria, and casts secondary to nephron ischemia and hypoxia. It can be seen in high-intensity runners and swimmers. These sports-related hematurias tend to clear after 48 hours. In cases of persistent bleeding, medical conditions such as carcinoma, von Willebrandís disease, and sickle cell disease should be considered.

C. RHABDOMYOLYSIS

Rhabdomyolysis is a condition of significant muscle breakdown leading to renal impairment. The typical cause is heat illness and dehydration, but underlying metabolic issues and supplement or alcohol use can be contributing factors. The athlete may present with "on field collapse" from severe muscle pain or the causative heat illness, but usually the presentation is subacute and will need to be evaluated with blood work that includes creatine phosphokinase (CPK), blood urea nitrogen (BUN), and creatinine as well as a urinalysis that includes myoglobin.

D. TESTICULAR TORSION

Testicular torsion is a medical urgency that should not be missed. It presents with unilateral pain and swelling that is exacerbated by lifting the testes above the pubic symphasis. (This is in contrast to epididymitis, in which pain is relieved by this maneuver.) If diagnosis by examination is uncertain, an ultrasound or testicular scan (90% accurate) should be performed. Derotation can be attempted by turning the testes anteriorly and away from midline. If unsuccessful, surgical treatment within 4 hours provides better outcomes.

Musculoskeletal Injuries

"Collapse" of an athlete on the field is often the result of a musculoskeletal injury. The most common injuries and their evaluation and management are covered in other chapters in this book. Musculoskeletal injuries that can pose an immediate risk to the athlete are discussed here.

A. OPEN FRACTURES

Open fractures should be splinted in the position found after a sterile dressing has been placed. Urgent transport is necessary for definitive treatment.

B. DISLOCATIONS

Hip or knee dislocations can cause significant vascular injury, as can posterior sternoclavicular dislocations. Because of this, athletes with these injuries should be urgently transported to a hospital emergency department that has the ability to evaluate such problems. In the case of a joint dislocation with neurovascular compromise, a person with proper training should attempt reduction. Neurovascular status must be checked and documented before and after successful (or attempted) reduction. All reductions should have follow-up radiographs to rule out associated fracture in addition to further evaluation (eg, vascular) as necessary.

Environmental Issues

A. HEAT ILLNESS

Exertional heat syndromes form a continuum: heat stress → heat cramps → heat exhaustion → heat stroke → death (Table 1–7). Heat dissipation (ie, removal of heat) occurs by four methods: radiation, conduction, convection, and evaporation. If the environmental temperature is greater than 35°C (95°F), all heat loss must be through evaporation. Humidity of greater than 75% slows evaporation dramatically and sweating becomes inefficient. The body loses no heat when a temperature of greater than 35°C is combined with a humidity greater than 90%. Thermoregulation is under the control of the autonomic nervous system via the anterior hypothalamus. Thermoregulation failure, which can occur when there is no heat dissipation, can eventually lead to multiple organ system collapse and death. Factors that increase the risk of heat illness include vigorous physical activity, impermeable or wet clothing, poor muscle conditioning, lack of acclimation, obesity, extremes of age, diuretic beverages and supplements, or medications that affect the autonomic nervous system (eg, stimulants, anticholinergics, and α-adrenergics such as decongestants). It is important to note that heat illness and dehydration go hand in hand. Exertional heat syndromes can be prevented with adequate hydration in addition to education regarding dangerous environmental conditions (wet bulb globe temperature greater than 19°C), use of proper clothing and equipment, acclimation, and gradual physical conditioning.

B. COLD INJURIES

Cold-related injuries are most often associated with winter sports such as skiing, skating, and mountaineering, but can also be seen in other sports such as running, cycling, and swimming. Body heat is produced by four mechanisms: basal heat production is via normal metabolic processes, muscular thermoregulatory heat is produced by shivering and increases body heat three to five times basal level, increased muscular activity during mild to moderate exercise produces five times basal heat production, and high-intensity exercise can produce up to 10 times basal heat but can be sustained for only several minutes. Mechanisms of heat loss have been mentioned previously. To avoid illness and injury, the core temperature must be maintained within a narrow range. Heat conservation occurs by external sources, body insulation, and shunting of blood away from the body's surface area to the core (via peripheral vasoconstriction).

Medical problems that can be stimulated by cold exposure include cold-induced asthma or bronchoconstriction, cold urticaria, and Raynaud's phenomenon. Local cold injury ranges from mild frostnip to the much more severe injury, frostbite. Frostnip is reversible ice

Table 1–7. Continuum of exertional heat syndromes.

	Predominant Pathophysiology	Core Temperature	Symptoms	Treatment
Heat stress	Increased temperature	Normal	Increased blood pressure and heart rate, dizziness, fatigue	Mild cooling, oral hydration
Heat cramps	Total body Na$^+$ deficiency (predominant theory)	Normal	Increased heart rate, muscle cramps/spasm, weakness, fatigue, nausea/vomiting	Mild cooling, oral hydration with electrolyte solution (IV if vomiting), gentle stretching, ice
Heat exhaustion	Hypovolemia Dehydration Electrolyte loss	Normal to 40°C (104°F)	Orthostasis, syncope, dyspnea, weakness, profuse sweating, flushing and piloerection, headache, and irritability No significant central nervous system dysfunction	Moderate cooling, (move to cool environment, remove excess clothing, water and fans), oral versus IV hydration (depends on ability to take water PO)
Heat stroke	Hyperthermia Thermoregulatory failure	>40°C Poor prognosis with temperature >42°C	Change in mental status, +/– seizure and coma Hypotension, vomiting, diarrhea, sweating → hot, dry skin Can rapidly progress to rhabdomyolysis, neurologic injury, kidney and liver failure, diffuse intravascular dissemination, acute respiratory distress syndrome, death	Rapid cooling to core temperature 39°C (with the above methods + ice packs/bath), IV fluid challenge (monitor for pulmonary/cerebral edema), respiratory assistance and O$_2$, urgent transport

crystal formation on the skin's surface that is treated with gradual rewarming. Frostbite is caused by actual freezing of the skin and is classified as first to fourth degree based on the depth of soft tissue involvement. Factors that increase risk of frostbite include constricting clothing, smoking, atherosclerosis, diabetes mellitus, immobilization, and use of vasoconstrictive drugs. In severe injury, bullae or dry black eschar will form in previously waxy yellow or mottled blue areas, signifying that the tissue will eventually be lost. At extremes, mummification and autoamputation can occur. Treatment is aimed at prevention of further tissue damage. Rapid rewarming in a hot bath at 40°C is appropriate treatment, but only if there is a mechanism to maintain warmth, as thawing and refreezing result in increased injury. Dry heat and rubbing the affected areas are contraindications. Most cases require hospitalization and analgesic support.

Hypothermia is a potentially life-threatening systemic injury that occurs when the body core temperature decreases to less than 35°C (95°F) and is classified as mild, moderate, and severe. Symptoms progress from shivering, chills, and increased respiratory rate, to increased fatigue, loss of shivering, and peripheral numbness, and eventually to changing levels of consciousness. At core temperatures less than 90°F, respiratory rate, blood pressure, and pulse are depressed, and there is significant danger of pulmonary edema and fatal cardiac arrhythmia. Treatment is active rewarming with intravenous fluids, warmed peritoneal dialysis, etc under close monitoring. Prevention is through attention to nutrition and hydration needs, appropriate windproof and insulated layered clothing, avoidance of getting wet, and abstinence from alcohol.

C. Altitude Sickness

There is significant physiologic stress placed on the body when adapting to the lower barometric pressures and resultant hypoxia at high altitude (Table 1–8). Syndromes of high-altitude sickness are essentially maladaptations to this physiologic stress and range from mild, acute mountain sickness (AMS) to severe high-altitude pulmonary edema (HAPE) and high-altitude cerebral edema (HACE).

Armsey TD, Hosey RG: Medical aspects of sports: epidemiology of injuries, preparticipation physical examination, and drugs in sports. Clinics Sports Med 2004;23(2):255.

Lausanne Convention: Sudden cardiac death in sport. Lausanne, Switzerland, December 9–10, 2004.Maron BJ, Zipes DP: 36th Bethesda Conference: eligibility recommendations for competitive athletes with cardiovascular abnormalities. J Am Coll Cardiol 2005;45(8):1313.

Truitt J: Pulmonary disorders and exercise. Clinics Sports Med 2003;22(1).

Wexler RK: Evaluation and treatment of heat related illness. Am Fam Phys 2002;65(11):2307.

NONEMERGENT & CHRONIC MEDICAL ISSUES

Neurologic Disorders

A. Headache

Headaches are a common complaint in the general population as well as in the athlete. Specific exercises and sports-related headaches that must be considered in athletes are listed in Table 1–9.

Additionally, typical migraine, sinus, and tension headaches can be aggravated or induced by activity. In an athlete, a headache not only can impair performance, but may signal a more significant underlying medical problem and thus complaints should be taken seriously. Headache management can pose a challenge in this population because of side effects as well as restrictions on drug use by governing bodies. The workup for the athlete with headache starts with a detailed history and physical examination. The initial interview should include a search for a previous history of headaches as well as causative and precipitating factors. The physical examination should rule out neurologic deficits, cervical spine issues, and other contributing factors of concern. If an athlete presents with acute onset of severe headache, or if the headache is brought on by exertion, further workup is warranted. Findings of particular concern are shown in Table 1–10.

Exertional headaches occur in 12% of the general population and in up to 50% of athletes. Although most are benign in origin, studies show a 10–40% association with underlying illness that includes intracranial mass, bleeds, and other significant pathology. A thorough investigation, often including blood work and imaging, is necessary when an obvious precipitating factor cannot be determined. A diagnosis of "benign exertional headache" can be made once organic disease and inciting factors other than exertion have been ruled out. The initial treatment is usually indocin. Ergots and triptans are also effective, but their use may be limited because of untoward side effects in the athletic population. An athlete with headaches may return to full activity once underlying disease is ruled out and the pain is adequately controlled.

B. Epilepsy

Seizures, caused by an abnormal paroxysmal neuronal discharge in the brain, are relatively common in the general population (with a lifetime risk of 10% and 1–2% having a diagnosis of epilepsy). The prevalence in active individuals and specifically athletes has not been well studied. Trauma (ie, closed head injury) can cause transient seizure activity, but there is no evidence that this increases the overall risk of developing a chronic seizure disorder. Other factors associated with participation in sports can cause seizures and/or aggravate an underlying disorder, but the relative risk is believed to be low. Aerobic exercise has been shown, overall, to decrease seizure frequency, but it can also, at times, exacerbate a condition. Historically, seizure excluded people from participation in sports, but experience has dictated a more moderate approach in recent years. Current recommendations encourage physical activity and, in general, support involvement in athletics provided the seizure disorder is under adequate control. In counseling patients, the type of activity is clearly an important issue.

Table 1–8. High-altitude illness syndromes.

Syndrome[1]	Severity	Course	Altitude (feet)	Signs and Symptoms	Treatment and Prevention
AMS	Mild; self-limited	Very mild brain edema that occurs in the first 2–36 hours of arrival at moderate altitude	7,000–10,000	Mild to moderate headache, loss of appetite, lethargy, nausea, vomiting	Symptoms abate at the same altitude in 1–2 days without treatment Watch for worsening symptoms Prevent by slow ascent and/or acetazolamide (125 mg bid)
APE	With rapid treatment, all patients recover, but can rarely progress to death	Pulmonary edema, with onset at 2–4 days. Often preceded by AMS	>10,000	Dry cough, SOB, decreased exercise tolerance, hypoxemia leads to increased dyspnea, frothy pink sputum, and death (if untreated)	Treat with low flow O_2 when available and descent by 2000–3000 feet (if descent is not possible, a hyperbaric bag can temporize) Patient may be able to reascend once symptoms clear Prevent by slow ascent and/or nifedipine XL (30 mg qid)
ACE	Can be rapid in onset and fatal, but with acute treatment, most fully recover	Brain edema— severe end of AMS spectrum May occur with HAPE	>12,000	Severe headache, changes in mental status, ataxia, tachycardia, tachypnea	Treat with immediate descent, O_2, dexamethasone (10 mg IM followed by 4 mg PO qid) Patient cannot reascend Prevent with slow ascent

[1] AMS, acute mountain sickness; HAPE, high-altitude pulmonary edema; HACE, high-altitude cerebral edema.

Table 1–9. Differential diagnosis of exercise-related headaches.

Increased intracranial pressure
Traumatic: postconcussive, maxillofacial trauma
Metabolic: overtraining, hypoglycemia, anemia, acute mountain sickness, barotrauma (scuba diving), exercise-induced asthma
Muscle tension: temporomandibular joint, C-spine degenerative joint disease/strain, facet syndrome, postural (cycling, wrestling)
Equipment related: goggle headache, occipital neuralgia (overtight headgear)
Depression
Eye strain
Analgesic rebound
Benign exertional headache

Some groups recommend restrictions for certain sports, including sky diving, mountain climbing, and scuba diving, because of the potential for disaster should the athlete seize during the activity. Other cases of seizure and sports participation need to be evaluated on a case-by-case basis.

Pulmonary Disorders

A. Asthma

Asthma is characterized by airway obstruction (bronchospasm), inflammation, and hyperresponsiveness to stimuli such as allergens, chemicals, viral infections,

Table 1–10. Headache "red flags."

Severe headache reaches maximal intensity within a few seconds or minutes
"First or worst"
Preceding infection
Rapid onset after trauma or with exercise, cough, or sexual activity
Associated neck/shoulder pain
Change in mental status, personality, or level of consciousness
Focal neurologic signs and symptoms (with or without other signs of increased intracranial pressure, focal or infectious lesion)

cold air, or exercise. It affects approximately 10 million people in the United States. Once a contraindication to athletic participation, today, asthma should not prohibit participation in sports, with scuba diving as the exception, if adequate treatments are used.

Exercise-induced asthma (EIA) typically occurs 5–10 minutes following, but may occur during, strenuous exercise and usually resolves spontaneously within 20–30 minutes. Attacks are rarely life-threatening. Up to 20% of high-school athletes and up to 10% of world class athletes have been diagnosed with EIA. Although some athletes report wheezing, symptoms can vary widely and are often nonspecific, such as cough, shortness of breath, and chest tightness after exertion. Diagnosis is made by history and examination and with pulmonary function testing that reveals a decrease by at least 15% in forced expiratory volume in 1 second (FEV_1) after a free running challenge. Methacholine challenge testing is more sensitive than a running or ergometry challenge, but has a much lower specificity for EIA. Treatment of asthma and EIA should be individualized, but initial therapy is almost always with inhaled β-agonists. It should be noted that oral, long-acting β-agonists are banned by the NCAA and International Olympic Committee. Other pharmacologic treatments for prevention of attacks may include other bronchodilators (ie, anticholinergics) and antiinflammatories (glucocorticoids, khellin derivatives such as cromolyn, and leukotriene antagonists). Nonpharmacologic treatment can be useful in some cases. Approximately 50% of athletes with EIA are able to induce a "refractory period" following either 3–4 minutes of high-intensity exercise or about 1 hour of low-intensity warm-up. Although aerobic training may have some preventive benefit, there is no way to predict whether a person will be able to induce a refractory period or not.

B. Chronic Obstructive Disease

Exercise in patients with chronic obstructive pulmonary disease, chronic bronchitis, and cystic fibrosis has been shown to decrease dyspnea and fatigue and to increase endurance and overall quality of life. Patients with mild to moderate disease should be allowed to participate in athletics based on severity of symptoms. In patients with chronic obstructive pulmonary disease, care should be taken when environmental conditions can increase airway reactivity, specifically cold and windy or hot and humid conditions. Those with cystic fibrosis lose more sodium and chloride in their sweat and therefore need to be counseled about proper hydration practices in the heat.

Cardiovascular Disorders

A. Hypertension

Hypertension is the most common cardiovascular condition in adults, affecting over 50 million people in the United States. Cardiovascular endurance and resistance exercise programs have been shown to have beneficial effects on hypertension of all levels and in general should be encouraged. Despite a lack of evidence for increased risk of sudden death or even of end-organ damage, persons with severe hypertension are believed to require limitation of activity, primarily from sports with high static demands. There are no limitations of activity for athletes with mild and moderate hypertension. In a newly diagnosed athlete, a thorough evaluation, including history, physical examination, EKG, and blood work (for evidence of target organ damage), is appropriate. Exercise stress testing in all patients over the age of 35 years with hypertension (even in the absence of other cardiac risk factors) has been recommended, but the utility of this is debatable. Further evaluation may be necessary if a secondary cause is suspected.

Antihypertensive treatment should be implemented in athletes with the goal of minimizing organ damage just as in a nonathletic population, but many of the more commonly used medications can affect performance and may not be well tolerated. Diuretics may lead to dehydration and hypokalemia, especially in endurance athletes. β-Blockers may produce fatigue and decreased exercise tolerance. Both diuretics and β-blockers are banned by the International Olympic Committee. Angiotensin-converting enzyme (ACE) inhibitors and calcium channel blockers tend to be well tolerated and efficacious and should be considered first-line therapy in most athletes unless accompanying medical issues dictate otherwise.

B. Valvular and Congenital Disease

In an athlete with valvular or congenital disease, recommendations for participation in competitive sports are based on several factors including type and severity of lesion, ventricular function, presence of arrhythmias or altered hemodynamics, and presence of other cardiac abnormalities. Recommendations that have been set by the 36th Bethesda Conference are not based on precise information, but nonetheless are believed to follow prudent judgment. In general, full participation should be allowed in athletes with mild, asymptomatic disease. In the setting of mitral valve prolapse, mild stenosis (aortic, mitral, pulmonic), or mild to moderate regurgitation, it should be demonstrated that the athlete has normal exercise tolerance and no signs of ventricular enlargement, abnormal ventricular function, or arrhythmias before full clearance. Persons with small septal defects (atrial or ventricular), or those with small patent ductus arteriosus, can participate without restriction when there is no accompanying pulmonary hypertension, arrhythmias, or evidence of myocardial dysfunction. Athletes who have more significant disorders must be evaluated on an individual basis.

C. Arrhythmias

Arrhythmias that can potentially lead to sudden cardiac death, such as Wolff–Parkinson–White (WPW) and long-QT syndrome, have already been discussed briefly, but it is important to note that there are many cardiac arrhythmias that pose little if any threat to the athlete and therefore should not limit activity. Marked sinus bradycardia, first-degree and type I second-degree (Wenckebach type) atrioventricular (AV) block, and uniform premature ventricular contractions occur frequently in healthy athletes, often directly related to their conditioning. These individuals nonetheless require evaluation and periodic follow-up. The type and complexity of an arrhythmia, the presence of structural heart disease, associated ventricular dysfunction or ischemia, and the response of the arrhythmia to exercise determine its significance. A full evaluation of and recommendations for specific arrhythmias, which are beyond the scope of this chapter, can be referenced in the 36th Bethesda Conference report.

Endocrine Disorders

A. Diabetes Mellitus

Diabetes mellitus, characterized by relative or absolute insulin deficiency, is extremely common in the general population, affecting approximately 17 million people in the United States (1 million with type I and 16 million with type II). Most patients with diabetes mellitus can safely exercise and even participate in elite level competitive sports. Adequate glucose control is extremely important to minimize risk and optimize performance. Although it is recommended that athletes with diabetes with complications such as nephropathy, neuropathy, and retinopathy refrain from certain high-intensity sports, in general, regular physical activity should be encouraged. In addition to the desirable affects seen in nondiabetics, this population often sees even more profound improvements in overall well being, weight control, lipid profile, and other cardiac risks. Improved glycemic control leads to a reduction in microvascular complications, diabetes-related deaths, and all-cause mortality (35%, 25%, and 7% reduction, respectively, for each percentage point reduction in hemoglobin (Hgb)A_{IC}. This is usually the result of moderate caloric restriction and regular exercise, and is enhanced by exercise-induced weight loss and resultant improved insulin sensitivity.

The benefits of regular exercise can be dramatic, but there are serious risks as well. The major risks for most athletes with diabetes involve complications in metabolic control, specifically hypoglycemia. Hypoglycemia can occur during or after exercise if caloric intake and/or medications have not been properly adjusted. Patients on insulin or sulfonylureas tend to be at higher risk for this complication. Symptoms of hypoglycemia are variable, but often include dizziness, weakness, blurred vision, confusion, diaphoresis, nausea, cool skin, and/or parasthesias of the tongue or hands. Recommendations for minimizing the risk of hypoglycemia in the active individual are listed in Table 1–11.

Table 1–11. Minimizing hypoglycemic risk.[1]

Closely monitor glucose levels before, during, and after activity

Daily morning exercise (as opposed to sporadic exercise) facilitates medication and caloric adjustments

Ensure immediate access to glucose (oral carbohydrates or SQ/IM 1 mg glucagon injection) if necessary

Adjust medications/food intake

    Insulin adjustments before exercise

        Avoid insulin injection into exercising extremity—abdomen is preferred site

        Decrease short-acting insulin based on planned minutes of exercise as follows: decrease dose by 30% for <60 minutes, by 40% for 60–90 minutes, and by 50% for >90 minutes of planned exercise; intense exercise may require even further reductions

        Decrease intermediate insulin (neutral protamine Hagedorn; NPH) by one-third (33%)

        Consider using Lispro (faster onset, shorter duration)

        For insulin pumps, decrease basal rate by 50% 1–3 hours before and during exercise

        If exercise is planned immediately after a meal, reduce premeal bolus by 50%

    Food intake adjustment

        Eat a well-balanced meal 2–3 hours prior to exercise

        Take a carbohydrate snack just before exercise if glucose is <100 (15 g of carbohydrates raises glucose approximately 50 mg/dL)

        Eat 30–60 g carbohydrate/hour of activity (when >1 hour)

        Maintain adequate hydration

---

[1] Note that these are general recommendations. Each patient-athlete needs individualized assessment and adjustments.

Delayed-onset hypoglycemia often occurs at night, 6–15 hours after exercise and therefore can potentially be even more dangerous. It is usually brought on by inadequate replenishment of glycogen stores immediately after exercise and in the ensuing hours. Delayed-onset hypoglycemia may develop as long as 30 hours after exercise, reflecting continued exercise-heightened insulin sensitivity with increases in glucose uptake and glycogen synthesis in skeletal muscle. Glycogen is repleated more slowly in liver than in muscle, so carbohydrate requirements may be increased for up to 24 hours after prolonged exercise.

Hyperglycemia is also a potential danger secondary to increased hepatic glucose production. This is seen with a rise in counterregulatory hormones: epinephrine, norepinephrine, glucagon, cortisol, and growth hormone. Diabetic ketoacidosis can result in patients with insulin-dependent diabetes and hyperosmolar coma can result in those with non-insulin-dependent diabetes mellitus.

Because of these risks, exercise should be avoided if glucose levels are greater than 250 mg/dL and ketosis is present. In the absence of ketosis, exercise may be allowed with glucose levels greater than 300 mg/dL, but extreme caution is recommended. Because of the significant cardiovascular risk associated with diabetes mellitus, physicians must have a heightened awareness of issues in this population and potentially a lower threshold for cardiac screening. The American Diabetes Association recommends exercise stress testing if moderate to high-intensity activity is planned in patients with any of the conditions listed in Table 1–12.

Finally, foot problems can be a major issue in active patients with diabetes. Although a full discussion of these foot problems will not be included here, it is important to mention them as a great source of morbidity. It is imperative that physicians working with patients with diabetes and promoting active life-styles must also educate patients regarding proper shoes that fit well, have a wide enough toe box, and cushioned mid-sole, moisture-wicking socks, and appropriate foot hygiene to avoid problems.

B. THYROID DISORDERS

Although they rarely limit athletic participation, thyroid disorders are quite common, affecting approximately 5% of the general population. Hypothyroidism results from insufficient thyroid hormone secretion and presents with

Table 1–12. American Diabetes Association recommendations for exercise stress testing.

Age >35 years

Diabetes mellitus I >15 years duration

Diabetes mellitus II >10 years duration

Known coronary artery disease

Additional coronary artery disease risk factors (hypertension, tobacco use, family history, cholesterol)

Presence of microvascular disease

Peripheral vascular disease

Autonomic neuropathy

---

decreased exercise tolerance, lethargy, muscle ache, constipation, and intolerance to cold. It may also be part of a syndrome of proximal muscle weakness and fatigue with elevated CPK levels that may initially be confused with rhabdomyolysis. Hyperthyroidism causes hypermetabolism due to excessive hormone secretion. Patient-athletes complain of tremors, nervousness, palpitations, fatigue, proximal muscle weakness, and intolerance to heat. Women may present with oligo/amenorrhea. Diagnosis of a thyroid disorder is made by laboratory history, physical examination, and laboratory testing for thyroid-stimulating hormone (TSH) and thyroxine (T_4). Hypothyroidism is treated with hormone replacement. Hyperthyroidism is treated with antithyroid medications, radioactive iodine, or surgery. The effects of exercise on thyroid function are not clear, therefore, guidelines for return to play after treatment have not been established. In general, there are no absolute restrictions, but the athlete should be medically stable and able to tolerate the intensity of exercise demanded by the sport. It may be prudent to require several weeks of a persistent euthyroid state, especially in patients who have suffered cardiac manifestations, before allowing progression to intense activity. The athlete should then be followed clinically and through laboratory testing on a regular basis.

Gastrointestinal Problems

Gastrointestinal problems are common in the general population and up to 60% of competitive athletes complain of symptoms. The problems vary widely according to the specific sport, condition of the athlete, level of intensity, and other factors.

A. Nausea and Vomiting

Nausea and vomiting are frequent occurrences in athletes. They are very common in athletes who simply exceed their exertional capacity, but can also be seen with anxiety, heat illness, hypoglycemia, head injury, and other significant issues. In females, pregnancy should be considered. In the absence of other etiology, treatment consists of rest and rehydration (occasionally with intravenous fluids if the athlete is unable to take fluids orally). In some extreme cases antiemetics (compazine, tigan, thorazine) are useful adjuncts.

B. Gastroesophageal Reflux Disease

Studies have shown that vigorous exercise can induce gastroesophageal reflux disease (GERD) even in normal subjects. Running and swimming seem to cause the majority of the problems related to esophageal sphincter relaxation. Although there are no good studies on the treatment of exercise-related GERD, it is accepted that most young people with symptoms such as belching, heartburn, and regurgitation can be treated without further diagnostic

workup. The initial treatment consists of limiting food intake in the several hours preceding exercise, avoiding foods that delay gastric emptying (fatty foods), and using non-magnesium-containing antacids. If this is unsuccessful, H2 blockers should be used; proton pump inhibitors may be necessary in refractory cases. Individuals who have persistent problems, or those who experience abnormal symptoms such as dysphagia or weight loss, must be evaluated with further diagnostic studies.

C. Abdominal "Stitch"

Transient, sharp, subcostal pain, referred to as a "stitch," is well known by athletes. It is an entity of unclear etiology, possibly attributed to gas, ischemia, or muscle spasm. It is most often experienced by runners, is exacerbated by deep breathing, and is decreased by rest. Frequency tends to decline with endurance training and does not typically require further investigation unless pain persists.

D. "Runner's Diarrhea"

Among endurance athletes, cramps, urgency, diarrhea, and incontinence are some of the most common and bothersome of symptoms experienced. It is speculated that the repetitive jarring of foot-strike during running may stimulate mass movements in the colon. This "runner's diarrhea" often occurs during or immediately following high-intensity exertion. Initial management is dietary adjustment (eg, limiting high-lactose and high-fructose foods). If non-exercise-related causes (infection, irritable bowel disease, malabsorption, cancer) are ruled out and dietary changes are ineffective, use of a prophylactic antidiarrheal 1 hour prior to activity can be considered.

E. Gastrointestinal Bleeding

Although it has been shown that up to 20% of marathon runners have occult blood in their stools following competition, gastrointestinal (GI) bleeding is in general relatively uncommon in otherwise healthy athletes. Positive guiac testing in endurance athletes has been thought, in many cases, to be related to use of nonsteroidal antiinflammatory drugs, but there are no studies to date showing a correlation. Other theories include GI ischemia secondary to decreased splanchnic blood flow and simple biomechanical trauma from repetitive jarring during running. Most cases are self-limited, but athletes with GI bleeding should, nonetheless, be considered for further medical evaluation to rule out pathologic causes.

Genitourinary Issues

A. Chronic Renal Failure

Research regarding chronic renal disease and exercise has not been at the forefront (in contradiction to cardiac, pulmonary, and neurologic issues). Despite the lack of aggressive prospective trials, there have been many studies suggesting improvement in gait speed, strength, muscle mass, hematocrit, and overall function in patients with chronic renal failure who participate in regular physical activity. This is believed to be particularly important in the preservation of muscle mass for those on a low-protein diet. Although there are significant obstacles in many patients including anemia, severe muscle fatigue (with vitamin D deficiency and secondary hypoparathyroidism, androgen abnormalities), and steroid myopathies, dramatic benefits from strength and aerobic training have been obtained by patients who are predialysis, on chronic dialysis, and even posttransplant. It is therefore routinely recommended that these patients engage in a low-to-moderate intensity regular workout program keeping individual limitations in mind.

B. SINGLE-ORGAN ATHLETE

The overall risk of losing a kidney due to contact sports is very low, but nonetheless, a major consideration in competitive athletes with one functional kidney. Current recommendations are that these athletes avoid all collision sports. Limited-contact sports are felt to be safe if the solitary kidney is normal in anatomy and function. Protective equipment (eg, a flak jacket) may improve this safety even further and, when appropriate, should be used. The athlete with one abnormal kidney (pelvic, multicystic), however, should likely be precluded from contact sports. In the athlete with a single testicle, most contact and collision sports are felt to be safe if a protective cup is worn. In all cases of single organs, proper education regarding risks is imperative.

Infectious Diseases

A. UPPER RESPIRATORY INFECTION

Acute infections are associated with a variety of immune system responses that are triggered by cytokines and are correlated with fever, muscle pain, fatigue, and anorexia, along with other signs and symptoms. Acute viral and bacterial illness can potentially hinder exercise ability by affecting multiple body systems, including cardiopulmonary function, fluid status, and temperature regulation. Current recommendations regarding exercise and participation in sports follow a "neck check" approach. Because of potentially detrimental effects, patient-athletes with symptoms "below the neck" (ie, fever, chills, chest congestion, ongoing diarrhea, or nausea/vomiting) should refrain from intense exercise. However, in patient-athletes with has symptoms only "above the neck" (ie, nasal congestion, sore throat), continued participation in sports as tolerated is reasonable. Because no research offers clear evidence-based guidelines regarding exercise during viral infections, degree and manifestation of illness, as well as type of sport, intensity of training, potential risk of spreading disease, and other factors, should be considered in each case.

B. MYOCARDITIS

Myocarditis is an inflammatory condition of the myocardial wall most commonly caused by coxsackievirus B infection. It is a rare cause of sudden cardiac death in athletes. The typical clinical picture consists of fatigue, chest pain, dyspnea, and, occasionally, palpitations. There are no accurate predictors of risk of sudden death in patients with myocarditis, but because of the potential, the 26th Bethesda Conference guidelines take a conservative stance, recommending withdrawal from all competitive sports for about 6 months. Before returning to competition, the athlete should demonstrate normal ventricular function and dimensions on echocardiography and no signs of arrhythmia with ambulatory monitoring.

C. MONONUCLEOSIS

Infectious mononucleosis is caused by the Epstein–Barr virus and is typically characterized by fatigue, sore throat, tonsillar enlargement, lymphadenopathy, and splenomegaly. Activities are often self-restricted because of severe malaise and inability to perform hard physical exertion. The literature suggests that athletes may begin a noncontact exercise program as soon as they become afebrile without detrimental effects. Splenic involvement with mononucleosis and potential rupture are the primary concerns for most clinicians. Rupture occurs in 0.1–0.5% of cases. The majority are spontaneous and occur within the first 3 weeks from onset of illness when there is profuse lymphocytic infiltration putting the spleen in an enlarged and "fragile" state. There are no clear guidelines on whether to use palpation or an imaging technique (eg, ultrasound) to determine splenic size and therefore presumptive risk of rupture. Although it is well documented that palpation alone has a low sensitivity for splenic enlargement, return to play decisions are based on the ability to palpate the organ, implying that the rib cage can adequately protect even an enlarged spleen. Again, there is no evidence for or against this assumption. Although there have been only a few cases of splenic rupture associated with participation in sports reported in the literature, a prudent course is still recommended, particularly within the first few weeks of illness. The American Academy of Pediatricians recommends that a patient with an acutely enlarged spleen should avoid all sports and that a patient-athlete with a chronically enlarged spleen needs individual assessment before participation.

D. HEPATITIS

Viral hepatitis can present as a broad spectrum of clinical syndromes ranging from asymptomatic to fulminant and fatal. Common symptoms of acute infection include fatigue, myalgia, arthralgias, anorexia, and nausea. Liver dysfunction compromises energy availability during exercise by predisposing the patient to hypoglycemia and by altering lipid metabolism. Other physiologic disturbances include hormonal imbalances and coagulopathy.

Exercise can significantly alter liver hemodynamics, theoretically increasing the risk of complications. Although it is recommended that extreme exercise and competition be avoided until liver tests normalize and hepatomegaly resolves, available data suggest that moderate exercise and participation in sports can be safely permitted as tolerated, guided by the clinical condition of the patient-athlete with acute viral hepatitis.

E. HUMAN IMMUNODEFICIENCY VIRUS (HIV)

HIV is a chronic disease with a variable course and most infected persons will have years of a healthy life. Most HIV-infected patients are asymptomatic carriers, but the illness as well as the medications used to treat the retrovirus can cause dramatic fatigue and other problems that affect performance. There is no evidence that exercise is dangerous to the HIV-positive athlete and moderate activity may even improve overall immune function to a degree (in addition to the multiple other physiologic and psychological benefits) and should be encouraged. The decision to continue to play a sport must be made on a case-by-case basis, keeping in mind the patientís current state of health, the type of activity, and the potential for HIV transmission to others.

In general, the risk of transmission of HIV and hepatitis in the majority of sports is extremely low, such that currently, most agree that infection alone is insufficient to prohibit athletic competition. That said, there certainly are both medical and ethical questions to be answered regarding the potential increased risk of transmission in high-risk sports such as wrestling, boxing, and martial arts. It is, of course, of the utmost importance that confidentiality be maintained in all cases and that "universal precautions" be taken in dealing with any athlete.

Rheumatologic Disease

Many medical conditions can mimic traumatic and overuse musculoskeletal injuries. A full discussion of rheumatologic issues is beyond the scope of this chapter, but orthopedists and sports medicine physicians should be familiar with the differential diagnosis of polyarthropathies as listed in Table 1–13 to provide complete care for their patients. When there is a known rheumatologic diagnosis, exercise and participation in sports are not usually contraindicated, but there may be some limitations because of pain or other associated disease manifestations such as cardiac, pulmonary, or renal issues. Numerous studies have revealed the overwhelming benefits of exercise in patients with problems such as osteoarthritis, spondyloarthropathy (eg, ankylosing spondylitis), lupus (systemic lupus erythematosus), and rheumatoid arthritis. In general, a low-impact exercise and weight-training regimen should be recommended. Counseling regarding more intense exercise

Table 1–13. Major causes of polyarthritis.

Osteoarthritis
Crystal-induced arthropathy
Infectious arthritis: Lyme, bacterial endocarditis, viral illness
Seronegative spondyloarthropathies: reactive arthritis (enteric infection, rheumatic fever, Reiter's syndrome), ankylosing spondylitis, psoriatic arthritis, inflammatory bowel disease (IBD)
Systemic rheumatic illness: rheumatoid arthritis, systemic lupus erythematosus, vasculitis, sclerosis, poly/dermatomyositis, Still's disease, Behçet syndrome, relapsing polychondritis
Other systemic illnesses: sarcoidosis, malignancy, familial Mediterranean fever

and participation in sports needs to be done on a case-by-case basis.

Hematologic Issues

A. ANEMIA

Anemia is defined as a "decrease in red blood cell count or hemoglobin." This is caused by either decreased production, increased destruction/sequestration by the spleen, or by blood loss. The prevalence of anemia in the general population is estimated to be 2.5%. The true prevalence in athletes is unknown (Table 1–14). The clinical consequence of anemia in the athlete is a decreased O_2-carrying capacity that can lead to problems with endurance and fatigue, with decreased performance, and often increased risk of injury. A dilutional effect is the most common cause of low hemoglobin in athletes, but is not a true anemia. Iron deficiency is the most common cause of true anemia. These and other common etiologies, with their differentiating laboratory findings and treatments, are outlined in Table 1–14. The approach to the athlete with anemia begins with a thorough history and examination, evaluating for symptoms and signs of systemic illness, blood loss, disordered eating, and changes in training. Many anemias may be multifactorial, thus all contributing factors should be addressed. In general, an athlete's activity does not need to be limited unless the anemia is severe or the underlying illness is a contraindication to participation in sports (eg, acute mononucleosis infection).

B. SICKLE CELL DISEASE

Sickle cell disease is a genetic disorder affecting red blood cell (RBC) shape and flexibility that leads to

Table 1–14. Common anemias in athletes.[1]

Anemia	Causes	Laboratory	Treatment
Dilutional	Not a true anemia Secondary to plasma volume expansion that is proportional to amount and intensity of exercise	Normocytic Hgb: mildly decreased RBC mass, MCV, Fe: all normal	No treatment necessary To differentiate from other causes: Hgb will normalize with rest for 3–4 days
Iron deficiency	Nutritional (rarely) or second to blood loss from gastritis/ colitis (in endurance athletes or NSAID induced), menses, with low iron intake, or hematuria (trauma or renal tubular ischemia)	Microcytic, hypochromic Hgb, MCV, Fe: low (Fe <25)	Evaluate for underlying factors and address as necessary Supplementation with $FeSO_4$
Nutritional	B_{12} and folate deficiencies	Macrocytic (secondary to B_{12} and folate deficiency) Hgb low, Fe normal, MCV high	Consider medical conditions unrelated to exercise (inflammatory bowel disease, pancreatic insufficiency, etc)
	Anorexia	Anorexia often produces a normocytic anemia via an unknown mechanism	Supplementation and nutritional counseling as necessary
Hemolysis	Premature RBC destruction because of increased fragility (multifactorial: increased temperatures, "foot strike," etc) Inherited/ acquired causes of RBC fragility can be exacerbated (eg G6PD deficiency)	Mild macrocytic anemia MCV high, Fe normal, reticulocytes high, haptoglobin low	Treatment is aimed at reducing forces associated with footstrike (surface, intensity, technique, shoe wear)

[1] Hgb, hemoglobin; RBC, red blood cell; MCV, mean cell volume; G6PD, glucose 6-phosphate dehydrogenase; NSAID, nonsteroidal antiinflammatory drug.

aggregation and "sludging" within blood vessels and subsequent tissue ischemia. A person who carries both alleles (a homozygote) is at increased risk of sudden death and, therefore, participation in aggressive sports and extreme exertion are contraindicated. The prevalence of carriers (heterozygotes) for the sickle cell trait (SCT) is 6–8% in U.S. African-Americans and approximately one in 10,000 in American whites. These persons rarely have anemia or an abnormal blood smear. In general, there are few clinical consequences to SCT, but athletes are believed to have some increased risk of non-fatal events including rhabdomyolysis and heat illness, as well as splenic and renal infarcts (particularly at high altitude). The relative risk is unknown. There is also a possible association with increased risk of sudden death. There are no absolute restrictions to athletic participation, but fastidious compliance with fluid replacement, preseason gradual conditioning, and acclimatization are necessary preventive measures. Of note, there are no data to suggest performance deficits in these athletes.

C. Hematologic Manipulation

An artificial increase in hemoglobin has been shown to increase $\cdot\mathrm{Vo_2}$max and running time to exhaustion. Because of this, athletes have experimented with hematologic manipulation to enhance performance since the 1940s. Blood transfusions (doping) have in more recent times given way to use of pharmacologic agents that override the body's natural controls and stimulate erythrocytosis (ie, erythropoietin). These practices are extremely dangerous and have been linked to several deaths in endurance athletes. Complications from blood doping include infection and transfusion reactions. Both can cause polycythemia with increased viscosity and thrombogenicity, and subsequent deep venous, coronary, and cerebral thrombosis.

American Diabetes Association: Position statement on diabetes and exercise 2002. Diabetes Care 2002;25:S64.

Boule NG et al: Effects of exercise on glycemic control and body mass in type 2 diabetes mellitus: a meta-analysis of controlled clinical trails. JAMA 2001;286:1218.

Edelman JM et al: Oral montellukast compared with inhaled salmeterol to prevent exercise-induced bronchoconstriction. A randomized, double-blind trial. Exercise Study Group. Ann Intern Med 2000;132:97.

Johannsen KL et al: Muscle atrophy in patients receiving hemodialysis: effects on muscle strength, muscle quality, and physical function. Kidney Int 2003;63:291.

Maron BJ, Zipes DP: 36th Bethesda conference: eligibility recommendations for competitive athletes with cardiovascular abnormalities. J Am Coll Cardiol 2005;45(8):1313.

Shaskey DJ, Green GA: Sports hematology. Sports Med 2000;1:27.

Truitt J: Pulmonary disorders and exercise. Clinics Sports Med 2003;22(1).

Vasamreddy CR et al: Cardiovascular Disease in athletes. Clinics Sports Med 2004;23(3):455.

DERMATOLOGY

Infectious Disorders

A. Fungal Infections

Because sweating and heat predispose to the growth of dermatophytes on the feet and in intertriginous areas, fungal infections are very common in athletes. These infections most commonly present with pruritis and an erythematous, raised, advancing border. Occasionally skin may have a scaling, fissured, or even vesiculopustular appearance depending on location. Diagnosis and treatment can usually be based on physical examination alone, but if uncertain, potassium hydroxide (KOH) preparation will show microscopic hyphae (Figure 1–2). Tinea pedis ("athlete's foot") is the most common type of dermatophyte infection. An example is shown in Figure 1–3. Treatment is with topical imidazole creams for 3–4 weeks along with foot hygiene. *Staphylococcus aureus*, micrococci, and gram-negative bacteria can cause a superimposed infection and may need to be treated as well. Tinea cruris ("jock itch") is seen more commonly in warm summer months. If scrotal involvement is noted, *Candida* is the more likely causative agent. Intertrigo can also mimic tinea cruris, but tends to be limited to the body folds of obese patients. Tinea corporis ("ringworm"), as seen in Figure 1–4, occasionally produces an intense inflammatory response, and granulomatous or follicular variants may be seen. In these cases, oral medications (griseofulvin or antifungal agents) may be necessary. Close contact and abrasions that occur in wrestling predispose to widespread tinea infection known as tinea corporis gladiatorum. Topical or oral treatment may be considered depending on the extent of the lesions. Return to wrestling is allowed once an infected, exposed area has been treated for 72 hours and is able to be covered. Prevention with weekly oral antifungal medication may be considered in athletes who suffer recurrent infection.

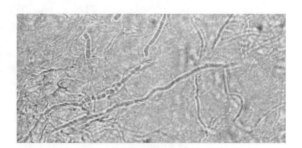

Figure 1–2. Potassium hydroxide preparation of skin scrapings showing septate hyphae. (Reproduced, with permission, from Fitzpatrick TB, Johnson RA, Suurmond D: Color Atlas & Synopsis of Clinical Dermatology, 4th ed. McGraw-Hill, 2001.)

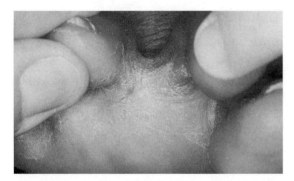

Figure 1–3. Interdigital tinea pedis. (Reproduced, with permission, from Fitzpatrick TB, Johnson RA, Suurmond D: Color Atlas & Synopsis of Clinical Dermatology, 4th ed. McGraw-Hill, 2001.)

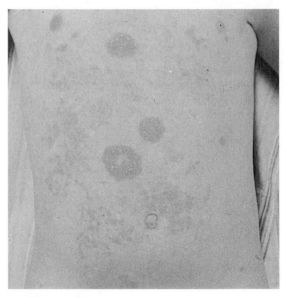

Figure 1–4. Tinea corporis. (Reproduced, with permission, from Fitzpatrick TB, Johnson RA, Wolff K, Suurmond D: Color Atlas & Synopsis of Clinical Dermatology, 4th ed. McGraw-Hill, 2001.)

B. BACTERIAL INFECTIONS

Staphylococci and streptococci bacteria may cause impetigo, characterized by honey-colored crusted lesions occurring in injured skin. Erythromycin or dicloxacillin is usually curative. *Staphylococcus* infection at hair follicle sites is also common and appears as a furuncle (Figure 1–5). Methacillin-resistant *Staphylococcus aureus* (MRSA) infection has recently become more common in the training room setting and has been most frequently documented in football players. MRSA presents with either solitary or multiple pustular lesions that have a "spider bite" appearance. A high level of suspicion is necessary.

Diagnosis should be made by wound culture and sensitivity. Treatment is diligent cleansing with antibacterial soap (Hibaclense) and topical mucipirocin. Oral antibiotics (trimethoprim-sulfamethoxazole) may be necessary in more disseminated cases, and, occasionally, intravenous

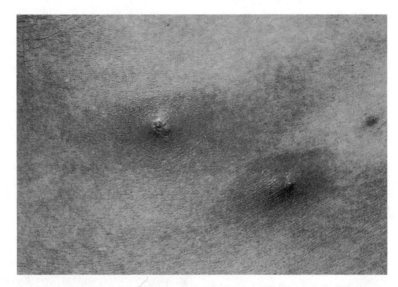

Figure 1–5. Furuncle. A common *Staphylococcus* skin infection with exquisitely tender discrete, hard nodules surrounded by a broad erythematous base. (Reproduced, with permission, from Fitzpatrick TB, Johnson RA, Polano MK, Suurmond D, Wolff K: Color Atlas & Synopsis of Clinical Dermatology, 2nd ed. McGraw-Hill, 1994.)

antibiotics (vancomycin, rifampin) are required. The need for and utility of nasal screening and/or treatment of teammates are under debate.

Erythrasma, caused by *Corynbacterium* presents as dull red plaques in the axillary or inguinal folds and therefore may be confused with tinea or *Candida*. The problem is usually eradicated with use of antibacterial soap, but topical erythromycin can be used.

C. Viruses

Viruses such as mulluscum contagiosum and herpes simplex virus (HSV) can be particularly problematic for athletes. Molluscum is a mildly pruritic infection induced by the pox virus. The skin colored, umbilicated lesions (Figure 1–6) are highly contagious and should be treated aggressively. Grouped vesicles on an erythematous base are the primary characteristic of HSV (Figure 1–7). This should be treated with antivirals (acyclovir 400 mg three times a day for 5 days, or other agents). Wrestlers with active lesions are disqualified since spread among competitors is common. This can lead to herpes gladiatorum,

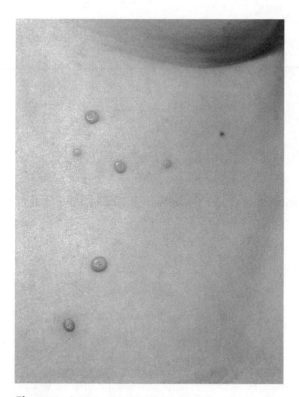

Figure 1–6. Molluscum contagiosum. Multiple, scattered, and discrete lesions. (Reproduced, with permission, from Fitzpatrick TB, Johnson RA, Suurmond D: Color Atlas & Synopsis of Clinical Dermatology, 4th ed. McGraw-Hill, 2001.)

in which skin abrasions or lacerations become inoculated with the virus, and often presents with associated systemic symptoms of headache, myalgias, and fever.

Infestations

Sexual contact is the most common mode of transmission of lice and scabies in adults; however, the sharing of towels, hair brushes, etc among teammates, in addition to close skin-to-skin contact in some sports, makes infestations with these organisms a potential issue for the athlete. Figure 1–8 shows an example of the erythematous nodules commonly produced by scabies infestation. This results in intense pruritis, whereas the presentation of lice infestation is more moderate. All bedding, clothing, towels, etc should be washed to avoid spread. In addition to meticulous cleaning, topical lindane or permethrin is used to eradicate the organisms. In most cases, all household members should be treated even if asymptomatic. Depending on the sport, teammates should be considered for treatment as well.

Environmental Dermatologic Issues

Sunburn is very common in fair-skinned athletes, causing discomfort and increasing risk of cutaneous malignancy, most importantly melanoma. Use of sunscreen has been shown to be very helpful in decreasing this risk. Gel, lotion, and spray products may be better tolerated by athletes who object to heavy or greasy products that can impede sweating. A broad-spectrum sunscreen with a skin-protection factor (SPF) of 15 or more that protects against ultraviolet A and B (UVA and UVB) should be applied 20 minutes prior to going out into the sun. Despite claims of being "waterproof," many sunscreens will have a decreased effect and require reapplication after vigorous exertion and substantial sweating. If sunburn develops, soothing compresses, NSAIDs, and topical emollients can help relieve symptoms. Corticosteroid ointments can help with irritation resulting from moderate to severe burns.

Pernio is characterized by erythematous, tender papules and nodules that occur on acral sites, most commonly the feet and toes of athletes. This results from prolonged exposure to cold and can be prevented by avoiding moisture and wearing properly insulated shoes and warm socks.

Mechanical Problems

A. Blisters and Corns

Blisters and corns are ubiquitous in athletes. Attention to properly fitting footwear and minimizing moisture in shoes are the key to preventing these foot problems. Blisters should be left intact when possible. When necessary, however, the blister can be drained with a syringe and 18-gauge needle. Use of a small amount of zinc ointment, antibiotic

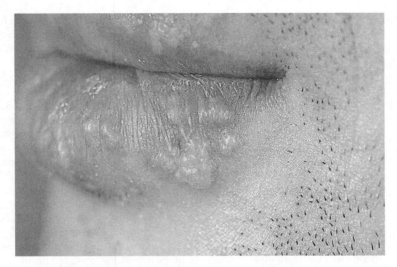

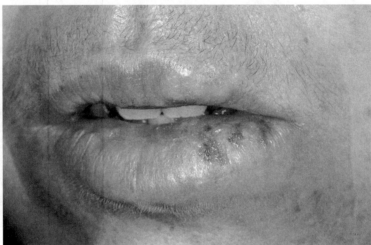

Figure 1–7. Herpes simplex virus. Grouped vesicles on an erythematous base. **A:** Day 1. **B:** Day 5. (Reproduced, with permission, from Fitzpatrick TB, Johnson RA, Suurmond D: Color Atlas & Synopsis of Clinical Dermatology, 4th ed. McGraw-Hill, 2001.)

ointment, or hydrocolloid dressing may help minimize the risk of superimposed infection and potentially enhance healing. Corns may be gently debrided and lotions with lactic acid, urea, or propylene glycol can be helpful. Intracorneal hemorrhage may occur, particularly in athletes engaged in sports with rapid starts and stops such as tennis and basketball. This is referred to as "talon noir." Athletes may be concerned about the dark discoloration, confusing it with melanoma, but gently paring the skin should easily remove the pigment and reassure the athlete.

B. "JOGGER'S NIPPLE"

The nipple is a common site of abrasion injury in athletes. This is especially true for women involved in running or other sports in which the activity leads to strong

repetitive rubbing. The resultant irritation and excoriation are characteristic of "jogger's nipple," so named because it often occurs in runners. Exposure to cold wind further promotes bleeding, raw, severely painful nipples. This can be an issue in events such as cycling, crew, and multisport competitions. Prevention includes coating the nipples with petroleum jelly or applying bandages before activity, avoiding cold and wind exposure by wearing appropriate clothing, and for women, using a properly fitted sports bra.

C. CAULIFLOWER EAR

A shear force applied to the external ear can result in the formation of a painful hematoma. This is seen most commonly in sports such as wrestling and rugby. If left untreated,

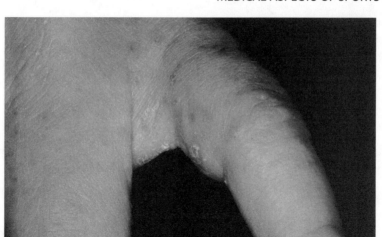

Figure 1–8. Scabetic nodules. (Reproduced, with permission, from Fitzpatrick TB, Johnson RA, Suurmond D: Color Atlas & Synopsis of Clinical Dermatology, 4th ed. McGraw-Hill, 2001.)

the result is a deformed appearing "cauliflower ear." Early treatment involves aspiration of the hematoma and subsequent application of a pressure dressing. Antibiotics are recommended after drainage to prevent chondritis.

Contact Dermatitis & Urticaria

A. Contact Dermatitis

Contact dermatitis in active individuals is often the result of exposure to common "outdoor" allergens such as poison ivy, poison sumac, and poison oak. Athletes may, alternatively, have an allergic reaction to adhesives, metal used on equipment, or even clothing dyes. The most important issue is identifying the offending allergen, which may be obvious or may require patch testing. Treatment is with cool compresses and topical corticosteroid cream. Occasionally, oral steroids can hasten recovery.

B. Urticaria

Hives (urticaria, as seen in Figure 1–9) can result from either allergic or physical triggers. Common physical triggers include sun exposure, cold, and pressure. Acute urticaria (present less than 6 weeks) can typically be treated symptomatically with antihistamines and soothing lotions. Persistent urticaria deserves further workup. Exercise-induced urticaria and cholinergic urticaria can both be brought on by exertion, but must be differentiated from one another. Cholinergic urticaria presents with pruritis, punctate urticaria, warmth, and occasionally wheezing, but tends to be mild. Hot water can also be a trigger. Exercise-induced urticaria, with its large, greater than 1 cm, lesions frequently progresses to laryngeal angioedema and exercise-induced anaphylaxis. This can be life-threatening. Antihistamines do not prevent this progression, therefore, acute attacks must be treated with intramuscular epinephrine and corticosteroids.

Adams BB: Dermatologic disorders of the athlete. Sports Med 2002;32(5):309.

SPORTS NUTRITION

Basics of Nutrition

The goals of sports nutrition are to (1) provide adequate "fuel" to optimize health, energy, and athletic performance, (2) achieve/maintain ideal body mass and composition, (3) maintain proper hydration and electrolyte balance, (4) promote recovery from training, and (5) safely supplement the diet when there is a deficiency or need. Caloric needs vary depending on weight, age, gender, sport, and many other factors. In general, the minimum caloric requirement is approximately 18 × weight (in pounds) for females and 21 × weight (in pounds) for males. A well-balanced diet is recommended for most with 60–70% of calories coming from carbohydrates, 20–25% from fats, and 10–15% from protein. Because carbohydrates are the primary energy source for all types of exercise, a low carbohydrate dietary intake can cause fatigue, can impair performance, and may increase risk of injury. Recommendations for carbohydrate ingestion are listed in Table 1–15.

Many athletes, particularly those in "body conscious" sports, attempt to avoid all fat in the diet, often to their detriment. Fat is a necessary part of every diet and is an important energy source for low-intensity, prolonged activity. Inadequate intake can lead not only to poor athletic performance and fatigue, but also to low levels of certain vitamins, decreased intramuscular triglycerides, a lack of essential fatty acids, and low testosterone levels in males or menstrual dysfunction in females. Protein requirements vary from as low as 0.5 g/lb/day in a low-demand, recreational athlete, to 1.0 g/lb/day in teenage

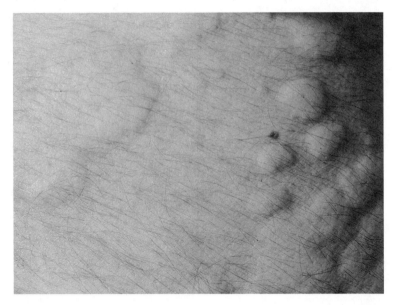

Figure 1–9. Urticarial lesions. (Reproduced, with permission, from Fitzpatrick TB, Johnson RA, Suurmond D: Color Atlas & Synopsis of Clinical Dermatology, 4th ed. McGraw-Hill, 2001.)

athletes and those building mass, the maximum a body can use. Although protein provides only 5–10% of fuel for exercise, strength-training athletes require protein to support increased mass and endurance athletes need protein for aerobic enzymes, for formation of myoglobin and RBC, and to replace protein stores. Inadequate protein intake can lead to decreased muscle mass, suppressed immunity, and fatigue, whereas excess protein can increase the risk of dehydration, increase calcium loss, and result in increased body fat stores.

Hydration

Fluid balance is essential for performance, recovery from injury, and mental functioning during athletic activity. More importantly, loss of fluid balance (ie, dehydration) can impair cardiovascular function and thermoregulation, putting the athlete at risk for injury and even death. The American College of Sports Medicine has produced guidelines for fluid intake, as thirst is an extremely poor indicator of need. These guidelines are listed in Table 1–16. Maintaining hydration with water alone seems adequate for activity that lasts less than 1 hour, but a drink that contains glucose and sodium (eg, sports drink, lemonade) is recommended for athletes engaged in more prolonged exercise.

Performance-Enhancing Substances & Nutritional Supplements

Nutritional supplementation has been a more than 15 billion dollar industry in each of the past 5 years, up from 3.3 billion dollars in 1990. Performance-enhancing substances including anabolic agents and stimulants have

Table 1–15. Carbohydrate intake recommendations.

	Preexercise	During Exercise (>1 hour)	Postexercise
Carbohydrate (grams)	1.8 g/lb 3–4 hours prior to exercise as part of a balanced meal 0.5 g/lb 1 hour prior to exercise	30–60 g/hour Examples: 5–10 oz sports drink every 15–20 minutes or 2 gels/hour (plus water) or gummy-type candy	50–150 g within 30 minutes: include glucose- or sucrose-containing foods

Table 1–16. American College of Sports Medicine guidelines for fluid intake during exercise.

16 oz at 2 hours and again 30 minutes prior to exercise
8 oz 5–10 minutes prior to exercise
4–8 oz every 15–20 minutes during exercise
24 oz/lb lost from exercise within 6 hours postactivity

been used by athletes for years to advance their performance to a "supranormal" level. Use of these substances not only raises moral and ethical questions, but also can be extremely dangerous from a health standpoint. Testosterone and synthetic anabolic steroids have shown efficacy in terms of increasing lean mass and strength. Recovery from high-intensity work is facilitated, leading to increased endurance and speed. Table 1–17 lists the known adverse affects of androgen use.

Sympathomimetic drugs have been shown to increase alertness and performance in a fatigued athlete. They may also increase utilization of free fatty acids during endurance work, prolonging time to exhaustion. These substances, which include amphetamines, Ephedra, and even caffeine at high doses, result in cardiac arrhythmias, anxiety, and dependency, among other adverse affects. Several recent instances of sudden cardiac deaths in athletes have been linked to the use of Ephedra.

Other supplements claim "ergogenic" potential, but there is little evidence for the efficacy of many commonly

Table 1–17. Adverse affects of androgens.

Increased risk of cardiac ischemic events and stroke
Increased blood pressure
Increased cancer risk: liver, kidney, prostate, testicular
Weakening of musculotendinous tissue leading to increased risk of injury
Psychosis, depression, and other psychological/behavioral changes
Masculinization of women
In men, gynecomastia, impotence, prostatic hypertrophy, infertility
Premature growth plate closure
Immune system dysfunction

used substances. No benefits have been demonstrated for amino acids, chromium, 1-*carnitine, or* 1-tryptophan and their safety is unknown. Human growth hormone has been touted as a "fountain of youth." It enhances both lean mass and strength in deficiency states, but studies in nondeficient states show mixed results at best. Side effects can be serious and include cardiac and diabetogenic issues as well as acromegaly and all of its implications. Steroid prohormones (eg, dehydroepiandrosterone, androstenedione) may confer anabolic effects and produce similar side effects, but have not definitively been shown to enhance performance or body composition.

Creatine (methylguanide-acetic acid) intake has been shown to enhance the bioavailability of phosphocreatine in skeletal muscle cells, allowing for faster adenosine triphosphate (ATP) resynthesis and thus quicker recovery from brief, high-intensity exercise. Phosphocreatine also buffers hydrogen ions that are produced during exercise and contribute to muscle fatigue. Both of these effects can confer significant performance enhancement with supplementation of 20–30 g of creatine per day. Potential hazards include severe muscle cramping and possible kidney damage when creatine is used in a dehydrated state, but there is only anecdotal evidence for this. It may cause unwanted weight gain and water retention in athletes who require speed and endurance. No studies have evaluated its long-term effects, but, in general, creatine is believed to be relatively safe with short-term use.

Low-risk supplements include protein bars, sports drinks, and vitamins. These may be safely used to augment, but not replace, a well-balanced diet. Occasionally, vitamin and mineral supplementation may be required by athletes who restrict energy intake, eliminate one or more food groups, or consume a high-carbohydrate, low-macronutrient diet. Overall, it is important that physicians who work closely with athletes have some understanding of the claims, efficacy, limitations, and risks of supplements that are commonly used.

American Medical Society for Sports Medicine: Drugs and performance-enhancing against in sport. Clin J Sport Med 2002;12:201.

Armsey TD, Hosey RG: Medical aspects of sports: epidemiology of injuries, preparticipation physical examination, and drugs in sports. Clinics Sports Med 2004;23(2):255.

King DS et al: Effect of oral androstenedione on serum testosterone concentrations in young men. JAMA 2000;283:779.

The National Center for Drug Free Sport Inc: Nutritional supplements available at www.drugfreesport.com. Accessed November 2004.

National Collegiate Athletic Association: Available at www.ncaa.org. Accessed October 2004.

National Federation of State High School Associations: Available at www.nfhs.org. Accessed October 2004.

Noakes TD: Fluid replacement during exercise. Clinics Sports Med 2003;22(1).

Hip & Pelvis Problems

2

Hussein Elkousy, MD, & Gregory Stocks, MD

HIP PAIN

Anatomy

Three joints make up the pelvic girdle: the hip joint, the sacroiliac joint, and the pubic symphysis. The pubic symphysis and sacroiliac joint allow little motion. The ball-and-socket configuration of the hip is designed to provide stability and mobility for the body.

Several bony prominences act as muscular origins and insertions in the hip and pelvis (Figure 2–1). The anterior superior iliac spine (ASIS) and greater trochanter are easily palpable in most athletes. The ASIS is the origin of the sartorius. The greater trochanter is the insertion of the gluteus medius. The anterior and posterior iliac crest, symphysis pubis, and ischial tuberosity can be palpated in most individuals. The hip adductors originate from the pubis and the hamstring tendons originate from the ischial tuberosity. The anterior inferior iliac spine (AIIS) is the origin of the direct head of the rectus femoris. The lesser trochanter is not palpable, but it is the site of insertion of the iliopsoas tendon.

Although there may be some overlap in the function of some of the muscles of the hip and pelvis, most have a specialized role. The primary hip flexor is the iliopsoas. The gluteus maximus is the most important hip extensor. The hip abductors are the gluteus medius and minimus. The tensor fascia lata and its extension, the iliotibial band, provide additional stability to the hip during single-leg stance. The hip is adducted by a large group of muscles that originates from the pubis and inserts onto the medial femur. These include the adductor longus, adductor magnus, and adductor brevis.

Several muscles cross the hip and knee joint. Muscles that cross two joints are generally more prone to injury. These are the rectus femoris, the hamstrings, and the iliotibial tract.

Several bursae in the hip and pelvis serve to reduce friction between tendons and surrounding structures. Some of the more important are the greater trochanteric, ischial, and iliopsoas bursae. These are common sites of irritation and pain with overuse.

The acetabular labrum is a cartilaginous structure that lines the periphery of the acetabulum and deepens the hip socket by 30%. However, its primary function is to provide squeeze film lubrication to the cartilage of the femoral head. It creates a vacuum phenomenon that contributes to hip stability. The ligamentum teres, which enters the fovea of the femoral head, is not an important source of blood supply to the femoral head in adults. It may, however, contribute to hip stability, limiting external rotation. The hip capsule is tightened in external rotation and extension.

Differential Diagnosis

Diagnosing the etiology of hip pain can be a daunting task. Pain felt in the hip and pelvis may originate from hip structures or it may be referred from structures in the torso or viscera. As such, the Differential Diagnosis is broad and includes pathology of the abdominal viscera, lumbar spine, or genitalia. Differential diagnoses that should be entertained when diagnosing hip pain include meralgia paresthetica, hernia, athletic pubalgia, and piriformis syndrome. This chapter will address only those pathologies directly related to athletic hip injuries: contusions, avulsions, bursitis, stress fractures, and articular derangements.

CONTUSIONS ABOUT THE HIP & PELVIS

ESSENTIALS OF DIAGNOSIS

- *Contusions occur from direct contact with another player or playing surface.*
- *Contusions usually occur over bony prominences.*
- *Pain is the primary cause of disability.*
- *Treatment focuses on pain control, maintenance of flexibility, and strength until symptoms resolve.*
- *Compartment syndrome and myositis ossificans may be early and late complications of contusions.*

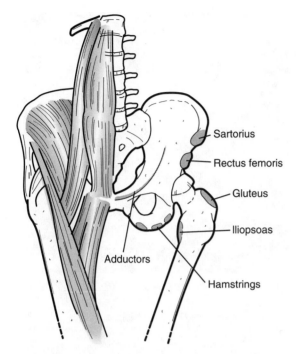

Figure 2–1. Bony prominences of the hip and pelvis and the muscular origins. (Reproduced, with permission, from Anderson K et al: Am J Sports Med 2001; 29:521.)

Sartorius

Rectus femoris

Gluteus

Iliopsoas

Adductors

Hamstrings

Prevention

Contusions about the hip and pelvis are an unavoidable consequence of contact sports. Because of the inherent risks involved in greater contact, certain sports, such as football, hockey, or lacrosse, result in more contusions. It is difficult to prevent these injuries. Of course, some measures may be implemented. In football, hockey, and lacrosse, players wear protective padding over hip and pelvic prominences. In addition, wearing other pads, such as shoulder pads, is less likely to result in a contusion to another player. The surface of play can also be a significant factor in injury. For example, although there are no data to support the assertion that fewer contusions occur on natural grass than on artificial turf, this seems to be a commonly held assumption.

Clinical Findings

A. Symptoms

Each sport and each specific site of injury differs in precise history, but all injuries share the common theme of direct trauma. The most common sites of injury are the bony prominences, although the soft tissue areas of the thigh can also be involved. The commonly affected bony prominences are the iliac crest, the pubic ramus, the greater trochanter, and the ischial tuberosity. Injuries to the iliac crest are often referred to as "hip pointers"and

injuries to the soft tissue of the thigh are referred to as a "charley horse."

The athlete complains of pain over the specific site that is aggravated by direct contact and, often, exacerbated by use of associated muscle groups. Pain may be localized to the hamstrings with ischial tuberosity injuries or to the quadriceps with anterior thigh contusions. Because most of the lower extremity muscles are involved in walking, many of these injuries result in the athlete walking with a limp.

B. Signs

The most reproducible sign is pain with palpation over the site of injury. This occurs with both superficial and deep injuries. Swelling and ecchymosis may be apparent. Patients may have pain with passive stretch of the involved or overlying muscle. Active resistance may also elicit pain. A contusion of the iliac crest, for example, may result in pain with active abduction or passive adduction of the hip. A contusion of the anterior thigh causes pain with knee extension or hip flexion.

C. Imaging Studies

Acutely, plain radiographs are generally obtained to rule out a fracture. Contusions will not yield any radiographic findings. The only other useful imaging technique is magnetic resonance imaging (MRI) (Figure 2–2). This may demonstrate a hematoma or an occult fracture not seen on plain radiographs. Generally, however, this is not useful acutely and may be reserved for patients who fail to improve after initial conservative management.

D. Special Tests

No special tests exist for diagnosing a contusion. However, compartment syndrome should be considered if swelling is profound. In these cases, compartment pressures should be measured. This applies in particular to the proximal thigh and even to the gluteal region. Elevated pressures that warrant treatment should follow general guidelines for compartment syndrome. These include a pressure above 30 mm Hg or a pressure within 30 mm Hg of the diastolic blood pressure. However, it should be noted that even with elevated compartment pressures, these injuries may be treated with observation with good results.

Complications

Complications with contusions are rare. Compartment syndrome may occasionally occur as mentioned. This may result in some muscle fibrosis with associated loss of range of motion. A second possible complication is the development of myositis ossificans (Figure 2–3). This may be avoided by minimizing the period of immobilization after the injury and minimizing the development of a hematoma. The resulting hematoma

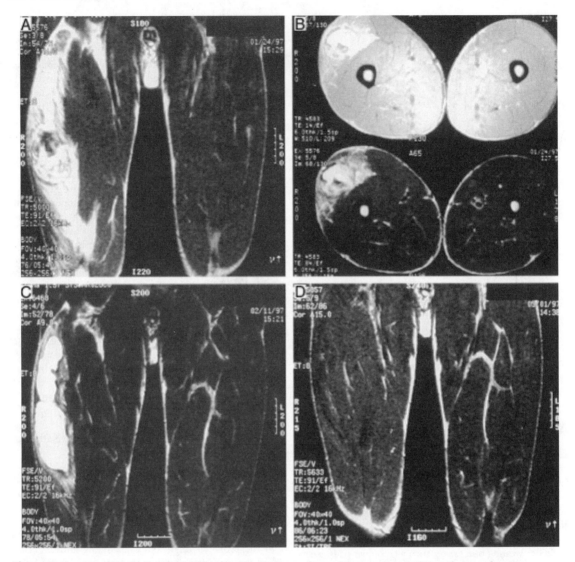

Figure 2–2. Coronal and axial magnetic resonance images of muscle contusion. ***A:*** Coronal view of acute hematoma and edema of vastus lateralis. ***B:*** Axial view of acute injury. ***C:*** Coronal view of injury at 3 weeks with hematoma replaced with fluid collection. ***D:*** Coronal view at 3.5 months demonstrating resolving injury. (Reproduced, with permission, from Diaz JA et al: Am J Sports Med 2003;31:289.)

may eventually form a calcified mass. This mass is best assessed with plain radiographs or a computed tomography (CT) scan. It is differentiated from a soft tissue sarcoma by the history of trauma as well as its radiographic appearance. Myositis ossificans develops in a centripetal fashion resulting in a peripheral rim of calcification that subsequently progresses centrally. If it does not cause significant symptoms, it may be ignored. However, if it is symptomatic, it may be resected after it has matured. Maturation is best assessed by bone scan and may require several months to occur.

Treatment

A. Rehabilitation

The goals of treatment are return of painless full range of motion and strength in a timely fashion. Initial management is conservative. This entails controlling pain and swelling. These can be managed initially with ice, nonsteroidal antiinflammatory medications, and relative rest. The relative rest may require the use of crutches if weight bearing or walking is painful. This should be done for the first 24–48 hours. The focus should then

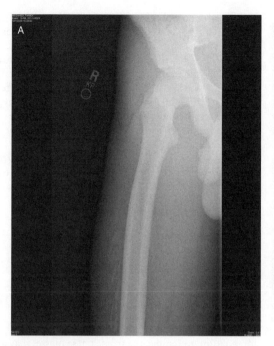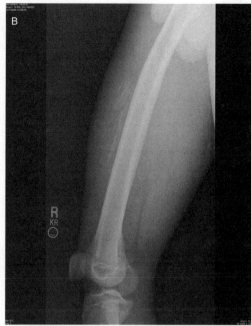

Figure 2–3. Myositis ossificans in a 15-year-old boy secondary to a deep anterior thigh contusion. **A:** Anteroposterior view of the proximal thigh. **B:** Lateral view of mid thigh.

shift to rehabilitation with restoration of range of motion with passive stretching. This may be started initially by immobilizing the involved muscle group in a lengthened or stretched position. This is most commonly done for a proximal quadriceps contusion by keeping the knee in a flexed position. Concomitantly, with the stretching regimen, the surrounding muscle groups are strengthened. Activity is gradually resumed as full range of motion and full strength are obtained.

B. Surgical

Surgery is generally not indicated for contusions. Occasionally, however, a hematoma may need to be surgically decompressed or a compartment syndrome may require fasciotomies.

C. Special Procedures

Some patients may have extensive swelling or may simply fail to progress with conservative management. These patients may have a large hematoma that prevents them from improving rapidly. In these cases, an MRI may be obtained and the hematoma may be aspirated.

Prognosis

The prognosis is excellent for most contusions about the hip and pelvis. The athlete can generally return to full sport activity without limitations.

Return to Play

The time to return to play is difficult to predict with contusions. It depends on the seriousness of the injury, the site of the injury, and the athlete's response to the injury. It ranges from no time off to several weeks off.

Anderson K et al: Hip and groin injuries in athletes. Am J Sports Med 2001;29(4):521. [PMID: 15297126]

Diaz JA et al: Severe quadriceps muscle contusions in athletes. A report of three cases. Am J Sports Med 2003;31(2):289. [PMID: 12642267]

AVULSIONS ABOUT THE PELVIS

 ESSENTIALS OF DIAGNOSIS

- *Avulsion injuries in adults involve tendinous origins.*
- *Equivalent injuries in the skeletally immature patient involve the apophyses.*
- *Common sites include the ischium, AIIS, ASIS, greater and lesser trochanters, iliac crest, and pubis.*
- *Most injuries occur from an eccentric muscle contraction.*
- *Most injuries may be managed nonoperatively.*

Prevention

No definitive data exist to prove that stretching provides any protective benefit against avulsion injuries. However, preparing the muscle–tendon unit for the large loads required to cause an avulsion injury may afford some benefit.

Clinical Findings

A. SYMPTOMS

Athletes describe an eccentric load to the injured muscle–tendon unit. Pain is acute and may be associated with a pop in a skeletally immature athlete. The mechanism of injury varies with the specific site of injury. For example, an avulsion of the ischium occurs from knee extension and hip flexion. Activities that classically result in these injuries include water skiing and running the hurdles. An avulsion of the AIIS occurs from eccentric hip extension or resistance against forceful flexion of the hip. This may occur with sprinting or kicking. An avulsion of the ASIS may occur from eccentric hip and knee extension.

The athletes complain of pain at the specific site of injury with direct contact and with use of the avulsed muscle–tendon unit. An ischial avulsion injury causes discomfort with sitting. An ASIS injury results in pain when standing erect. Pubic injuries result in groin pain.

B. SIGNS

Findings from the physical examination are similar to those for contusions. The history plays a large part in differentiating an avulsion injury from a contusion. All injuries may result in ecchymosis, swelling, and tenderness to palpation over the site of injury. Pain is reproduced with passive stretching or active contraction of the injured muscle–tendon unit.

An ischial avulsion injury is tender over the ischium. Pain is elicited with passive hip flexion and varying degrees of knee extension. Resisted knee flexion with an extended hip also causes pain. An avulsion of the AIIS or rectus femoris results in pain with passive hip extension and knee flexion or active hip flexion and knee extension. An avulsion of the ASIS or sartorius results in pain with simultaneous passive hip and knee extension or active hip and knee flexion. An avulsion of the gluteus medius or the greater trochanter results in pain with passive hip adduction or active hip abduction. An avulsion of the lesser trochanter or iliopsoas tendon results in pain with passive hip extension or active hip flexion.

C. IMAGING STUDIES

Plain radiographs are useful in the skeletally immature patient. They are usually normal in adult patients unless the injury is chronic or is a recurrence of a childhood injury. Avulsion injuries in skeletally immature patients generally result in apophyseal fractures. These can be seen on plain films (Figure 2–4A). In descending order, the most common avulsion fractures in the skeletally immature athlete are ischial tuberosity, AIIS, and ASIS avulsions (Figure 2–4B). Iliac crest, greater trochanter, lesser trochanter, and pubic avulsions are less frequently seen. The equivalent injury in an adult results in a soft tissue injury not apparent on a plain radiograph (see Table 2–1).

MRI is more useful for the skeletally mature patient. It may demonstrate the site of a muscle or tendon tear, the extent of the tear, and any associated edema or hematoma (Figure 2–5).

Complications

Complications of conservative management include weakness and the potential for reinjury. Specific injuries such as an ischial apophysis avulsion may result in a calcific mass at the site of injury (Figure 2–6). This mass may irritate the sciatic nerve or it may cause discomfort with sitting. This may necessitate surgical intervention to remove the mass. These masses may also form at other sites of injury and may also require delayed surgical removal. Often, a more sinister etiology, such as a malignant tumor, must be considered; therefore, at least a biopsy, and often complete surgical excision, is warranted.

Treatment

A. REHABILITATION

Most avulsion injuries are treated nonoperatively. Conservative management involves relative rest with comfortable positioning and the use of crutches for non-weight-bearing activities to minimize pain. Ice and pain medication may be used initially. A gradual stretching regimen is initiated with pain as a guide to the level of activity. As pain dissipates, weight bearing is allowed and full painless range of motion is restored. Isometric exercises are gradually implemented, followed by isotonic strengthening. Activities are gradually increased until full motion and strength are restored.

B. SURGICAL

Many reports have been published specifically addressing injuries in the skeletally immature patient. The consensus is that most injuries should be treated nonoperatively. However, in injuries with greater than 2 cm of displacement of the apophyseal fragment, in particular, injuries to the ischial apophysis, consideration should be given to surgical fixation. This procedure can generally be done using two screws to fix the avulsed apophysis to the ischium (Figure 2–7).

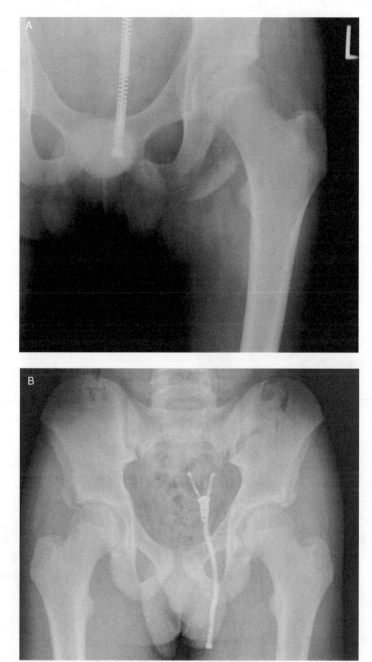

Figure 2–4. Apophyseal avulsion injuries. ***A:*** Left ischial avulsion in a 14-year-old track athlete. ***B:*** Right AIIS avulsion fracture in a 15-year-old male sustained while kicking a soccer ball.

Table 2–1. Avulsion injuries in the skeletally immature and skeletally mature individual.

Skeletally Immature	Skeletally Mature
Ischial tuberosity	Hamstring
Anterior superior iliac spine	Sartorius
Anterior inferior iliac spine	Rectus femoris
Greater trochanter	Gluteus medius
Lesser trochanter	Iliopsoas
Pubic symphysis	Adductor magnus

Soft tissue injuries in adults should also initially be treated nonoperatively. One notable exception, however, involves injuries to the hamstring origin. These have been shown to benefit from surgical repair. This can be done using suture anchors to fix the torn tendon end to the ischium (Figure 2–8).

Prognosis

The prognosis is good for a full recovery. Generally, ischial or hamstring injuries tend to recover more slowly and have a higher likelihood of recurring than injuries to other sites.

Return to Play

Injuries of the origins at the ASIS or AIIS generally recover in 4–6 weeks. Assuming no complications, the time between injury and return to full sport activity may range from several weeks to several months.

Klingele KE, Sallay PI: Surgical repair of complete proximal hamstring tendon rupture. Am J Sports Med 2002;30(5):742. [PMID: 12239012]

Moeller JL: Pelvic and hip apophyseal avulsion injuries in young athletes. Curr Sports Med Rep 2003;2(2):110. [PMID: 12831668]

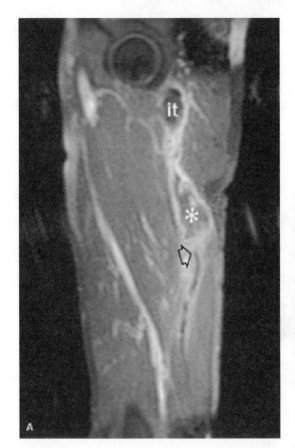

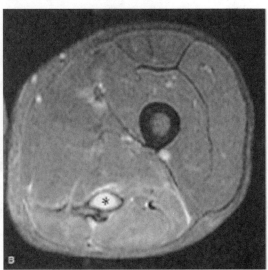

Figure 2–5. Hamstring avulsion. ***A:*** Sagittal view showing torn tendon end (***arrow***) and hematoma (***asterisk***) it, ischial tuberosity. ***B:*** Axial view showing hematoma (***asterisk***) and tendon void. (Reproduced, with permission, from Bencardino JT et al: Top Magn Reson Imaging 2003;14:145.)

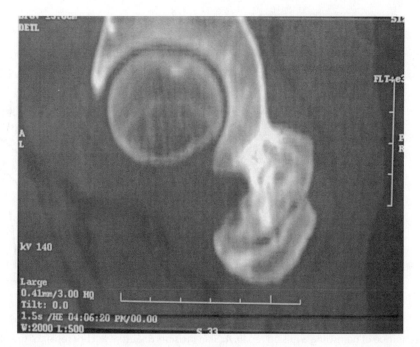

Figure 2–6. Sagittal CT reconstruction of a calcific mass at the level of ischial tuberosity secondary to an old avulsion fracture. The patient presented with pain when sitting.

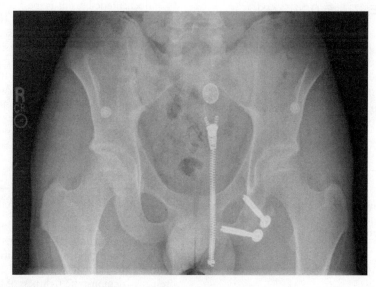

Figure 2–7. Open reduction and internal fixation of a displaced ischial avulsion fracture in a skeletally immature male. Preoperative radiograph is shown in Figure 2–4A.

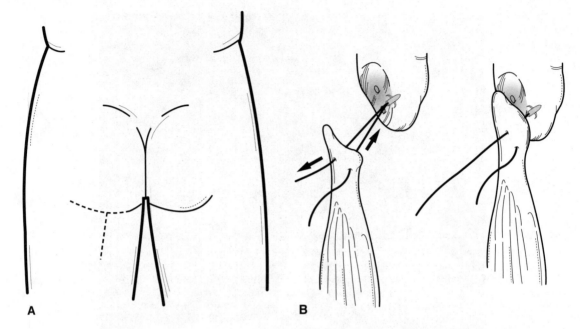

Figure 2–8. Technique of hamstring avulsion repair. **A:** Skin incision. **B:** Suture anchor repair of the tendon to ischial tuberosity. (Reproduced, with permission, from Klingele KE et al: Surgical repair of complete hamstring. *Am J Sports Med* 2002;30:743.)

TROCHANTERIC BURSITIS

ESSENTIALS OF DIAGNOSIS

- *Trochanteric bursitis may develop insidiously or from an acute injury.*
- *Most cases resolve with stretching, antiinflammatory drugs, and modification of activity.*
- *Modalities, injections, and surgical intervention may be necessary in refractory cases.*

Prevention

Adequate stretching of the iliotibial band and warm up prior to exercise may help prevent trochanteric bursitis, but no data exist to support this.

Clinical Findings

A. SYMPTOMS

Patients complain of lateral hip pain that may occasionally radiate along the distal lateral thigh. The pain may begin insidiously, but it may occasionally be acute. When it is acute, it can generally be traced to a specific fall or collision and it may be associated with a contusion. Patients may report a snapping sound or sensation in the hip as well.

Trochanteric bursitis is most common in female runners. Because females, in general, have a broader-based pelvis than their male counterparts, they are more susceptible to friction over the greater trochanter. Some runners may identify a causative factor for their symptoms such as an increase in their mileage or an increase in the level of difficulty of their training course. Additionally, if running is done on the road, often only one leg will be affected. This leg is generally the leg on the outer side of the road, which is affected by the drainage slope incorporated into the design of roads. Other provocative activities include lying on the affected side.

B. SIGNS

The patient is tender over the greater trochanter with direct palpation. Care should be taken to differentiate this from gluteus medius tendinitis. That pain is more proximal and is directly associated with active abduction. The most provocative positions for trochanteric bursitis are external rotation and adduction. The Ober test may demonstrate tightness of the iliotibial band.

C. IMAGING STUDIES

Imaging studies are useful only for differential diagnosis. If the diagnosis is straightforward by physical examination, imaging studies are not necessary. Magnetic resonance imaging may demonstrate fluid or inflammation in the bursa, but it is generally not needed to make the diagnosis.

Complications

The main complication of trochanteric bursitis is failure to resolve. This may eventually necessitate surgical management.

Treatment

A. Rehabilitation

Generally, trochanteric bursitis is managed nonoperatively. The first line of management includes relative rest from precipitating activities, iliotibial band and tensor fascia lata stretching, gluteal muscle strengthening, and antiinflammatories. The second line of treatment may include modalities such as iontophoresis and ultrasound. If these fail or if the patient cannot tolerate the symptoms, a steroid injection into the point of maximal tenderness may be of benefit. A majority of patients will improve with conservative management.

B. Surgery

Patients rarely require operative intervention for greater trochanteric bursitis. However, if the pain persists in spite of conservative management, surgery may be performed. Several procedures have been described with most focusing on releasing the iliotibial band with or without debridement of the trochanteric bursa. Reports in the literature indicate good success for these procedures with return to full sport activity over several months.

Most procedures involve a longitudinal incision over the greater trochanter. The iliotibial band, gluteus maximus, and tensor fascia lata are identified. The trochanteric bursa lies between the iliotibial band and the greater trochanter. It may be approached by creating a longitudinal incision in the iliotibial band and excising the bursa. Prior to closure of the wound, the iliotibial band may be Z-lengthened or an ellipse of tissue may be excised.

Prognosis

The prognosis is generally good for return to sport activity and resolution of symptoms with conservative management.

Return to Play

No published studies exist in the literature regarding trochanteric bursitis and return to sports. Generally, several days to several months may be required before the athlete is able to return to full uninhibited activity. The athlete can often continue to participate with some discomfort in spite of the symptoms.

STRESS FRACTURES OF THE PELVIS & FEMUR

ESSENTIALS OF DIAGNOSIS

- *Stress fractures may occur in the femoral neck, sacrum, pubic rami, ischium, acetabulum, or femoral head.*
- *Women are more commonly affected than men.*
- *Stress fractures are overuse injuries.*
- *Most stress fractures are treated with rest and modification of activity, but some require operative intervention.*

Prevention

Several factors contribute to the development of stress fractures. These can be divided into intrinsic and extrinsic factors. Extrinsic factors include footwear, running surface, and type or intensity of activity. Intrinsic factors include osteopenia and alignment abnormalities such as coxa vara. Many of these factors need to be addressed to prevent the occurrence or recurrence of stress fractures. For long distance running, using well-cushioned running shoes or running on more forgiving surfaces may minimize the incidence of femoral neck stress fractures. Gradually increasing the intensity of training rather than an abrupt increase can minimize the development of all types of stress fractures.

Intrinsic factors are less readily addressed. Alignment issues may be addressed with orthotics. Osteopenia is more common in women athletes and is associated with female athlete triad. This requires more extensive management using medications and diet.

Clinical Findings

A. Symptoms

Depending on the location of the stress fracture, patients typically complain of pain in the low back, buttock, groin, thigh, or even the knee. The pain is initially noticed after activity, but it may then progress to pain with activity or pain with weight bearing. Athletes usually seek medical advice when the pain interferes with their regimen of exercise or when it occurs with weight bearing. In general, the athlete will not remember any particular trauma.

B. Signs

The physical examination is limited. Patients will tend to walk with an antalgic gait. For sacral or pubic stress fractures, patients will be tender over the site of the fracture. For femoral neck stress fractures, there is no specific site of point tenderness. Range of motion of the hip may be reduced due to pain resulting from femoral neck stress fractures. Internal rotation, in particular, may be limited. Sacral stress fractures may be painful with the Patrick test. Pubic stress fractures may involve pain with pelvic compression.

C. LABORATORY FINDINGS

A metabolic workup to evaluate the female patient for osteopenia may be necessary.

D. IMAGING STUDIES

Plain radiographic changes may not appear for up to 4 weeks. Findings include cortical hypertrophy, sclerosis, or lucency. Radiographs for a sacral stress fracture would include, at a minimum, an anteroposterior radiograph of the pelvis, an inlet view of the pelvis, and a lateral view of the lumbosacral spine. Radiographs for a pubic stress fracture would require an anteroposterior view, inlet and outlet views, and Judet views of the pelvis. Radiographs for a femoral neck stress fracture would require an anteroposterior radiograph of the pelvis, an anteroposterior radiograph of the hip, and a frog leg view of the hip.

A CT scan of the hip or pelvis is useful for all stress fractures of the hip and pelvis. Coronal and sagittal reconstructions are helpful in identifying a fracture. Findings are the same as those expected on plain radiographs including sclerosis, cortical hypertrophy, and a lucent line. A bone scan is useful in identifying increased activity in stress fractures (Figure 2–9). Bone scans have a high sensitivity but low specificity in detecting stress fractures, with false-positive rates up to 30%. In addition, they may be used as a guide for healing and return to sport activity.

MRI is highly sensitive and specific in diagnosing stress fractures. Stress reactions may be differentiated from stress fractures. Both result in edema that is hypointense on T1-weighted images and have increased signal on fat-suppressed T2-weighted images. However, a stress fracture will have a low signal line within the edematous region that may extend to a cortex.

Complications

Femoral neck stress fractures must be considered early in the differential diagnosis and ruled out prior to considering other possibilities due to the potentially devastating results from a missed diagnosis. If the diagnosis is

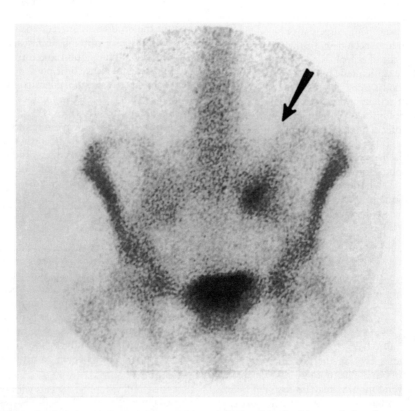

Figure 2–9. Bone scan of a left sacral stress fracture (***arrow***). (Reproduced, with permission, from Johnson AW et al: Am J Sports Med 2001;29:498.)

missed, the stress fracture may progress to a complete fracture. This is generally more difficult to correct and may require open reduction with internal fixation. Long-term sequelae include delayed union, nonunion, or avascular necrosis. These conditions may necessitate prosthetic replacement or osteotomy of the hip, which both yield a poor result in this active population.

Treatment

A. REHABILITATION

Most hip and pelvic stress fractures are managed conservatively. Depending on the site of the fracture and the level of symptoms, the athlete may initially require crutches for non-weight-bearing activities. As the symptoms subside, weight bearing is permitted. Activities are gradually increased with pain as the guide. Stress reactions are treated the same as stress fractures, but recovery is generally faster.

During the period of convalescence, non-weight-bearing conditioning is permitted. This includes swimming, pool exercises, and riding a stationary bicycle if these activities are not painful.

Management of femoral neck stress fractures is dictated by the type of fracture. Generally, they are divided into tension or compression sided fractures. Compression side fractures occur on the inferior cortical surface. Treatment is conservative because they are less likely to result in a complete fracture. Weight bearing is limited depending on the level of pain. Patients who have pain with weight bearing should be placed on crutches and not permitted to bear weight. This may have to be continued for up to 6 weeks. They are then gradually progressed to weight bearing as tolerated if it is painless. The decision to progress to more strenuous activity is difficult and is based on level of pain. Surgery may be indicated in patients who fail to improve with prolonged nonsurgical management.

B. SURGERY

Tension-sided fractures have a greater potential to progress to a complete fracture. Radiographically, these are found on the superior cortex of the femoral neck. Fractures that progress to a complete fracture are more likely to displace; therefore, they are treated with surgical fixation. Fixation may generally be done percutaneously for incomplete unicortical fractures or for nondisplaced complete fractures. Fluoroscopy is used to place three cannulated screws through the lateral cortex into the femoral head. These screws may range in diameter from 6.0 to 7.3 mm depending on the size of the patient. Typically the screws are placed in a triangular configuration for maximum stability. After internal fixation, the screws may be removed at 6 months to 1 year. This may avoid a more complicated removal at a later time.

Prognosis

The prognosis is good for return to full sport activity for most hip and pelvic stress fractures. The notable exception is tension side femoral neck stress fractures. These must be treated as described above with a guarded prognosis initially.

Return to Play

It may require up to 6 months to return to full sport activity for some athletes with femoral neck fractures. Repeat radiographs or bone scans may be helpful to determine if the fracture has healed sufficiently to allow a return to sport activity. As the weight-bearing status is advanced, radiographs are obtained to ensure that the fracture does not progress.

Bencardino JT et al: Magnetic resonance imaging of the hip: sports-related injuries. Top Magn Reson Imaging 2003;14(2):145. [PMID: 12777887]

HIP PAIN WITH MECHANICAL SYMPTOMS

Anatomy

The iliopsoas tendon and the anterior acetabular labrum lie within several millimeters of each other. The iliopsoas tendon lies immediately anterior to the anterior hip capsule and labrum (Figure 2–10). These two structures lie in such close proximity that there is a bursal communication between the hip joint and the iliopsoas tendon sheath in 20% of individuals. The acetabular labrum is continuous with the hyaline articular cartilage of the acetabulum (Figure 2–11). In fact, the bony acetabulum and its tidemark extend into the labrum.

Differential Diagnosis

Hip pain associated with mechanical symptoms or snapping has been classified as external, internal, and intraarticular. External snapping hip pain occurs at the greater trochanter and may be associated with trochanteric bursitis. External snapping hip and trochanteric bursitis are described above and will not be discussed further in this section. Internal and intraarticular causes of a snapping hip are discussed in the following sections.

Causes of groin pain other than the iliopsoas tendon and the acetabular labrum should also be considered. These include inguinal hernia, nerve entrapment, lumbar radiculopathy, osteitis pubis, stress fractures of the pelvis or femoral neck, and hip instability. Idiopathic hip instability has been described as a cause of groin pain associated with snapping. Patients with symptomatic hip instability have an abnormal gait. They walk with the leg abducted and externally rotated. Hip pain that is associated with mechanical symptoms of clicking, popping,

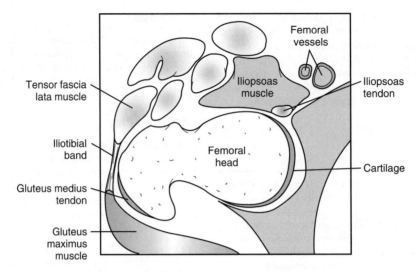

Figure 2–10. Note the close proximity of the iliopsoas tendon and the anterior acetabular labrum, two structures that can be responsible for hip pain felt in the groin associated with mechanical symptoms. (Reproduced, with permission, from Pelsser V et al: AJR Am J Roentgenol 2001;176:67.)

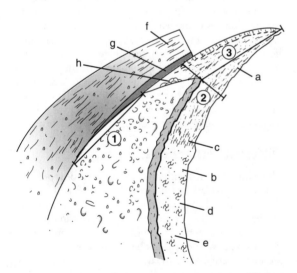

Figure 2–11. Cross section of a normal acetabular labrum. The articular edge of the labrum blends into the hyaline cartilage of the acetabulum. There is a limited blood supply to the periphery of the labrum. (a) Labrum; (b) articular hyaline cartilage; (c) articular cartilage–labrum transition zone; (d) bony acetabulum; (e) tide-mark; (f) hip capsule (cut); (g) capsular recess; (h) group of vessels. (1) Capsular recess; (2) thickness of labrum; (3) width of labrum. (Reproduced, with permission, from Seldes et al: Clin Orthop Relat Res 2001;382:232.)

catching, locking, or giving way is often caused by intraarticular pathology or snapping of the iliopsoas tendon. Intraarticular pathology includes tears of the acetabular labrum, loose bodies, synovial chondromatosis, and arthritis. Another source of intraarticular pathology is a "lateral impaction injury," which may result from a hard fall directly onto the greater trochanter. The force transmitted from the impact can result in full-thickness loss of the articular cartilage of the femoral head or chondronecrosis of the superomedial acetabulum. MRI will show an altered signal within the femoral head that can mimic osteonecrosis and it may occasionally reveal a chondral defect.

Symptoms from an internal snapping hip are usually of insidious onset, often following a change in workout routine. Repetitive activities involving high hip flexion can be provocative. Plain radiographs of the hip are usually normal. Groin pain with mechanical symptoms in an athlete caused by a labral tear usually follows an acute injury. Pain that does not follow an acute injury can occur in an athlete with a degenerative labral tear, or with an underlying developmental abnormality of the hip such as dysplasia (Figure 2–12) or femoral–acetabular impingement (Figure 2–13). These abnormalities are often apparent on plain radiographs.

Byrd JW: Lateral impact injury. A source of occult hip pathology. Clin Sports Med 2001;20(4):801. [PMID: 11675888]

Kelly BT et al: Hip arthroscopy: current indications, treatment options, and management issues. Am J Sports Med 2003;31(6):1020. [PMID: 14623676]

Seldes RM et al: Anatomy, histologic features, and vascularity of the adult acetabular labrum. Clin Orthop 2001;Feb(382):232. [PMID: 11153993]

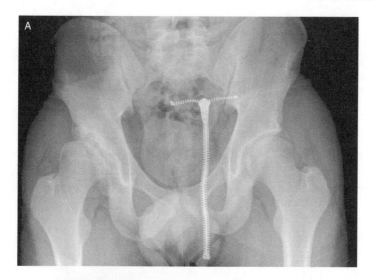

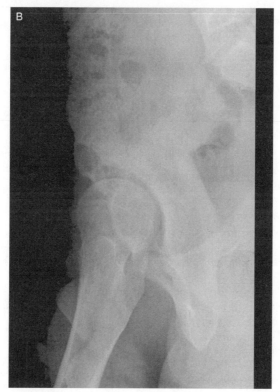

Figure 2–12. An (*A*) anteroposterior pelvis and (*B*) false profile view of a 20-year-old male who forfeited a college baseball scholarship due to right hip pain. There is severe acetabular dysplasia of the right hip. The mild dysplasia of the left hip is asymptomatic.

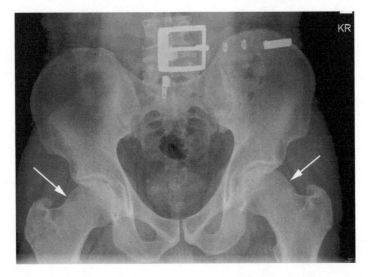

Figure 2–13. A 24-year-old right-footed soccer player with right groin pain due to femoral–acetabular impingement. There are typical radiographic findings of loss of the normal concavity of the superior femoral neck. There are also subchondral cysts (**arrows**) at the junction of the femoral head with the neck.

SNAPPING HIP (INTERNAL COXA SALTANS)

 ESSENTIALS OF DIAGNOSIS

- Groin pain or hip flexor dysfunction is caused by iliopsoas tendinitis.
- Iliopsoas tendon is irritated by repetitive hip flexion.
- Athletes experience a dull, deep catch or clunk in the groin.
- It is difficult to distinguish snapping hip from an acetabular labral tear.
- The distinction is made by physical examination and confirmed by special tests.
- MRI and ultrasound can confirm the diagnosis.
- Treatment consists of activity and training modification, nonsteroidal antiinflammatory drugs (NSAIDs), and physical therapy.
- Cortisone injection is reserved for pain refractory to conservative treatment.
- Surgical recession of the iliopsoas tendon is rarely required.

Prevention

Repetitive activities involving high hip flexion are the most common inciting factor leading to a painful internal snapping hip. Elimination of training exercises involving high hip flexion will often allow symptoms to improve. Stretching hip flexors prior to activity may be helpful. Although prevention of an internal snapping hip can be difficult, early recognition of the exacerbating activities, and elimination of these activities from the training routine can decrease the duration and extent of symptoms.

Clinical Findings

A. SYMPTOMS

Symptoms of a snapping hip usually begin insidiously with a dull, deep catch or "clunk" in the groin with flexion and extension of the hip. The pain can be located anywhere below the ASIS to the hip flexion crease, and is often centered about the AIIS. The symptoms can be described as an uncomfortable vibration, catching, or locking. Runners often describe weakness or dysfunction that is particularly noticeable as they advance the trailing leg. With severe irritation of the iliopsoas tendon, athletes will use their hands to lift the leg as they get onto the examination table or into a car.

A careful history including the specifics of training activities and any change in the workout routine can be helpful in distinguishing a snapping hip from other causes of groin pain. In particular, a labral tear is more often associated with an acute injury or underlying morphologic bony abnormality that is usually evident on plain radiographs.

B. Signs

Reproduction of snapping or clunking while taking the hip from a flexed, abducted, externally rotated (FABER) position to extension and neutral rotation is diagnostic of an internal snapping hip (Figure 2–14). This maneuver creates tension in the iliopsoas tendon as it is stretched across the iliopectineal eminence of the pelvis and femoral head and neck. The groin pain and clunk are often reproduced with each repetition of this maneuver. In addition to being perceived by the patient, snapping can often be heard and palpated in the groin by the examiner. Repetition of this maneuver will cause soreness in the groin, often characteristic of the athlete's pain.

Groin pain from an anterior labral tear or femoral–acetabular impingement occurs with the opposite maneuver of taking the hip from extension and neutral rotation to flexion, adduction, and internal rotation (FADIR). This maneuver brings the anterior superior femoral head and neck into proximity with the anterior superior acetabular labrum.

C. Imaging Studies

MRI of the hip can demonstrate abnormalities of the iliopsoas tendon and bursa, anterior hip capsule, and musculature of the iliopsoas mechanism. Findings are often subtle, so a high strength magnet that provides excellent resolution and imaging of both hips for comparison can be helpful.

Dynamic ultrasound can be diagnostic of snapping hip. This test is operator dependent.

Complications

Tendon rupture following paratendinous iliopsoas cortisone injection has not been reported. Temporary

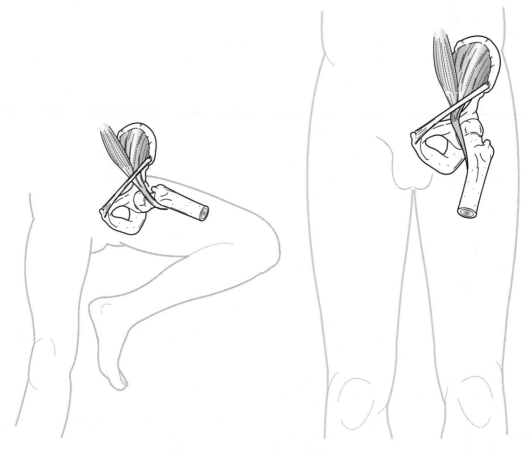

Figure 2–14. **A, B:** Clunking or snapping with the pictured maneuver can occur at the lesser trochanter, femoral head, superior pubic ramus, or sacroiliac joint. The underlying problem with internal snapping hip is excess tension or inflammation of the iliopsoas mechanism. (Reproduced, with permission, from Dobbs et al: Surgical correction of the snapping iliopsoas tendon in adolescents. *J Bone Joint Surg Am* 2002;84:420.)

exacerbation of symptoms following injection can occur. If symptoms persist following injection the treating physician should consider other causes of groin pain with mechanical symptoms caused by intraarticular pathology. Investigation with MR arthrography may be warranted in this circumstance.

Care must be taken during open surgical intervention for a snapping hip to avoid direct injury to the femoral nerve. When the iliopsoas tendon has been identified, it should be tested with a nerve stimulator prior to recession. The lateral femoral cutaneous nerve is in the field of dissection. The patient should be warned that numbness in the anterior thigh is not uncommon following surgery. Weakness of hip flexion following recession of the iliopsoas tendon is expected, but should be temporary and disappear with rehabilitation. Prolonged weakness has been reported with complete release of the tendon from the lesser trochanter. For this reason, other surgical approaches should be considered in athletes.

Treatment

Avoidance of precipitating activities, particularly hip flexion greater than 90°, and NSAIDs are the mainstay of treatment.

A. REHABILITATION

A physical therapy program including stretching can be helpful. Modalities such as cryotherapy and electrical stimulation have been reported to be effective.

B. SPECIAL PROCEDURES

Steroid injection can relieve the symptoms of a snapping hip. The injection can be done with ultrasound, CT, or fluoroscopic guidance. A mixture of 40 mg of triamcinolone acetonide (Kenalog), 0.5 mL of 1% lidocaine, and 0.5 mL of 0.5% bupivicaine injected into the tendon sheath has been recommended. The procedure is done under local anesthetic. The spinal needle is placed over the superior medial quadrant of the femoral head and directed into the region of the iliopsoas tendon sheath and underlying bursa. Repeat injection can be performed if the first injection is partially or temporarily effective.

C. SURGICAL

Surgery for a snapping hip is rarely necessary. When conservative measures fail and symptoms warrant, surgical intervention should be considered. The goal of surgery for a snapping hip is to decrease the tension in the iliopsoas tendon as it moves across the front of the hip joint and pelvis during flexion and extension of the hip. A secondary goal of surgery is to maintain the strength of the hip flexors.

Surgical strategies that have been recommended include open release near the insertion of the iliopsoas tendon to the lesser trochanter, open recession of the tendinous portion of the musculotendinous junction proximal to its insertion, and arthroscopic recession at either location. Release at the lesser trochanter has been associated with prolonged weakness of hip flexion. Arthroscopic recession proximal to the lesser trochanter by working through the anterior capsule of the hip joint to access the iliopsoas tendon has been described.

Prognosis

Symptoms from a snapping hip usually improve rapidly if the exacerbating drill or activity is avoided. With modification of activity, NSAIDs, and stretching, the athlete may be able to return to participation within 1–4 weeks. If rapid improvement does not occur, a steroid injection should be considered. The prognosis to full return to activity within 1–2 weeks following injection is good.

Return to Play

Return to elite athletic performance has been reported following surgical recession of the iliopsoas tendon. Recovery of strength sufficient for high level athletic activity is expected to take up to 6 months.

Dobbs MB et al: Surgical correction of the snapping iliopsoas tendon in adolescents. J Bone Joint Surg Am 2002;84-A(3):420. [PMID: 11886912]

Gruen GS et al: The surgical treatment of internal snapping hip. Am J Sports Med 2002;30(4):607. [PMID: 12130417]

Wahl CJ et al: Internal coxa saltans (snapping hip) as a result of overtraining: a report of 3 cases in professional athletes with a review of causes and the role of ultrasound in early diagnosis and management. Am J Sports Med 2004;32(5):1302. [PMID: 15262657]

LABRAL INJURIES

ESSENTIALS OF DIAGNOSIS

- Labral injuries are analogous to meniscal injuries of the knee.
- Pain is in the groin, buttock, or "C-sign" location.
- Pain is often associated with popping, clicking, and catching.
- Tears can be acute or degenerative.
- Degenerative tears are more common in sports that involve high hip flexion, such as ballet, football kicking, or rock climbing, or that involve repetitive twisting, such as golfing, figure skating, or martial arts.

- *Degenerative tears are also common in athletes with underlying developmental hip abnormalities such as dysplasia or femoral–acetabular impingement.*
- *Hips with acetabular dysplasia have hypertrophy of the acetabular labrum, which is more prone to tearing.*
- *Hips with a "pistol-grip" deformity (loss of concavity of the superior and anterior femoral neck) are prone to femoral–acetabular impingement.*
- *Femoral–acetabular impingement leads to labral tears and predisposes the hip to arthritis.*
- *Surgical treatment of acetabular labral tears is less predictable than treatment of meniscal tears.*
- *The prognosis depends on the location and severity of the tear, cause of the tear (traumatic versus degenerative), presence of underlying abnormalities, and degree of associated chondromalacia.*

Prevention

The best way to avoid degenerative labral tears is to avoid repetitive activities that bring the femoral neck in forceful contact with the labrum (Figure 2–15). This is not possible for some athletes whose sports involve extremes of flexion, abduction, or rotation of the hip. Competitive golfers, figure skaters, martial artists, cheerleaders, dancers, and gymnasts cannot avoid these activities during training or competition.

Acute labral tears have been seen in high force or ballistic activities in an undertrained individual such as a high school dancer performing a jump-split or an unconditioned individual performing a leg press with heavy weights. Proper training, with a gradual increase in extreme positions or weights, may help to avoid traumatic labral tears.

It is not uncommon for female athletes to have acetabular dysplasia. The increased hip motion associated with dysplasia may help gymnasts and ballerinas to excel. These athletes may be more prone to injury from

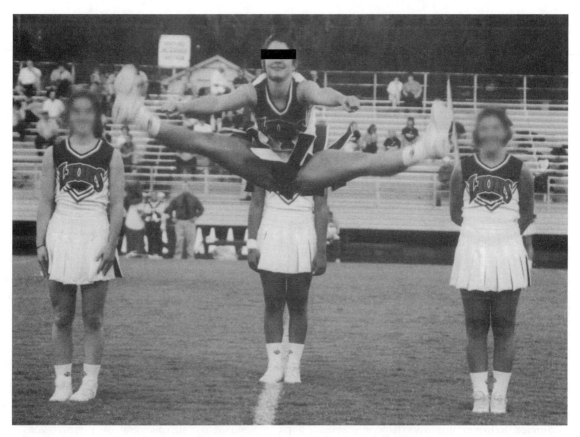

Figure 2–15. A 17-year-old high school cheerleader with a labral tear of the left hip.

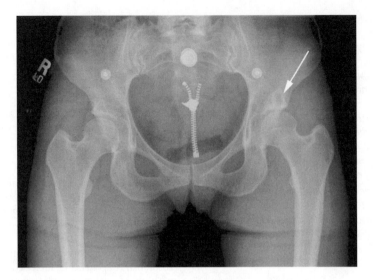

Figure 2–16. A 36-year-old former elite competitive gymnast with left hip pain. Note the mildly dysplastic acetabulum with a large superior-lateral acetabular cyst. This is indicative of separation of the labrum from the hyaline cartilage of the acetabulum. Slight narrowing of the cartilage space is also present. The potential for arthritic deterioration is high.

repetitive activities with extreme ranges of motion in a hip with a hypertrophic labrum and possibly some instability. Labral tears can progress to or be associated with arthritic deterioration of the hip joint, particularly in athletes with underlying dysplasia (Figure 2–16) or femoral–acetabular impingement (Figure 2–17).

Clinical Findings

A. SYMPTOMS

Pain from a labral tear is usually felt in the groin or anterior hip. Athletes often indicate that their pain is located in front of and around the side of their hip by using the

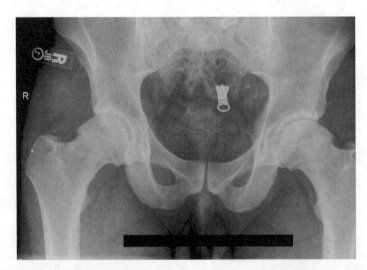

Figure 2–17. A 27-year-old National Football League lineman with right groin pain and difficulty getting down into his stance. There is underlying femoral–acetabular impingement that has caused a labral tear. There are signs of hip arthritis, including narrowing of the cartilage space, osteophytes, and loose bodies.

extended thumb and index finger or hand to grab the front and side of the hip. This has been called a "positive C-sign" because the extended thumb and index finger make a "C." Pain from a labral tear can also radiate to or be felt in the buttock or posterior lateral hip region. Anterior labral tears are most common. There may be a correlation between anterior labral tears causing anterior (groin) pain and posterior labral tears causing posterior (buttock) pain.

Hip pain from a labral tear is often associated with mechanical symptoms of painful clicking or popping. Catching and locking can also occur with a torn labrum. As with other hip pathologies, the pain from a labral tear can radiate down the leg, most often from the groin down the anterior thigh toward the knee. It can also radiate down the medial thigh along the adductor muscle group.

Pain from a torn labrum can range from subtle, dull, activity-induced, positional pain that fails to improve with rest to severe constant pain that interferes with activities of daily living. Athletes with a torn labrum will seldom walk with a significant limp or require crutches for ambulation. They will frequently avoid certain positions or activities that provoke symptoms. Provocative positions usually involve flexion, abduction, and rotation of the hip. The positional pain frequently interferes with athletic performance.

Specific traumatic events such as twisting, falling, or other loads on the leg may precede the onset of symptoms. A traumatic labral tear can be caused by the application of force to the hyperextended, externally rotated hip. At times, the onset of symptoms is more insidious, without a sentinel event, particularly with degenerative labral tears. An athlete may experience lingering symptoms from a "groin pull" that are actually caused by a torn labrum.

B. Signs

Physical examination will usually allow the examiner to distinguish athletes with a torn labrum from those with a snapping hip. With the athlete supine, symptoms from a torn labrum are reproduced by bringing the hip into FADIR. This maneuver, which brings the femoral neck into contact with the labrum, is termed the "impingement test."

Joseph McCarthy has described a variation of the Thomas test that is analogous to McMurray's test for a meniscal tear of the knee. With the athlete supine, both hips are flexed, locking the pelvis. The painful hip is then extended with the hip first in external rotation, then in internal rotation. Reproduction of a painful click constitutes a positive McCarthy sign. Groin pain with a rise in a resistive straight leg has been described as evidence of a labral tear. This test is not specific for a torn labrum however, and can be positive with other causes of intraarticular hip pathology.

C. Imaging Studies

It can be challenging to confirm the presence of a torn acetabular labrum with radiographic imaging. Plain radiographs of the hip should be reviewed. An anteroposterior view of the pelvis allows comparison of the affected hip to the opposite side. A frog lateral view of the involved hip should be ordered. In a hip with normal morphology these radiographs will often be normal. These views should be screened for the presence of acetabular dysplasia. Intraosseous cysts, seen in patients with long-standing labral tears, are usually indicative of associated chondromalacia or separation of the junction of the labrum and acetabular cartilage (Figure 2–16). These cysts are most commonly located at the superior lateral edge of the acetabulum.

The most common radiographic abnormality in a hip with femoral–acetabular impingement is a "pistol-grip" deformity, or loss of concavity of the superior and anterior femoral neck (Figure 2–13). This developmental abnormality is associated with degenerative labral tears. Intraosseous cysts in the femoral head located at the anterior superior junction of the head and neck (herniation pits) can be seen in hips with impingement. One study from the Mayo Clinic found that at least one structural abnormality of the hip was detectable on conventional radiographs in 87% of patients with acetabular labral tears. This review included all patients seen over a 6-year period of time and was not specific for labral tears sustained during sport.

Plain MRI is unreliable either in confirming the presence of a torn labrum or in ruling it out. A paralabral cyst is, however, strong indirect evidence of a torn labrum. Accuracy is improved significantly with MR arthrography, the diagnostic test of choice. MR arthrography is technique dependent (Figure 2–18). An arthrogram of the hip with gadolinium should be followed by an MRI done with surface coils, with a high-resolution scanner. A protocol specific for imaging the labrum, with cuts in the oblique sagittal plane of the femoral neck, is helpful (Figure 2–19).

CT scans and bone scans are generally not helpful in confirming the diagnosis of a torn acetabular labrum. Because of the significant false-negative rate of radiographic imaging techniques, including MR arthrography, it is reasonable to recommend hip arthroscopy for an athlete with symptoms and a physical examination suggestive of labral tear, even with a normal MR arthrogram, or without performing MR arthrography.

D. Special Tests

A hip block, injection of the hip joint with a local anesthetic under fluoroscopic guidance, can be helpful in deciding whether an intraarticular source of pain exists. Temporary relief of typical pain is supportive of intraarticular pathology as the source of the athlete's symptoms (Figure 2–18).

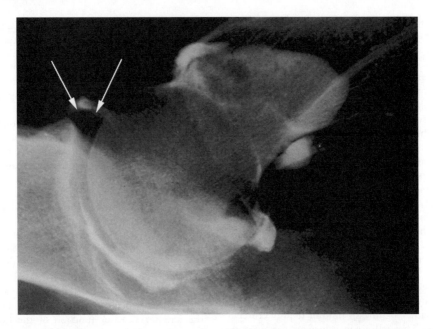

Figure 2–18. Hip arthrogram performed with fluoroscopic guidance using isovue and gadolinium. The superior lateral edge of the labrum is shown with arrows. Note the dye in the medial acetabular fossa that tracks along the articular cartilage of the hip. Addition of local anesthetic can be useful to confirm the presence of intraarticular pathology. Steroids can be injected at the time of the arthrogram, if clinically indicated. This athlete had a torn labrum that is not seen on the arthrogram, but was visible on the subsequent MRI.

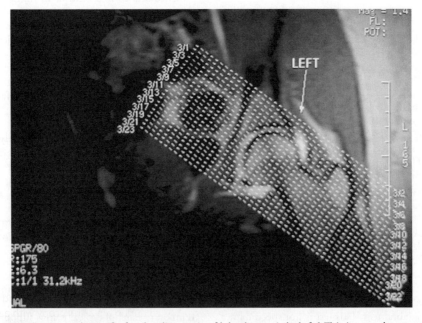

Figure 2–19. An MRI protocol specific for the diagnosis of labral tears is helpful. This image demonstrates sagittal cuts that are taken in the oblique plane of the femoral neck.

E. Special Examinations

Clinical examination is the most accurate way to diagnose intraarticular pathology in the hip. The diagnostic accuracy of a clinical examination has been compared with MRI, MR arthrography, intraarticular injection, and arthroscopy. With arthroscopy as the gold standard, clinical assessment had a 98% accuracy rate in detecting intraarticular abnormality. MRI demonstrated a 42% false-negative and a 10% false-positive rate and MR arthrography had an 8% false-negative and 20% false-positive rate. Response to intraarticular injection as an indicator of intraarticular abnormality had a reliability of 90%. The study was not specific for labral tears, but included all intraarticular pathology.

Complications

There is no information in the literature regarding the natural history of labral tears. The risk for progressive arthritic deterioration of the hip joint with or without arthroscopic treatment is not known. For this reason, surgical treatment should be reserved for athletes in whom symptoms or restriction of activity are intolerable, or athletic performance is significantly impaired. The mere presence of a torn labrum on MR arthrography does not indicate the need for hip arthroscopy.

Complications associated with hip arthroscopy include the risk of surgery with general anesthesia. Iatrogenic injury to the labrum and articular cartilage can occur. Instrument failure or breakage is possible. Traction must be applied to the leg during hip arthroscopy. This places the nerves of the leg at risk for traction injury. Direct injury to the sciatic and lateral femoral cutaneous nerves from portal placement is possible.

Treatment

A. Rehabilitation

Labral tears usually do not respond to conservative treatment. Physical therapy can be helpful if there is significant associated muscle spasm or gait abnormality. NSAIDs can reduce associated inflammation, which at times will decrease symptoms. Neither will improve the underlying source of inflammation and mechanical symptoms. Definitive treatment for a torn labrum is hip arthroscopy.

B. Surgical

Hip arthroscopy allows visualization of the labral tear, confirming the diagnosis (Figure 2–20). The goal of arthroscopic treatment of a torn labrum is to relieve pain by eliminating the unstable flap tear that causes discomfort (Figure 2–21). The surgeon seeks to debride all torn tissue and leave as much healthy labrum intact as possible (Figure 2–22). Hip arthroscopy also allows

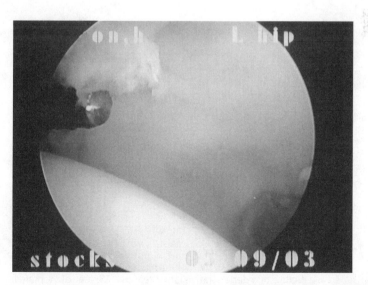

Figure 2–20. An arthroscopic view of the hip demonstrating an anterior labral tear in the cheerleader pictured in Figure 2–15. A posterior superior flap tear of the labrum was debrided during hip arthroscopy with a shaver and flexible thermal probe. (The femoral head is pictured on the bottom, the acetabular fossa is in the lower right-hand corner, the acetabular cartilage is in the middle, and the labrum is on the top left.)

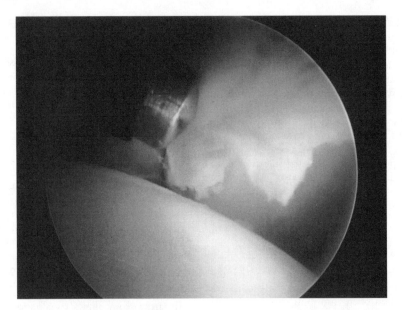

Figure 2–21. Picture from hip arthroscopy of a 26-year-old physician's assistant with an anterior superior labral tear sustained while rock climbing. (The femoral head is on the bottom, the hip capsule to the left, and the labrum on the right.)

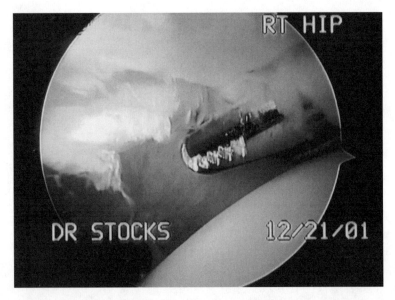

Figure 2–22. An arthroscopic picture of a degenerative labral tear in a 33-year-old female former National Collegiate Athletic Association volleyball player. (The femoral head is on the lower right, the labrum is on the top, and the labral tear is to the left.)

visualization of other sources of hip pain and mechanical symptoms, including the articular cartilage of the acetabulum and femoral head, the ligamentum teres, and the capsule.

C. SPECIAL PROCEDURES

For an athlete with severe and constant hip pain, indicating an inflamed hip joint, there is occasionally a role for intraarticular steroid injection. This is usually a temporizing measure.

Prognosis

The prognosis for arthroscopic treatment of isolated, acute traumatic labral tears is good. Good to excellent results have been reported in 80–90% of patients. Return to competition, even at the elite level, is possible. Persistent popping, particularly with certain positions or activities, is common, even following otherwise successful hip arthroscopy. The athlete facing hip arthroscopy for a torn labrum should be forewarned of this possibility.

The prognosis for athletes with degenerative tears, those associated with repetitive high-risk activities, is relatively poor for return to high level competition. The prognosis is significantly worse if chondromalacia is seen at arthroscopy.

Following hip arthroscopy, athletes remain touchdown weight bearing for a short period of time, usually from 2 days to 2 weeks. Range of motion exercises are emphasized during the first 2–6 weeks following arthroscopy. Return to full athletic activity can usually occur from 6 to 12 weeks following hip arthroscopy.

There is limited information in the literature regarding the prognosis following arthroscopic treatment of a labral tear in an athlete with an underlying bony abnormality. Persistent symptoms would be expected with significant acetabular dysplasia or retroversion, or femoral–acetabular impingement. Surgical treatment to address these problems, such as periacetabular osteotomy (Figure 2–23) or surgical dislocation of the hip, has been described. Surgical dislocation, requiring a trochanteric osteotomy, can also allow repair of a bucket-handle labral tear (Figure 2–24).

Return to Play

There is no information in the literature on return to competitive athletics following these surgical procedures.

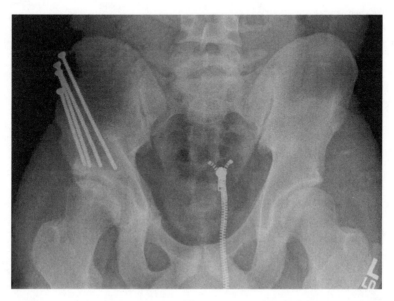

Figure 2–23. Following successful periacetabular pelvic osteotomy, the now 22-year-old male pictured in Figure 2–12 is pursuing a minor league baseball career. The screws were removed and the osteotomy solidly healed before release to full activity.

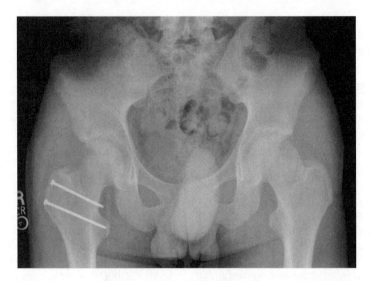

Figure 2–24. A 17-year-old soccer player and football kicker following surgical dislocation of the right hip, removal of the femoral neck impingement lesion, and repair of a bucket-handle labral tear. Right hip pain and popping improved, but the patient was unable to return to sports due to left hip pain. Note the loss of concavity of the left superior femoral neck, and improved concavity of the superior femoral neck of the right hip following surgery for femoral–acetabular impingement.

Byrd JW, Jones KS: Diagnostic accuracy of clinical assessment, magnetic resonance imaging, magnetic resonance arthrography, and intra-articular injection in hip arthroscopy patients. Am J Sports Med 2004;32(7):1668. [PMID: 15494331]

O'Leary JA et al: The relationship between diagnosis and outcome in arthroscopy of the hip. Arthroscopy 2001;17(2):181. [PMID: 11172248]

Siebenrock KA et al: Abnormal extension of the femoral head epiphysis as a cause of cam impingement. Clin Orthop 2004;Feb(418):54. [PMID: 15043093]

Wenger DE et al: Acetabular labral tears rarely occur in the absence of bony abnormalities. Clin Orthop 2004;Sep(426):145.

Knee Injuries

Lee Kaplan, MD, Nicholas Honkamp, MD, Ryan Kehoe, MD, Jonathon Tueting, MD, & Patrick J. McMahon, MD

Knee Pain with Mechanical Symptoms

Injury to the knee from athletic activities, daily living, or trauma is becoming more common. Children continue to participate in athletics and more adults than ever remain active. As our society becomes increasingly active, injuries to knee cartilage, meniscus, ligament, or bone will continue to increase.

Our ability to accurately and acutely diagnose knee injuries is critical. There are many diagnoses for knee pain, but most involve one or a combination of the following: meniscal tear, cartilage damage, osteochondral fracture, or ligamentous injury. These injuries may present in a similar fashion, but with a precise history and physical examination combined with appropriate imaging tests, the correct diagnosis can be obtained.

MENISCAL TEARS

Anatomy

A thorough understanding of meniscal anatomy is required for both the recognition of meniscal injury as well as its treatment. Beginning in the late 1800s, the menisci were thought of as "functionless remnants" of leg muscles. However, the realization of the important function of menisci in the knee has since stimulated extensive study. Grossly, the medial meniscus is C-shaped whereas the lateral meniscus is more semicircular shaped. Both are composed of fibrocartilage with bony attachments at the anterior and posterior aspects of the tibial plateau. Additionally, the medial meniscus has an extensive attachment at its periphery to the capsule, referred to as the coronary ligament. The thickening of this midportion of its capsular attachment is the deep portion of the medial collateral ligament. This extensive attachment of the medial meniscus to the capsule and plateau makes it relatively less mobile compared to the lateral meniscus.

The lateral meniscus covers a larger portion of the lateral tibial articular surface and is more semicircular shaped than the medial meniscus. Variants of the lateral meniscus, which have broader coverage of the tibial plateau than normal, have been termed "discoid" variants and have been reported to have an incidence of 3.5–5%. The more semicircular shape of the lateral meniscus places the anterior and posterior bony attachments of the lateral meniscus closer together. The anterior cruciate ligament (ACL) attachment is just medial to the anterior horn of the lateral meniscus. Ligaments attaching the posterior horn of the lateral meniscus to the medial femoral condyle course in front of and behind the posterior cruciate ligament and are termed the ligaments of Humphrey and Wrisberg, respectively (Figure 3–1). Discoid menisci can be classified into complete (covering the entire lateral plateau), incomplete, and Wrisberg variants. A Wrisberg variant discoid meniscus has an absent posterior horn bony attachment, and the posterior meniscofemoral ligament of Wrisberg is the only stabilizing structure.

Posterolaterally, the popliteus tendon emerges in the joint via the popliteal hiatus. Small fasciculi attach the popliteus tendon to the meniscus and are thought to have a stabilizing effect. The capsular attachments to the lateral meniscus are much less developed than the medial side, causing increased translation of the lateral meniscus compared to its medial counterpart.

Collagen bundles make up the microstructure of the normal meniscus. These collagen bundles form both circumferential and less numerous, radial bundles within the menisci. The radial bundles are mainly found at the surface of the meniscus forming a crossed meshwork of fibers thought to be important in resisting surface sheer stresses. The circumferential bundles make up the majority of the midsubstance of the menisci, and their orientation allows them to disperse the compressive loads applied though the knee. Approximately 60–70% of the dry weight of the menisci is composed of collagen, with 8–13% noncell proteins and 0.6% elastin. The majority of the collagen is type I, with lesser amounts of types II, III, V, and VI.

At birth, the entire meniscus is vascularized, but by 9 months of age the inner third of the meniscus is

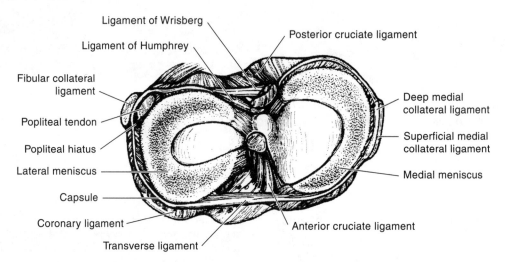

Figure 3–1. The anatomy of the tibial plateau showing the medial and lateral menisci with their associated intermeniscal ligaments. The lateral meniscus is not attached in the region of the popliteus tendon. (Reproduced, with permission, from Scott, WN: *Ligament and Extensor Mechanism Injuries of the Knee: Diagnosis and Treatment.* St. Louis, Mosby-Year Book, 1991.)

avascular. By adult age, only the outer 10–30% of the meniscus is vascular, with the main blood supply arising from the medial and lateral genicular arteries. There is also a relative avascular zone of the meniscus occurring at the popliteal hiatus secondary to the entrance of the popliteal tendon into the joint. Cell nutrition to the inner two-thirds of the menisci occurs through diffusion and cell pumping of synovial fluid. The anterior and posterior horns as well as the periphery of the meniscus have neural elements present, and these are thought to play a role in proprioceptive feedback during knee range of motion.

The function of the meniscus involves load sharing, shock absorption, distribution of contact stresses, stabilization, limiting extremes of motion, and proprioception. Primary among these is its affect on loading sharing, shock absorption, contact stresses, and stabilization. The menisci transmit approximately 50–70% of the load in extension, and 85% of the load with 90° of knee flexion. A total medial meniscectomy decreases the femoral contact area by 50–70% with a 100% increase in the contact stress. Similarly, a total lateral meniscectomy decreases the femoral contact area by 40–50% and increases the contact stress by 200–300%. Such increases with meniscectomy often lead to joint space narrowing, osteophytes, and squaring of the femoral condyles seen on radiographs. In addition, cartilage function is also affected with meniscectomy. The menisci are 50% as stiff as cartilage and thereby function as significant shock absorbers in the knee. Loss of the meniscus leads to a loss of this shock absorbency and increased demands on the cartilage. Finally, the medial meniscus functions as a secondary stabilizer to anterior

translation of the knee. In an ACL-competent knee, loss of the medial meniscus does little to affect the anterior to posterior motion of the knee. However, in an ACL-deficient knee, loss of the medial meniscus leads to a greater than 50% increase in anterior translation at 90° of flexion. In general, the inner two-thirds of the menisci are important for maximizing contact area and shock absorption, whereas the outer one-third is essential for load transmission and stability.

Pathogenesis

The incidence of meniscal tears is 60–70 per 100,000 persons, and affects males more frequently at a 2.5–4:1 ratio to females. The peak incidence of acute tears occurs in the 20- to 30-year-old age group, whereas degenerative chronic tears are more common in 40- to 60-year-old males. Female meniscal pathology is relatively constant after the second decade.

Younger patients often have an acute event as the cause of their meniscal tear. Approximately one-third of patients with an acute ACL tear will have a concomitant meniscal tear. Because of the relative increase in mobility of the lateral meniscus and lateral knee compartment, lateral meniscal tears are about four times as common as medial meniscal tears in ACL injuries. Because of its role as a secondary stabilizer to anterior translation in an ACL-deficient knee, medial meniscal tears are more prevalent in chronic ACL-deficient knees. Additionally, meniscal tears can occur in up to 47% of tibial plateau fractures, and are frequently observed in patients with a femoral shaft fracture and a concomitant knee effusion.

Allen CR et al: Importance of the medial meniscus in the anterior cruciate ligament-deficient knee. J Orthop Res 2000;18:109.

Garrick JG (editor): *Orthopaedic Knowledge Update: Sports Medicine 3.* American Academy of Orthopaedic Surgeons, 2004.

Greis PE et al: Meniscal injury: I. Basic science and evaluation. J Am Acad Orthop Surg 2002;10:168.

Clinical Findings

A. SYMPTOMS

Acute traumatic tears of the menisci are often caused by axial loading combined with rotation. Patients typically report pain and swelling. Patients with smaller tears may have a sensation of clicking or catching in the knee. Patients with larger tears in the meniscus may complain of locking of the knee as the meniscus displaces into the joint and/or femoral notch. Loss of knee motion with a block to extension often involves a large bucket-handle tear that has displaced into the femoral notch. In acute tears involving an associated ACL injury, the swelling may be more significant and acute. ACL injuries often involve a lateral meniscal tear as the lateral compartment of the knee subluxates forward trapping the lateral meniscus between the femur and tibia.

Conversely, chronic or degenerative tears of the menisci often present in older patients (>40 years old) with a history of an insidious onset of pain and swelling with or without an acute increase superimposed. Often no identifiable history of trauma is obtained, or the inciting event may be quite minor such as a bending or squatting motion. Symptoms of catching or locking may also derive from chondral or patellofemoral damage.

B. SIGNS

A thorough physical examination of the knee involving the entire leg is essential. Assessing hip range of motion and irritability is useful, especially in children, as referred pain from the hip to the knee area is common. Examining for quadriceps atrophy and the presence of a knee effusion should also be done. Any joint line swelling or deformity may be a clue to a meniscal cyst. Measurement of range of motion may reveal a loss of terminal extension seen in meniscal tears. Assessing for tenderness of the femoral condyles, joint lines, tibial plateaus, and patellofemoral joint may provide clues as to a possible osteochondral lesion, meniscal lesion, fracture, or chondrosis, respectively. Ligamentous testing including varus and valgus stress testing at full extension and 30° of flexion, Lachman, anterior drawer, and posterior drawer testing should be done to assess stability.

The most important physical examination finding in a patient with a meniscal tear is joint line tenderness. Other specialized tests including the McMurray, flexion McMurray, and Apley grind test have also been studied. The McMurray test is performed with the patient lying supine with the hip and knee flexed to about 90°. While one hand holds the foot and twists it from external to internal rotation, the other hand holds the knee and applies compression. A positive test elicits a pop or click that can be felt by the examiner when the torn meniscus is trapped between the femoral condyle and the tibial plateau (Figure 3–2). A variation of this test is the flexion McMurray, in which the knee is held as for the McMurray test. To test the medial meniscus, the foot is externally rotated and the knee is maximally flexed. A positive test occurs when the patient experiences pain over the posteromedial joint line as the knee is gradually extended. The Apley grind test involves placing the patient prone with the knee flexed to 90°. The examiner applies downward pressure to the sole of the foot while twisting the lower leg in external and internal rotation. A positive tests results in pain at either joint line (Figure 3–3).

Many studies have attempted to quantitate the reliability of various physical examination findings. In a prospective study comparing preoperative joint line tenderness to arthroscopic findings of meniscal tears, the sensitivity of joint line tenderness was found to be 86% and 92%, with an overall accuracy rate of 74% and 96% for the medial and lateral meniscus, respectively. Another study found similar results, with joint line tenderness having a sensitivity of 74%. The only significant McMurray sign to correlate with a meniscal injury was a "thud" elicited on the medial joint line with a medial meniscal tear. However, the McMurray and Apley tests were found by others to have less than 75% sensitivity for diagnosing meniscal tears.

In the setting of an acute ACL injury, joint line tenderness was found to be less useful in defining a meniscal injury preoperatively. In addition, misdiagnoses occurred with chondromalacia patella, plica, fat pad impingement, and chondral lesions.

Overall, joint line tenderness remains the most accurate finding by which to diagnose a meniscal tear. Despite the poor reliability of other examination findings taken individually, a thorough history and a physical examination using multiple tests combined with plain radiographs were 95% and 88% sensitive for detecting medial and lateral meniscal tears, respectively.

Eren OT: The accuracy of joint line tenderness by physical examination in the diagnosis of meniscal tears. Arthroscopy 2003;19(8):850.

C. IMAGING STUDIES

1. Radiography—The next step in the workup of a patient with mechanical knee symptoms involves obtaining weight-bearing plain radiographs of the knee, including 45° posteroanterior flexion views of both knees, a lateral view, and a patellofemoral view such as a Merchant view. The posterior femoral condyles often show earlier and more advanced wear, and corresponding joint space

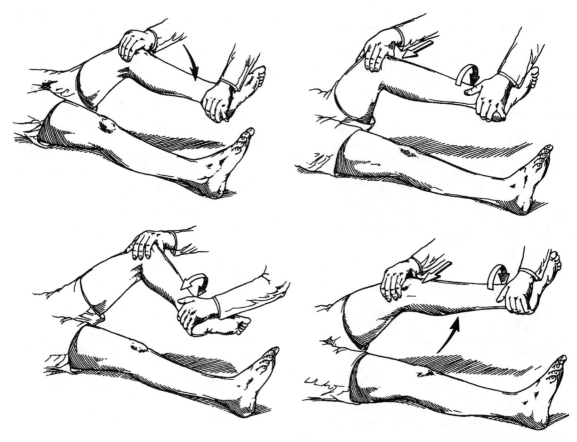

Figure 3–2. McMurray test.

narrowing on a 45° weight-bearing view is often seen. This would not necessarily be seen on a non-weight-bearing radiograph, and is the principal reason that non-weight-bearing radiographs have no role in the workup of mechanical knee pain (Figure 3–4). Patients with knee pain and significant joint-space narrowing on radiographs should be cautioned that extensive meniscal and chondral damage may be present that is unlikely to respond to arthroscopic partial meniscectomy. A patellofemoral radiograph is essential to help exclude patellofemoral chondrosis as the source of knee pain. Additionally, plain radiographs will not make the diagnosis of a meniscal tear, but will help eliminate concurrent problems such as an osteochondral lesion, fracture, patellofemoral malalignment, or loose body.

2. Magnetic resonance imaging—Magnetic resonance imaging (MRI) has contributed greatly to the accurate diagnosis of meniscal tears. Its advantages include the ability to image the meniscus in multiple planes and its lack of ionizing radiation. In addition, the ability to

evaluate other articular and extraarticular structures is particularly useful in patients with a nondiagnostic history and physical examination, or in patients with associated injuries that make physical examination difficult. Its disadvantages include its high cost and the possibility of misinterpretation and a false-positive result leading to further evaluation. The normal meniscus has a uniform low-intensity signal on all pulse sequences. Because of increased vascularity in children, the appearance of a child's meniscus on MRI may have an increased intrameniscal signal. In older adults, an increased intrameniscal signal may be a sign of degeneration.

The appearance of the meniscus on MRI is done on a four-grade system. Grade 0 is a normal meniscus. Grade I has a globular increase in signal within the meniscus that does not extend to the surface. Grade II has a linear increase in signal within the meniscus that does not extend to the surface. Grade III has an increased signal that abuts the free edge of the meniscus. Only Grade III, where an increased signal reaches the

MRI has also been used to assess meniscal repair. It has been found to be equal or superior to contrast arthrography in assessing a repaired meniscus, as well as the ability to discriminate partial versus complete meniscal healing.

Fu FH et al (editors): *Knee Surgery*. Williams & Wilkins, 1998.

Kocabey Y et al: The value of clinical examination versus MRI in the diagnosis of meniscal tears and anterior cruciate ligament rupture. Arthroscopy 2004;20:696.

D. Tear Classification

Meniscal tears can be classified either by etiology or by their arthroscopic and MRI appearance. Etiologic classification divides tears into either acute (excessive force applied to an otherwise normal meniscus) or degenerative (normal force applied to a degenerative structure).

Classification should describe the tear location and its associated vascularity, morphology, and stability. Tear location is described by the location of the tear in the anteroposterior plane (anterior, middle, or posterior) and its circumferential location with respect to its vascularity. The common vascular zones include the most peripheral red/red zone near the meniscocapsular junction, the intermediate red/white zone, and the most central white/white zone. As tears occur more centrally, the vascularity as well as the associated healing rates decrease.

Tear morphology describes the orientation of the tear within the meniscus and includes vertical or horizontal longitudinal, radial (transverse), oblique, and complex (including degenerative) tears (Figures 3–5 and 3–6). Most acute tears in younger patients involve vertical longitudinal or oblique tears, whereas complex and degenerative tears occur more commonly in older patients. Vertical longitudinal, or bucket-handle tears, can be complete or incomplete and usually start in the posterior horn and continue anteriorly a variable distance. Long tears can cause significant mobility of the torn meniscal fragment allowing it to displace into the femoral notch and cause a locked knee. This more commonly occurs in the medial meniscus, possibly due to its decreased mobility, which leads to increased sheer stresses. Oblique tears commonly occur at the junction of the middle and posterior thirds. They are often smaller tears, but the free edge of the tear can catch in the joint and cause symptoms of catching. Complex or degenerative tears occur in multiple planes, are often located in or near the posterior horns, and are more common in older patients with degenerative menisci. Horizontal longitudinal tears are often associated with meniscal cysts. They usually start at the inner margin of the meniscus and extend toward the meniscocapsular junction. They are thought to result from sheer stresses and, when associated with meniscal cysts, occur in the medial meniscus and cause localized swelling at the joint line.

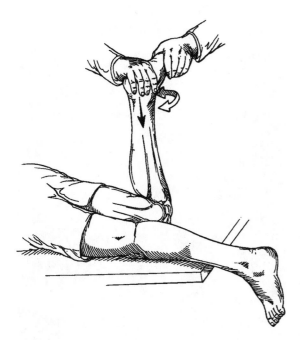

Figure 3–3. Apley test.

meniscal surface, is considered a true meniscal tear. MRI is approximately 90–95% accurate in diagnosing a meniscal tear, particularly when two consecutive images show an increased meniscal signal touching the surface of the meniscus. The meniscal shape can also be important in the diagnosis of a meniscal tear. Generally, sagittal images through the meniscus give the meniscus a "bowtie" shape. Loss of the bowtie shape may indicate a meniscal tear. Also, the "double posterior cruciate ligament" sign indicates a torn and displaced meniscus that is adjacent to the posterior cruciate ligament in the femoral notch.

Common misinterpretations of normal structures include the popliteal hiatus posteriorly and the intermeniscal ligament anteriorly. There is often difficulty in determining a tear of the anterior horn of the meniscus, an uncommon finding. False-positive results of meniscal tears seen on MRI in asymptomatic patients do occur and the incidence increases with age. This emphasizes the importance of taking the entire clinical and radiographic picture into perspective when evaluating a patient. A recent study documented a 5.6% incidence of meniscal tears diagnosed by MRI in asymptomatic patients between the ages of 18 and 39 years with a normal physical examination. A second study found 13% of asymptomatic patients younger than 45 years old and 36% of those older than 45 years old had MRI scans read as positive for meniscal tears.

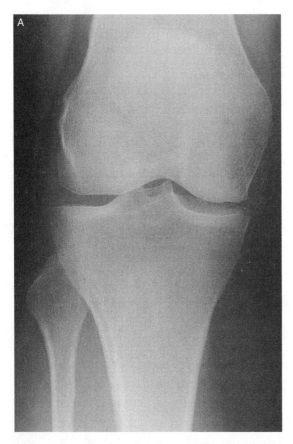

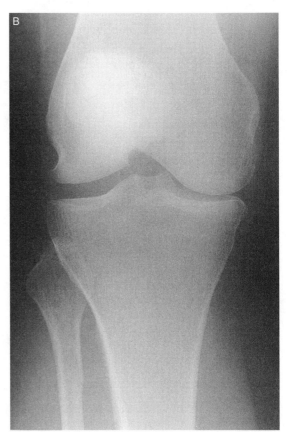

Figure 3–4. Advantages of the Rosenberg x-ray. **A:** No joint space narrowing can be seen in a weight-bearing view with the knee straight. **B:** With flexion and weight bearing, significant narrowing of the medial compartment is demonstrated. (Reproduced, with permission, from Anderson J: *An Atlas of Radiography for Sports Injuries.* McGraw-Hill, 2000.)

Treatment

Treatment options for meniscal tears include nonsurgical, meniscectomy (partial or complete), and meniscal repair. Advances in arthroscopy and technical skills have recently made meniscal transplant a more common procedure.

A. NONSURGICAL

Nonsurgical treatment of meniscal tears is generally limited to smaller, incomplete tears involving the posterior horns. These tears may be painful but do not catch in the joint so the patient does not feel popping or catching. Such tears are usually found in stable knees. Treatment includes modification of activity to avoid cutting and pivoting sports that may aggravate symptoms, stretching, and quadriceps and hamstring strengthening. Such treatment often works best in older individuals as arthritis rather than the meniscal tear may be the cause of their symptoms. Small (<10 mm) stable longitudinal tears, partial-thickness tears on the superior or inferior surface, or small (<3 mm) radial tears may heal spontaneously or remain asymptomatic.

B. SURGICAL

The indications for arthroscopic meniscal surgery are persistent pain with an effusion that does not respond to nonsurgical treatment, and catching or locking. Catching and locking are referred to as mechanical symptoms. These may interfere with activities of daily living. Physical examination should reveal joint effusion and joint line tenderness. Patients may also have limitations of knee motion and provocative signs such as pain with McMurray or Apley tests. Finally, other possible causes of knee pain should be ruled out through a thorough history, physical examination, and imaging studies.

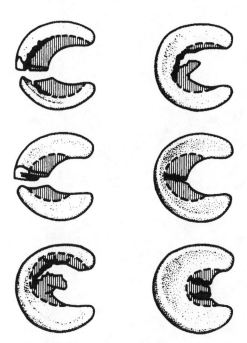

Figure 3–5. Types of meniscal tears: bucket-handle, flap, horizontal cleavage, radial, degenerative, and double radial tear of a discoid meniscus. (Reproduced, with permission, from Scott WN: *Arthroscopy of the Knee*. Philadelphia: WB Saunders, 1990.)

1. Meniscal resection—Open or arthroscopic removal of the entire meniscus, termed meniscectomy, was initially thought to be a benign procedure, but long-term outcome was poor and gender related: 75% of males and less than 50% of females had good or excellent results. But less than 50% of the males and only 10% of the females were symptom free. Results were poorer when surgery was done on younger compared to older individuals. Also, 75% of the patients had arthritis compared to only 6% of age-matched controls. The arthritis often did not manifest in many of the patients until more than 15 years after surgery. Lastly, degenerative changes occurred more rapidly after lateral compared to medial meniscectomy. With improved understanding of the importance of the knee menisci, advances in technique and instrumentation have allowed surgeons to perform a meniscal repair or a partial meniscectomy.

Deciding when to partially resect rather than repair a partially torn meniscus is difficult. There are many factors influencing outcome that need to be considered. For example, large partial meniscectomy that extends through the circumferential bands at the periphery of the meniscus yields poor results. Violation of these circumferential fibers significantly hinders the meniscus in distributing hoop stresses at its periphery. Also, when

the mechanical axis of the knee joint falls within the side of the knee that has had a meniscectomy, there are poorer results. Lastly, associated pathology in the knee, specifically, the amount of chondral damage and the presence of associated ligamentous instability, is associated with poorer results. Other factors to consider include the patient's age, tear pattern (geometry, size), vascularity, tissue quality, and knee stability. New repair techniques and the technical skills of the surgeon may also influence the decision. Most importantly, the expected outcome and rehabilitation must fit the patient's individual goals. Partial meniscectomy has good or excellent results in nearly 90% of patients when there is no knee arthritis and the knee is stable. Results are satisfactory in only two-thirds of patients when arthritis or ACL injuries are present. Overall, radiographic progression of degenerative changes occurs with follow-up beyond 10 years, although radiographic changes do not necessarily correlate with patient symptoms. Again, medial meniscal tears generally have better results than lateral tears, and an intact meniscal rim and intact cartilage surfaces are associated with a better prognosis.

Aglietti P et al: Arthroscopic meniscectomy for discoid lateral meniscus in children and adolescents: 10-year follow-up. Am J Knee Surg 1999;12:83.

Anderson-Molina H et al: Arthroscopic partial and total meniscectomy: long-term follow-up study with matched controls. Arthroscopy 2002;18:183.

Chatain F et al: The natural history of the knee following arthroscopic medial meniscectomy. Knee Surg, Sports Trauma, Arthrosc 2001;9(1):15.

Chatain F et al: A comparative study of medial versus lateral arthroscopic partial meniscectomy on stable knees: 10 year minimum follow-up. Arthroscopy 2003;19(8):842.

2. Meniscal repair—Because of the importance of the meniscus in knee stability and protection of chondral surfaces, surgeons often recommend meniscal repair in young, active individuals and those undergoing ACL or chondral reconstruction. Commonly accepted criteria for meniscal repair include a complete, vertical, longitudinal tear greater than 10 mm in length, a tear of the peripheral 10–30% of the meniscus or within 3–4 mm of the meniscocapsular junction, a peripheral tear that can be displaced toward the center of the plateau by probing, the absence of secondary degeneration of the meniscus, and a tear in an active patient or one undergoing concurrent ligament or chondral reconstruction.

Multiple factors affect the success of meniscus repair. Although no absolute age limit exists, patients younger than 40 years old are thought to have a better chance of healing. Knees with associated ligamentous instability, particularly ACL instability, have inferior rates of meniscus healing because of abnormal meniscus stresses from tibiofemoral instability. The location of the tear and the time lapsed from injury to treatment are also important.

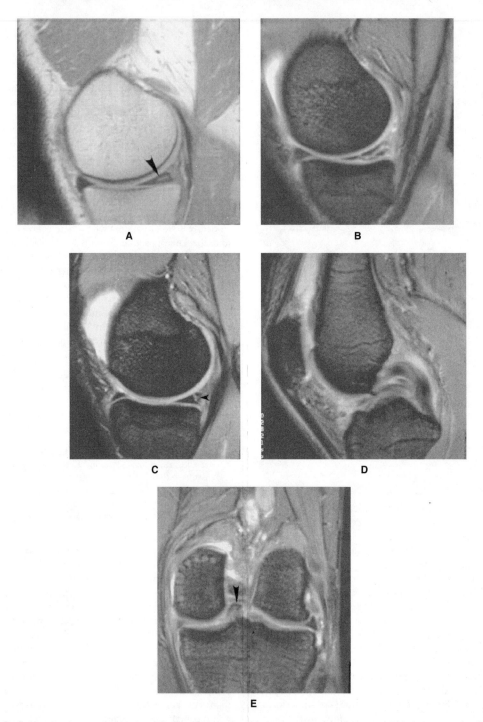

Figure 3–6. Meniscal tears. **A:** Meniscal degeneration should not be mistaken for a tear. This is a common finding of doubtful clinical significance, appreciated on MRI as an area of high signal that does not extend to the auricular surface. **B:** Complex tear of the posterior horn of the medial meniscus. **C:** Vertical peripheral tear in the posterior horn of the medial meniscus. **D:** Bucket-handle tear with flipping of the loose meniscal fragment into the intercondylar notch, producing a "double posterior cruciate ligament" sign on this sagittal MR image. **E:** The same bucket-handle tear in **D** shown in coronal section. (Reproduced, with permission, from Anderson J: *An Atlas of Imaging in Sports Medicine.* McGraw-Hill, 1999.)

Acute tears located in the peripheral red/red or red/white zone have better healing ability than chronic tears located in the red/white or white/white zones. Tears 5 mm or more from the periphery are considered avascular (white zone), tears between 3 and 5 mm are variable in vascularity (red/white), and tears in the peripheral 3 mm are considered vascular (red). In areas with marginal vascularization, abrasion of the meniscocapsular junction or use of a fibrin clot may be employed. It is thought that a vascular pannus forms from the abraded tissue, which aids in meniscus healing. Finally, the stability of the meniscus repair is a factor, with vertical mattress sutures generally considered the gold standard.

Meniscus repair is successful in up to 90% of meniscus tears when done in conjunction with ACL reconstructions, as compared to approximately 50% in patients with stable ACLs who had meniscus repairs.

Types of repairs include the traditional open repair and arthroscopic repairs that can be done with inside-out, outside-in, or all-inside techniques. Inside-out and outside-in repairs require a mini-incision and securing of the meniscus to the capsule with sutures. The all-inside technique has many device options including both absorbable and nonabsorbable arrows, tacks, darts, and fasteners. Regardless of the type of repair chosen, adequate preparation of the tear site is required. The tear edges should be debrided or abraded with a shaver or rasp to stimulate bleeding. Restoration of biomechanical function is encouraged by anatomic apposition of the tear edges to ensure good healing potential.

Greis PE et al: Meniscal injury: II. Management. J Am Acad Orthop Surg 2002;10:177.

Medvecky MJ, Noyes FR: Surgical approaches to the posteromedial and posterolateral aspects of the knee. J Am Acad Orthop Surg 2005;13:121.

Noyes FR, Barber-Westin SD: Arthroscopic repair of meniscal tears extending into the avascular zone in patients younger than twenty years of age. Am J Sports Med 2002;30(4):589.

Noyes FR, Barber-Westin SD: Arthroscopic repair of meniscus tears extending into the avascular zone with or without anterior cruciate ligament reconstruction in patients 40 years of age and older. Arthroscopy 2000;16:822.

a. Open—Open repair of meniscus tears has had successful long-term results. The technique involves making a small incision through the subcutaneous tissue, capsule, and synovium to directly visualize the tear. Open repair is most useful in peripheral or meniscocapsular tears, often performed in conjunction with open repair of a collateral ligament injury or a tibial plateau fracture. Follow-up studies of 10 years or longer have shown survival rates of repaired menisci of 80–90%, in part influenced by the peripheral nature of the tear and the associated hemarthrosis present in ligament tears or fracture repair cases.

Muellner T et al: Open meniscal repair. Am J Sports Med 1999;27:16.

b. Arthroscopic—

(1) Inside-out—Arthroscopic inside-out meniscus repairs are performed using long needles introduced through cannula systems with attached absorbable or nonabsorbable sutures passed perpendicularly across the tear from inside the knee to a protected area outside the joint capsule. These sutures are able to obtain consistent perpendicular placement across the meniscus tear, which gives this method an advantage over other repair techniques. Improved suture placement is gained at the expense of possible neurovascular injury from passing the needle from inside the knee to outside the joint. This technique requires a posteromedial or posterolateral incision to protect the neurovascular structures and safely retrieve the exiting needles. Secondary to its ability to gain vertical mattress suture fixation, this technique remains the gold standard for many surgeons. Numerous retrospective and prospective studies using second-look arthroscopy or arthrography to evaluate healing of the meniscus repairs have consistently shown rates of success of 70–90% in isolated repairs, and greater than 90% when done in conjunction with an ACL reconstruction. This technique is ideal for posterior and mid-posterior horn tears. There is difficulty in passing needles in mid- to anterior horn meniscus tears.

Elkousy H, Higgins LD: Zone-specific inside-out meniscal repair: technical limitations of repair of posterior horns of medial and lateral menisci. Am J Orthop 2005;34:29.

Spindler KP et al: Prospective comparison of arthroscopic medial meniscal repair technique: inside-out versus entirely arthroscopic arrows. Am J Sports Med 2003;31:929.

(2) Outside-in—The arthroscopic outside-in repair was developed in part to decrease the neurovascular risk associated with the inside-out technique. The outside-in technique involves passing a needle from outside the joint, across the tear, and into the joint. Two options then exist for repair of the meniscus tear. One option is to retrieve the suture through an anterior portal, tie a knot outside the knee joint, and then bring the knot back in through the anterior portal placing the knot against the reduced meniscus body fragment. A second option is to use parallel needles and retrieve the suture through the second needle. This can be done using a suture relay. A knot is then tied outside the joint over the capsule. This method is useful for tears in the anterior horn or body of the menisci, but does not work for tears in or near the posterior horn. Results of the outside-in technique using MRI, arthrography, or second-look arthroscopy to assess healing have shown complete or partial healing in 74–87% of meniscus repairs. As expected, results were not as good for posterior horn tears and tears in unstable knees.

Rodeo SA: Arthroscopic meniscal repair with use of the outside-in technique. J Bone Joint Surg A 2000;82:127.

Yiannakopoulos CK et al: A simplified arthroscopic outside-in meniscus repair technique. Arthroscopy 2004;20:183.

(3) All-inside—The popularity of the all-inside repairs has increased as numerous devices and techniques have been introduced in the past few years. This is due in part to the fact that these repairs do not require accessory incisions, thereby saving operative time, and they avoid more technical arthroscopic techniques required in other types of repairs. However, because of the speed of their introduction, their documented clinical effectiveness compared to more traditional techniques has lagged behind their use.

The initial devices introduced in the early 1990s included biodegradable meniscus arrows, meniscus darts, and simple suture devices such as the T-Fix. There was a good initial experience with these devices, particularly the meniscus arrows, which were the first to be introduced. Early studies showed success rates of 80% or higher at 1–2 year follow-ups. However, complications with these first-generation devices began to be reported, including retained fragments, foreign body reactions, inflammation, chronic effusions, and articular cartilage injuries. Additionally, mechanical testing of these first-generation devices showed pull-to-failure strengths closer to that of horizontal, not vertical, sutures.

Updated first-generation and second-generation devices were developed in response to these biomechanical strength concerns and to address the early complication rates. Implant design modifications included a change to smaller or rounded heads on the meniscus arrow and darts, polymer composition changes to decrease their resorption times, and the introduction of suture-based implants that did not require arthroscopic knot tying. Examples included contoured and headless arrow designs and suture-based implants such as the FasT-Fix and RapidLoc devices.

It is difficult to compare studies for these updated first- or second-generation devices, but in general studies can be classified into two groups: follow-up clinical studies on human implanted devices and biomechanical cadaveric or animal studies. Secondary to their earlier introduction into clinical use, long-term follow-up studies are most prevalent for updated first-generation meniscus arrow devices. First reported in 1993, multiple studies have shown 60–90% clinical success rates using either second-look arthroscopy or clinical examination evaluations. Some have even been comparable to traditional open suture techniques. Complications, including inflammatory reactions and articular cartilage damage, remain a concern for sutureless devices that may migrate from their original implanted meniscus tear position.

Biomechanical studies on second-generation devices have also been recently published. A follow-up to the initial T-Fix device, the second-generation FasT-Fix suture device, has shown superior results. Its biomechanical performance in load to failure, stiffness, and cyclic displacement tests has been equivalent to the gold standard of vertical mattress sutures. Other devices including other suture devices and various meniscus arrows or screws have biomechanical performance equivalent to that of horizontal mattress sutures. It is generally believed that the superiority of vertical mattress over horizontal mattress sutures is derived from the ability of vertical mattress sutures to capture the strong circumferential fibers of the meniscus. Additionally, suture devices in general have a lower risk of loose body reactions as their fixation device is extracapsular. However, there is a learning curve associated with placement of suture devices that may cause their fixation strength to be suboptimal until the technique is mastered.

Caution should be exercised in interpreting biomechanical studies of meniscus repair devices. Most larger studies involve porcine, bovine, or canine models secondary to increased cost and availability issues in obtaining human cadaveric menisci. Studies involving human menisci should also be evaluated for the source of their menisci, as older samples taken from arthritic total joint patients may not accurately reflect in vivo conditions. It is also not known if in vitro load-to-failure or cyclic loading testing is applicable to the in vivo stress environment.

In general, however, multidevice studies have shown that (1) vertical are superior to horizontal mattress sutures, (2) arrows and other nonsuture devices have 40–70% of the pull-to-failure strength and cyclic load displacement of vertical mattress sutures, and (3) suture devices such as the FasT-Fix have biomechanical profiles similar to vertical mattress sutures. What remains to be determined, however, is the minimal strength that meniscus repair devices need to provide for meniscus healing to occur in vivo.

Repairable meniscus tears often occur with an ACL tear. Stabilizing the knee with ACL reconstruction protects the repaired meniscus from abnormal knee motion; this results in a higher rate of success than if the knee is left unstable.

Anderson K et al: Chondral injury following meniscal repair with a biodegradable implant. Arthroscopy 2000;16:749.

Barber FA, Herbert MA: Load to failure testing of new meniscal repair devices. Arthroscopy 2004;20(1):45.

Borden P et al: Biomechanical comparison of the FasT-Fix meniscal repair suture system with vertical mattress and meniscal arrows. Am J Sports Med 2003;31(3):374.

Klimkiewicz J, Shaffer B: Meniscal surgery 2002 update. Arthroscopy 2002;18(suppl 2):14.

Miller MD et al: Pitfall associated with FasT-Fix meniscal repair. Arthroscopy 2002;18(8):939.

Miller MD et al: All-inside meniscal repair devices. Am J Sports Med 2004;32(4):858.

Petsche T et al: Arthroscopic meniscus repair with bioabsorbable arrows. Arthroscopy 2002;18:246.

Sgaglione NA et al: Current concepts in meniscus surgery: resection to replacement. Arthroscopy 2003;19(10; suppl 1):161.

Shaffer B et al: Preoperative sizing of meniscal allografts in meniscus transplantation. Am J Sport Med 2000;28:524.

Rath E et al: Meniscal allograft transplantation: two to eight-year results. Am J Sports Med 2001;29:410.

Zantop T et al: Initial fixation strength of flexible all-inside meniscus suture anchors in comparison to conventional suture technique and rigid anchors: biomechanical evaluation of new meniscus refixation systems. Am J Sports Med 2004;32(4):863.

3. Meniscal transplantation—Meniscal transplantation is now a viable option for selected patients with meniscal-deficient knees. Recent advances in surgical technique and clarification in the indications for the procedure have improved the clinical outcome. Meniscal transplantation is indicated for patients with symptoms referable to a meniscal-deficient tibiofemoral compartment. Contraindications to meniscal transplant include patients with advanced articular cartilage degeneration, instability, or malalignment of the lower limb.

Fresh-frozen, cryopreserved, and irradiated allografts have all been used. Based on early reports, fresh-frozen grafts may give superior results. Graft sizing is a critical factor in the success of meniscal transplantation. Currently, more sophisticated techniques such as MRI have not proved more accurate than plain radiographic tibial plateau measurements. Improved techniques to accurately size meniscal allografts to within 2 mm of the actual meniscal dimensions are still needed.

Lateral meniscal transplants are usually done using a common bone bridge that connects the anterior and posterior horn insertions, whereas medial meniscal transplants typically use separate anterior and posterior bone plugs. The reason for the differing techniques involves the close proximity of the anterior and posterior horns of the lateral meniscus, which makes the placement of a common bone bridge technically easier. The medial or lateral meniscal allograft is then sutured to the surrounding capsule. The use of both capsular sutures as well as bone plugs has been shown to be biomechanically superior to capsular sutures alone.

The long-term success (>10 years) of meniscal transplantation, particularly with the use of fresh-frozen allografts, is promising. Successful results have been shown in both isolated meniscal transplants as well as transplants combined with ACL reconstruction. Functional scores in activities of daily living after surgery have shown significant improvements over scores before surgery. Currently, it is not recommended that meniscal transplant patients return to high-level athletic activities.

Allen CR et al: Importance of the medial meniscus in the anterior cruciate ligament-deficient knee. J Orthop Res 2000;18:109.

Fukushima K et al: Meniscus allograft transplantation using posterior peripheral suture technique: a preliminary follow-up study. J Orthop Sci 2004;9(3):235.

Rijk PC: Meniscal allograft transplantation—part I: background, results, graft selection and preservation, and surgical considerations. Arthroscopy 2004;20(7):728.

OSTEOCHONDRAL LESIONS

There is much confusion about the nomenclature and etiology of juvenile and adult osteochondral lesions (OCLs) of the knee. Initially, an inflammatory etiology for the condition was suggested. Further inquiry attributed the condition to an ossification abnormality. Still others thought that avascular necrosis may be responsible for the lesions. However, work in basic science, histopathology, and vascular studies did not support any of these etiologies as the cause of OCLs. Currently, OCLs are defined as potentially reversible idiopathic lesions of subchondral bone resulting in possible delamination or fragmentation with or without destruction of the overlying articular cartilage. OCLs are subdivided into juvenile and adult forms depending on the presence of an open distal femoral physes. In children, a combination of etiologies is now thought to be responsible for OCLs. For example, a stress fracture may develop in the subchondral bone of the distal femoral condyle. Such an injury may provoke further vascular compromise, which results in injury to the subchondral bone that was initially covered with normal articular cartilage. Loss of support from the subchondral bone may result in damage to the overlying articular cartilage. The majority of adult OCLs are thought to have arisen from a persistent juvenile OCL, although new lesions in adults are possible as well.

Both adult and juvenile lesions that do not heal have the potential for further sequelae including degenerative osteoarthritis. Juvenile OCLs generally have a better prognosis than adult lesions. The classic location of an OCL is the posterolateral aspect of the medial femoral condyle, which accounts for 70–80%. Lateral condyle lesions are seen in 15–20% of patients, and patellar involvement ranges from 5% to 10%. The increased use of MRI and arthroscopy over the past decade may have resulted in greater recognition of OCLs.

Clinical Findings

A. SYMPTOMS

A common presentation of a patient with an OCL is aching and activity-related anterior knee pain that is poorly localized. Pain may worsen with stair climbing or running. Patients with early or stable lesions usually do not complain of mechanical symptoms or knee instability. Mechanical symptoms are more common in patients with unstable or loose OCLs. Parents may note a limp in their child, and patients may complain of knee swelling with possible crepitus.

B. SIGNS

An antalgic gait may be observed as the patient enters the room. An effusion may be variably present, but generally crepitus or pain with range of motion is absent in patients with stable lesions. Tenderness with palpation of the femoral condyle may be observed with various degrees of knee flexion. Loss of range of motion or quadriceps atrophy may be noted in more long-standing cases.

Patients with unstable lesions may have crepitus and pain with range of motion, and an effusion is typically present. Involvement is bilateral in up to 25% of cases, so both knees should be evaluated regardless of symptoms.

C. IMAGING STUDIES

Initial evaluation should include anteroposterior, lateral, and tunnel views of both knees. The goal of a plain radiographic evaluation is to exclude any bony pathology, evaluate the physes, and localize the lesion (Figure 3–7). Lesion location and an estimation of size should also be determined.

An MRI is frequently obtained once the diagnosis has been confirmed on plain radiographs. MRI can provide an estimation of the size of the lesion, the condition of the overlying cartilage and underlying subchondral bone, the extent of bony edema, the presence of a high signal zone beneath the fragment, and the presence of any loose bodies. There are four MRI criteria on T2-weighted images: a line of high signal intensity at least 5 mm in length between the OCL and underlying bone, an area of increased homogeneous signal at least 5 mm in diameter beneath the lesion, a focal defect of 5 mm or more in the articular surface, and a high signal line traversing the subchondral plate into the lesion. The high signal line was the most common sign in patients found to have unstable lesions; for these patients nonsurgical treatment was most likely to fail. Patient maturity and lesion size were also important predictors of failure of nonsurgical treatment.

Equivocal prognostic value has been found in the use of intravenous gadolinium in the diagnosis of OCLs. Technetium bone scans were initially proposed to monitor the presence of healing. However, MRI eliminates ionizing radiation and is fast, so bone scans are no longer widely used.

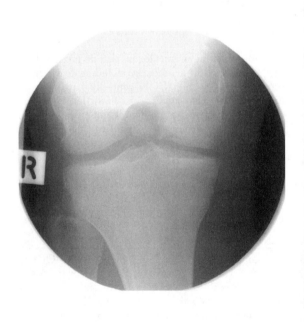

A

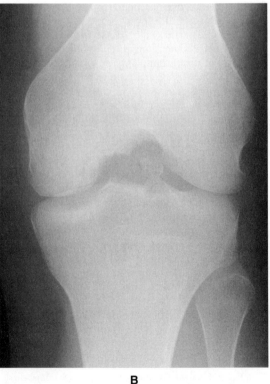

B

Figure 3–7. Osteochondritis dissecans. ***A:*** Fragmentation has occurred at the lateral aspect of the medial femoral condyle. A loose body has separated from the condyle and lies within the intercondylar notch. ***B:*** A subchondral bone defect at the medial femoral condyle shows a good cortical margin at its rim and appears healed. A displaced ossicle lies in the intercondylar notch. (Reproduced, with permission, from Anderson J: *An Atlas of Imaging in Sports Medicine.* McGraw-Hill, 1999.)

Treatment

A. NONSURGICAL

Nonoperative management should be pursued in children with open physes who present with a stable OCL. The goal of nonoperative treatment is to obtain a healed lesion before physis closure so as to prevent osteoarthritis. Even if patients are within 6–12 months of physeal closure, a trial of nonoperative treatment is warranted. Because failure of the subchondral bone precedes failure of the overlying articular cartilage, most orthopedists recommend some modification of activity. Debate exists as to whether this should include immobilization with a cast or brace. The tenet of nonoperative treatment is to reduce the activity level to a point at which pain-free activities of daily living are possible.

Patients should at least be non-weight bearing or partial weight bearing with crutches for 3–6 weeks or until they are pain free. Repeat radiographs are obtained at approximately 6 week intervals. Physical therapy with full weight bearing, which may be initiated once patients are pain free, should focus on low-impact quadriceps and hamstring strengthening. If patients remain asymptomatic during this phase, up to at least 3 months postdiagnosis, they may slowly advance to higher impact activities such as running or jumping. Any recurrence of symptoms or pain or any progression of the OCL on plain radiographs should prompt repeat of the non-weight-bearing period and possible immobilization for a longer period. Obvious patient frustration and lack of compliance, especially in adolescents, are common and a full discussion on the risks and benefits of nonoperative or operative treatment is required.

B. SURGICAL

Operative treatment should be considered in the following instances: (1) detachment or instability of the fragment while the patient is under treatment, (2) persistence of symptoms despite nonoperative treatment in a compliant patient, (3) persistently elevated or worsening radiographic appearance (plain radiographs or MRI), or (4) near or complete epiphyseal closure. Goals of operative treatment should include a stable osteochondral fragment that maintains joint congruity and allows early range of motion.

For stable lesions with an intact articular surface, arthroscopic drilling of the lesions is preferred. This creates channels for potential revascularization through the subchondral bone plate. Options include transarticular drilling versus transepiphyseal drilling. Multiple studies have shown radiographic healing and relief of symptoms in 80–90% of patients with open physes. This decreases to 50–75% in patients with closed physes.

Management of patients with flap lesions or partially unstable lesions should depend on the status of the subchondral bone. Fibrous tissue between the lesion and subchondral bone should be debrided. If significant subchondral bone loss has occurred, packing of the autogenous bone graft into the crater prior to fragment reduction and fixation is advised. If significant subchondral bone remains attached to the fragment such that an anatomic fit into its donor site is possible, fixation should be attempted. Various fixation methods have been described including Herbert or cannulated screws and bioabsorbable screws or pins. Complications, however, have been associated with these treatments.

Simple excision of the larger fragments has shown poor results with more rapid progression of radiographic osteoarthritic changes. For lesions greater than 2 cm², drilling or microfracture methods that depend on replacement of the defect with fibrocartilage have also shown inferior results. Results also tend to deteriorate with time as indicated by worsening radiographic changes. For these larger lesions, transplantation of autologous osteochondral plugs or autologous chondrocyte implantation has been tried. Disadvantages of autologous osteochondral plugs or mosaicplasty include donor site morbidity and incongruent articular fit. Advantages include biological fixation of autogenous material. Longer-term results in young adult patients show successful clinical outcomes in up to 90%. However, additional larger and longer-term follow-up studies are needed.

Bentley G et al: A prospective, randomized comparison of autologous chondrocyte implantation versus mosaicplasty for osteochondral defects in the knee. J Bone Joint Surg B 2003; 85:223.

Flynn JM et al: Osteochondritis dissecans of the knee. J Pediatr Orthop 2004;24:434.

Friederichs MG et al: Pitfalls associated with fixation of osteochondritis dissecans fragments using bioabsorbable screws. Arthroscopy 2001;17:542.

Kocher MS et al: Diagnostic performance of clinical examination and selective magnetic resonance imaging in the evaluation of intra-articular knee disorders in children and adolescents. Am J Sports Med 2001;29:292.

Kocher MS et al: Functional and radiographic outcome of juvenile osteochondritis dissecans of the knee treated with transarticular arthroscopic drilling. Am J Sports Med 2001;29:562.

Peterson L et al: Treatment of osteochondritis dissecans of the knee with autologous chondrocyte transplantation: results at two to ten years. J Bone Joint Surg A 2003;85(suppl 2):17.

Pill SG et al: Role of magnetic resonance imaging and clinical criteria in predicting successful nonoperative treatment of osteochondritis dissecans in children. J Pediatr Orthop 2003;23: 102.

■ WEAKNESS ABOUT THE KNEE

The differential diagnosis of weakness about the knee is vast and often overwhelming. It is helpful to think of the various causes in a systematic way, thereby simplifying the approach. The causes of weakness about the knee may be subdivided into those stemming from muscular (strains, contusions, tears), ligamentous (sprains, partial or complete tears), tendinous, neurologic (central or peripheral), vascular, and bony sources. This section will focus on muscular, tendinous, and bony causes of weakness about the knee.

QUADRICEPS CONTUSION

Traumatic contusion of muscle is one of the most common causes of soft-tissue injury and weakness. Up to 90% of all sports injuries are contusion or strain injuries. Muscle contusion injuries can occur from direct trauma, including laceration or blunt force, and indirect trauma or tensile overload. Tensile overload typically causes muscle failure at the musculotendinous junction or tendon insertion, whereas blunt force trauma is the most common cause of muscle contusion. The quadriceps is the most common site for muscle contusion, and this discussion will be limited to injuries sustained in this muscle from blunt force trauma.

Muscles are known to work optimally within a set temperature range. Additionally, fatigued muscle is known to decrease the ability of stretched muscle to withstand injury. Therefore, adequate rest and a warm-up period prior to exertion reduce the incidence of injury.

Clinical Findings

A. SYMPTOMS

Quadriceps muscle contusions are common after being struck from the front or side with the muscle compressed against the femur. Patients will often have a history of direct trauma, which is common in many sports including football, hockey, lacrosse, rugby, soccer, and the martial arts. The injury is associated with acute swelling, pain, and a decreased active and passive range of motion of the hip and knee. Patients may or may not be able to continue with their activity. If seen late, bruising may be evident on the skin overlying the quadriceps.

B. SIGNS

Tenderness to palpation over the quadriceps and a decreased range of motion of the hip and/or knee are the most common findings on examination. If severe, a palpable mass may be present indicating a possible hematoma. Also, a palpable gap may be present if significant muscle tearing has occurred.

C. IMAGING STUDIES

Quadriceps contusion injuries may be a diagnosis of exclusion, but are usually readily apparent given a history of direct trauma and the associated clinical findings. Plain radiographs may be obtained to rule out associated fracture, although this is uncommon. Ultrasound or measuring the size of any muscle gap and associated hematoma can differentiate acute hematoma from diffuse swelling. The use of MRI in diagnosing and following contusion injuries is not well defined.

D. SPECIAL STUDIES

If the patient exhibits pain out of proportion to the clinical findings or the clinical findings show severe swelling in a thigh compartment, compartmental pressure monitoring may be indicated. Pressures greater than 30 mm Hg have been suggested as thresholds for emergent fasciotomies.

Metaplasia of the severely contused muscle may result in ossification within the muscle, termed myositis ossificans. The risk of developing myositis ossificans is directly related to the severity of the injury, and has been reported to be as high as 9% following deep thigh contusions. Serial plain radiographs or computed tomography (CT) may be needed to follow the progression of ossification within the muscle. Generally, surgery is not recommended for this condition unless the ossification is severely limiting. A delay of at least 6 months after injury is recommended to allow the abnormal bone formation to mature, thereby limiting further surgery-induced ossification.

Treatment

The goal of treatment for quadriceps contusion injuries focuses on symptomatic pain relief, maintenance of knee motion and quadriceps strength, and prevention of myositis ossificans. Protocols have been developed for optimal rehabilitation and treatment. This includes an initial immobilization period not to exceed 48 hours, followed by progressive leg and gravity-assisted range of motion exercises. Decreased quadriceps muscle contraction has been found to occur when patients are immobilized with the hip and knee in flexion according to pain tolerance. Indomethacin or other nonsteroidal antiinflammatory drugs (NSAIDs) have been advocated to decrease the risk of myositis ossificans. These medications may have beneficial short-term effects on pain modulation, but their effect on early and late muscle healing and regeneration is not clear.

Beiner JM, Jokl P: Muscle contusion injuries: current treatment options. J Am Acad Orthop Surg 2001;9:227.

Diaz JA et al: Severe quadriceps contusions in athletes. Am J Sports Med 2003;31:289.

PATELLAR TENDON RUPTURES

Rupture of the patellar tendon is a rare but serious knee injury with a peak incidence in males during the third or fourth decade. It is typically seen in more active patients, and the injury may be the end result of repetitive microtraumatic injuries. A typical healthy adult tendon is extremely resistant to rupture. Patients who rupture their patellar tendons typically exhibit some form of tendinopathy clinically or pathologically. Dysfunction of the patellar tendon may exist across a degenerative spectrum, with younger patients exhibiting clinical symptoms of "jumpers knee" or patellar tendinitis and older patients exhibiting pathologic changes resulting in an end-stage tendon rupture due to a degenerative tendinopathy. Although unilateral ruptures are more common, bilateral ruptures have been described. Risk factors for bilateral ruptures include systemic diseases that weaken collagenous tissues such as rheumatoid arthritis, diabetes mellitus, chronic renal failure, or systemic lupus erythematosus. Chronic steroid use or previous major knee surgery, such as total knee arthroplasty or anterior cruciate reconstruction with patellar tendon autograft, is also a risk factor.

The patellar tendon should more accurately be named the patellar ligament, as it is a continuation of the quadriceps expansion over the patella distally to the tibial tubercle. For this discussion, however, it will be referred to as the patellar tendon. The quadriceps consists of the rectus femoris, vastus intermedious, vastus lateralis, and vastus medialis muscles. Portions of the vastus medialis and lateralis muscles extend distally to contribute to the quadriceps tendon and, ultimately, the patellar tendon. Tendinous expansions of the vastus lateralis and medialis, however, extend past the patellar to the proximal tibia and are referred to as the lateral and medial reticulum, respectively. Blood supply to the patellar tendon arises from the infrapatellar fat pad as well as the reticular structures through anastomoses from the inferior genicular arteries. The proximal and distal aspects of the patellar tendon attachment are watershed areas of vascularity where many ruptures typically occur.

With increasing knee flexion, the contact point of the patella within the femoral trochlear groove moves proximally, giving the patellar tendon a longer lever arm and a greater mechanical advantage with respect to the quadriceps tendon. Additionally, the greatest strain or tensile load deformation occurs at the insertion sites as opposed to the mid-tendon substance. Therefore, most ruptures occur with deep knee flexion at the distal pole of the patella.

Clinical Findings

A. Symptoms

Patellar tendon ruptures typically occur in patients 40 years of age or younger, often during athletic activities. Although a patient of any age can sustain a patellar tendon rupture, patients older than 40 years typically tear their quadriceps tendon. The history is that of a sudden, forceful quadriceps eccentric contraction on a flexed knee such as landing from a jump or stumbling on a stair. Patients describe a sudden pain and a popping or tearing sensation in the knee which leads to an inability to continue their activity. Weight bearing is often difficult and requires assistance.

B. Signs

Patients usually present with a knee effusion or a hemarthrosis. In a complete tear through the tendon and adjacent reticula, the patella is displaced proximally by the pull of the quadriceps tendon. Extensor function is absent or greatly decreased, with patients unable to actively extend their knee or passively maintain an extended knee position. In incomplete patellar tendon tears or complete patellar tendon tears with sparing of the reticula, patients may have some active extension against gravity. However, maintenance of extension against force is not possible. A palpable gap may be present.

In a patient with a delayed presentation, organizing hematoma or fibrosis may obscure the tendon defect. These patients, however, will typically have a classic history and will often have quadriceps atrophy, weakness in knee extension, and an antalgic gait.

C. Imaging Studies

1. Radiographs—Plain radiographs consisting of anteroposterior and lateral views are essential. The lateral view may show patella alta, with the entire patella located proximal to Blumensatt's line. The Insall–Salvati ratio (the length of the patella tendon divided by the length of the patella) will be greater than 1.2 signifying patella alta. An avulsed bone fragment in the distal pole of the patella may be seen. A patellar view and a flexed knee view may be helpful to rule out other intraarticular pathology such as patella fractures or osteochondral injuries. Comparison views of the contralateral knee may also be helpful to compare patellar height.

2. Ultrasound and magnetic resonance imaging— High-resolution ultrasonography has been utilized as an effective means of imaging the patellar tendon. Its advantages include its relatively low cost, lack of ionizing radiation, and quick availability and results. Its main disadvantage is that it is highly operator and reader dependent, which makes it unavailable or unreliable in many areas. MRI is very accurate in diagnosing patellar tendon tears. It is particularly helpful in patients with chronic tears and questionable partial versus complete tears, and in patients suspected of having additional intraarticular pathology. For most acute cases, MRI is not necessary for diagnosis.

Treatment

A. Surgical

No widely accepted classification system exists for patellar tendon ruptures. Various classification schemes based on the chronicity of diagnosis and treatment, the tear configuration, and the level of tendon rupture have been described. The only classification system that has been found to have a correlation with clinical outcome is that of Siwek and Rao, who grouped their patients into two categories: immediate repair (defined as less than 2 weeks) and delayed repair (defined as greater than 2 weeks). Subsequent studies have shown that patellar rupture repairs done acutely (2–4 weeks) generally have a better prognosis than repairs done on a delayed or chronic basis (>4–6 weeks). Repairs performed on a delayed basis are hampered by quadriceps contraction and fibrous adhesions that make restoration of tendon length and repair more difficult.

Thus, surgical restoration is necessary to reestablish the extensor mechanism in most patients, both athletes and nonathletes, with complete tears. Surgical repair should be done in a timely fashion, making accurate diagnosis essential. Nonoperative treatment is ineffective and has few indications.

The knee is approached anteriorly through a longitudinal incision from the mid-patella to the tibial tubercle. To avoid complications to wound healing, thick flaps of tissue are maintained during the exposure. The ruptured tendon ends and reticula are identified and debrided. Often, the rupture occurs so close to the patella that sufficient soft tissue on the patella is not present. If the tendon rupture is more mid-substance, primary end-to-end repair of both the tendon and reticula is done using heavy, nonabsorbable sutures. A strong stitch such as a Bunnell or Krackow is used. Typically, as the tendon rupture is adjacent to the inferior pole of the patella, the repair is accomplished by passing the suture from the patella tendon through two or three longitudinal, transpatellar drill holes. A circumferential reinforcing suture is often added to the repair. This suture is passed through a drill hole in line with and posterior to the tibial tubercle, and then brought proximally and passed transversely through the quadriceps tendon. Prior to tying, the sutures are tensioned, and a single lateral radiograph of the knee is obtained to assess patellar height. A contralateral radiograph is used for comparison. Once the appropriate patellar height is recreated by proper tensioning of the sutures, the sutures are tied over the superior pole of the patella. The circumferential reinforcing suture is then also tied. The knee flexion angle at which sufficient tension is present across the repair can be assessed to help guide postoperative physical therapy rehabilitation. The suture line can be oversewn with a smaller nonabsorbable suture depending on surgeon preference.

Careful attention to restoring the patellofemoral alignment can improve patellofemoral tracking and clinical outcome. Restoration of patellar tendon length and patellar height has been shown to improve results and diminish later patellofemoral symptoms. This can cause difficulty in the repair in delayed or chronic cases.

Such cases may require preoperative traction on the patella to restore length, intraoperative lysis of adhesions around the extensor mechanism, and the use of allograft or autograft tissue augmentation.

B. Postsurgical

Initially, most patients were immobilized in extension postoperatively for 6 weeks in either a brace or cylinder cast. This was thought to allow tendon healing without tension, and good results were reported. As evidence mounted that controlled movement after repair positively influenced tendon nutrition and healing, use of early range of motion has been reported to produce comparable results. A common protocol involves starting isometric quadriceps/hamstring exercises on the first postoperative day, with active flexion and passive extension added at 2 weeks postoperatively and active knee extension added at 3–4 weeks postoperatively. Patients are allowed toe-touch weight bearing immediately postoperatively, and are advanced to full weight bearing without crutches by 6 weeks postoperatively as quadriceps function and leg control return.

The most common complications following this injury are persistent loss of quadriceps strength and loss of full knee flexion. This is thought to be associated with the injury itself. This emphasizes the need for an aggressive postoperative physical therapy protocol emphasizing range of motion and strengthening. Manipulation under anesthesia and arthroscopic lysis of adhesions are typically not needed when such a protocol is instituted.

Complications

Surgical complications are infrequent, but include wound infection or dehiscence, a persistent hemarthrosis, rerupture, and patellofemoral pain. In a circumferential repair, breakage of the wire cerclage has also been reported. Wound complications can be reduced by maintaining thick skin flaps and using a slightly lateral incision away from the tibial tubercle. Rerupture is typically seen in patients who return to sport prior to obtaining full knee motion and adequate (85–90%) quadriceps and hamstring strength. Assessing the alignment and height of the patella on a lateral radiograph in comparison to the contralateral side can help in restoring proper patellofemoral mechanics.

Prognosis

Multiple studies detailing the results of patellar tendon rupture repairs have been reported in the literature. To date, the only factor correlated with a positive clinical outcome is acute repair. Additionally, younger and more athletic patients with an isolated injury tend to have better results compared to older or multitrauma patients. Siwek and Rao compared acute (<7 days) versus delayed (>7 days) repairs and found that acute repairs did significantly better in terms of range of motion and strength. Although some quadriceps atrophy and slight motion loss (<10°) may persist postoperatively, good and excellent reports have been shown to occur in 66–100% of patients, although a smaller percentage of recreational athletes return to their preinjury athletic level. Most studies reported use of some circumferential augmentation in the form of either a suture or wire. A retrospective comparison of polydioxanone suture to wire augmentation found no significant differences.

Patellofemoral arthritis or incongruity has not been shown to be associated with outcome. Although most patients with poorer outcomes tend to have patellofemoral complications, many patients without symptoms also have radiographic findings of incongruity or arthrosis. Thus, articular incongruity may not alone be the cause of poor outcomes. Despite evidence indicating the benefits of early motion, no study has found significant improvement in outcome in patients undergoing delayed versus immediate postoperative therapy. Overall, patients with acute treatment, higher level athletes or those involved in diligent postoperative rehabilitation, and athletes without significant quadriceps atrophy seem to achieve better postoperative outcomes.

There are only a few case reports or case series on the results of delayed reconstruction. Multiple reconstructions have been described including primary repair augmented with autogenous fascia lata or hamstring grafts; allografts have also been used. Patients repaired on a delayed basis who require preoperative traction or the use of allograft or autograft augmentation seem to have inferior results.

Kasten P et al: Rupture of the patellar tendon: a review of 68 cases and a retrospective study of 29 ruptures comparing two methods of augmentation. Arch Orthop Trauma Surg 2001; 121:578.

QUADRICEPS TENDON RUPTURES

Rupture of the quadriceps tendon typically occurs in patients over 40 years of age. Injuries usually occur from indirect mechanisms and require a previously weakened tendon prior to rupture. As in patellar tendon ruptures, bilateral ruptures do occur and are more likely in patients with underlying systemic conditions such as chronic steroid use, systemic lupus erythematosus, diabetes, or chronic renal failure.

The quadriceps tendon is formed by a convergence of the tendons of the rectus femoris, vastus intermedius, vastus lateralis, and vastus intermedius muscles approximately 3 cm proximal to the patella. Portions of the vastus medialis and lateralis extend adjacent to the patella and insert directly into the proximal tibia, forming the medial and lateral reticulum, respectively. The anatomic location of the muscles contributing to the quadriceps tendon is reflected in the distinct planes that make up the tendon. The superficial plane is composed of fibers from the rectus femoris, the middle plane from the vastus lateralis and medialis muscles, and the deep plane from the vastus intermedius. Adherent to the deep surface of the tendon is the capsule and synovial lining of the knee joint, which often tears with complete rupture of the quadriceps tendon, causing the acute hemarthrosis seen with such an injury.

A tendon from a normal, healthy adult is extremely resistant to rupture. When subjected to supramaximal loads, the extensor mechanism will fail at other weaker points such as the osteotendinous or musculotendinous junctions. Thus, for a rupture of the quadriceps tendon to occur, it is generally believed that a weakened tendon state must be involved. Alternations in the normal collagen structure of tendons do occur normally with age; however, despite this, quadriceps rupture is still a rare event. Other concurrent pathologic processes must be present to alter the structure of the tendon. Such processes may accelerate fatty or mucoid degeneration, decrease the collagen content, or disrupt the vascular supply. Conditions such as chronic renal failure, rheumatoid arthritis, gout, systemic lupus erythematosus, steroid use, or hyperparathyroidism have all been implicated as causative factors.

Clinical Findings

A. SYMPTOMS

In older patients traumatic ruptures of the quadriceps tendon generally occur during daily activities with the knee in a semiflexed state and the quadriceps firing in an eccentric fashion. Typical mechanisms include stumbling while walking, stair climbing, or, less likely, exertion during an athletic event. Patients typically complain of rapid swelling, an inability to ambulate, and lack of knee extension after such an injury. They may also describe a tearing sensation or pop in their knee with pain.

B. SIGNS

The diagnostic hallmarks of a quadriceps tendon rupture are an inability to actively extend the knee and a suprapatellar gap. Although active knee flexion remains intact, patients are typically unable to actively extend the knee or maintain extension in a passively flexed knee (ie, demonstrate an extension lag sign). Patients with partial ruptures or complete tendon ruptures with intact retinacula may demonstrate some active extension, but typically still demonstrate an extension lag. A palpable depression superior to the patella, known as the suprapatellar gap sign, is pathognomonic.

Failure to diagnose the injury, observed in up to 50% of cases, delays subsequent treatment. In patients with an acute hemarthrosis, the suprapatellar gap may be obscured. A helpful maneuver to elicit this sign involves having the patient actively flex the hip, which shortens the rectus femoris muscle thereby drawing the quadriceps tendon more proximally and widening the defect at the rupture site. Additionally, comparison with the contralateral leg for both palpation as well as active extension is essential.

C. Imaging Studies

Anteroposterior and lateral radiographs should be obtained on any patient suspected of having a quadriceps tendon injury. Four radiographic signs may be present in plain radiographs in patients with quadriceps tendon ruptures: obliteration of the quadriceps tendon shadow, a suprapatellar mass (retraction of the ruptured tendon), suprapatellar calcific densities (dystrophic calcifications or avulsed bone fragments), and an inferiorly displaced patella.

Ultrasound is highly sensitive and specific in assessing partial and complete quadriceps ruptures. It can also be used to assess the tendon after repair. It is a relatively cheap modality and spares the patient ionizing radiation. Ultrasound is, however, highly operator dependent and therefore is not available in all areas. MRI is also highly sensitive and specific in the diagnosis of quadriceps tendon ruptures. It is particularly helpful in patients with massive swelling, which may preclude a good physical examination, as well as in patients suspected of having additional intra-articular injuries. Because of its cost, MRI is generally not used in straightforward, acute cases of quadriceps tendon rupture.

Treatment

A. Nonsurgical

Management and treatment of quadriceps ruptures should initially be based on whether the rupture is partial or complete, as determined by physical examination and/or additional imaging. Partial ruptures can generally be managed nonoperatively with the knee braced or casted in near full extension for 6 weeks, followed by progressive range-of-motion and strengthening exercises. There are no data, however, concerning the percentage of tendon ruptures that can be effectively treated nonoperatively.

B. Surgical

Complete rupture of the quadriceps tendon is an indication for surgical treatment. The nonoperative management of complete ruptures results in long-term disability secondary to quadriceps weakness and extensor lag. In cases of delayed patient presentation or diagnosis, the repair can be more difficult due to retraction of the torn tendon ends making apposition difficult. Early intervention (less than 72 hours if possible) is recommended to optimize results.

Multiple methods of repair have been described, and no published data are available comparing the results of different types of repairs. Generally, repair proceeds in a similar fashion as described below. For midsubstance tears in which there is ample tendon tissue on both ends of the rupture, a primary end-to-end repair may be done. Typically, two heavy nonabsorbable sutures are placed in a running fashion (eg, Krakow or Bunnell) in each end. Similarly, smaller nonabsorbable sutures are placed in apposition to the torn reticula ends. These are opposed but not tied until the tendon sutures are tied. In ruptures near the osteotendinous junction of the superior patellar pole (a common place for rupture), a similar suture technique is used to secure the tendon end. The superior pole of the patella is debrided of remaining soft tissue and roughened to bleeding bone in preparation for tendon approximation. Three 2-mm longitudinal drill holes are then placed through the patella, and the free ends of the sutures are passed through the holes with a Keith needle and tied distally over the inferior pole of the patella with the knee in near full extension.

Circumferential augmentation, similar to what is done in patellar tendon ruptures, can be added. Options include wire, Mersilene tape, or a nonabsorbable suture. Another option to repair or augment acute ruptures includes the Scuderi technique, in which a partial-thickness triangular flap is excised from the anterior surface of the proximal quadriceps tendon, approximately 2 inches wide and 3 inches on each side. This flap is then folded down distally over the rupture site and sutured into place.

Bilateral ruptures should be treated in a similar fashion to unilateral ruptures. Additionally, an evaluation for known systemic diseases that cause tendon degeneration should be conducted. These patients are at increased risk for delayed presentation as they are often seen by nonorthopedists or their disabilities are attributed to other causes such as various arthritides or neurologic disorders.

Chronic ruptures of the quadriceps tendon can involve more difficult repairs, particularly when tendon retraction has occurred. Retraction typically requires lysis of adhesions between the tendon and underlying femur to gain appropriate length. When tendon ends can be reapproximated, a standard repair as described previously can be used. When significant gapping exists despite maximal mobilization of the tendon ends, a Codivilla lengthening procedure may be required. This involves making a partial thickness, V-shaped cut from the distal aspect of the proximal quadriceps tendon stump. The apex of the V-shaped cut points cephalad. The flap is then reflected distally on its attached base and sewn to the distal tendon stump. The upper portion is then sutured closed in a side-to-side fashion.

C. POSTSURGICAL CARE

The knee is splinted or braced in extension until the wound has sealed and any drains placed intraoperatively have been removed. Although data have shown improved tendon healing with gentle early range of motion, a comparison of patients immobilized in extension for 6 weeks versus those started on early range-of-motion exercises did not show a difference. For patients immobilized for 6 weeks, immediate weight bearing in extension is allowed. Range-of-motion exercises are started at 4–6 weeks and slowly advanced. Once adequate quadriceps function and leg control are obtained, the brace can be discontinued at 6–12 weeks. Patients on more aggressive rehabilitation protocols may start isometric quadriceps/hamstring contractions with active flexion and passive extension at 2–3 weeks, and progress to active extension at 6 weeks postoperatively. Complete range of motion should be seen at 12 weeks, with most patients returning to full activities by 4–6 months postoperatively.

Complications

The most common complications following quadriceps tendon repair are an inability to regain full knee flexion and continued quadriceps weakness. An extensor lag is also a known complication, but can usually be overcome with appropriate physical therapy. Other less common but known complications include wound infection or dehiscence, persistent hemarthrosis, and patella baja or patellar incongruity. Wound complications can be minimized by placing sutures or wires away from the incision, and maintaining thick skin flaps during surgical dissection. Postoperative drains may decrease the rate of hemarthrosis. Finally, attention to the patellar height and congruity of the patellofemoral articulation intraoperatively may help decrease patellofemoral complications.

Prognosis

Several studies have shown improved results of acute repair over chronic repair, although other studies have not shown such a correlation. In general, acute repairs result in excellent clinical outcomes in 83–100% of patients. No differences have been found in repair technique or postoperative protocols. Range of motion is generally within 5–10° of the uninjured side, with strength losses of approximately 10% or less. Over 90% of patients are generally satisfied, although one study showed only 51% were able to return to their presurgery level of recreational activity. Perhaps the high satisfaction rating and good clinical results may be attributable to the older age group and subsequent lower activity demands.

Ilan DI et al: Quadriceps tendon rupture. J Am Acad Orthop Surg 2003;11:192.

O'Shea K, Kenny P: Outcomes following quadriceps tendon ruptures. Injury 2002;33:257.

Shak MK: Outcomes in bilateral and simultaneous quadriceps tendon rupture. Orthopedics 2003;26(8):797.

AVULSION OF THE TIBIAL TUBERCLE

Developmentally, the tibial tubercle begins proximal on the tibia, and descends distally to a point just distal to the proximal tibial growth plate. A vertical component of the tibial growth plate appears under the tubercle. Progressive replacement of the immature fibrocartilage to mature bone occurs in a proximal-to-distal direction. Complete epiphysiodesis occurs in boys at about 17 years of age and in girls at about 15 years of age.

Clinical Findings

A. SYMPTOMS

Acute tibial tubercle avulsions occur almost exclusively in boys between the ages of 12 and 17 years. The history is often that of a sudden, forceful quadriceps contraction (eg, jumping) or an eccentric quadriceps contraction against a passively flexing knee (eg, landing from a jump). Competitive jumping sports such as basketball or high jumping or contact sports such as football are commonly involved.

Patients present with focal proximal tibial swelling and anterior knee pain. They may or may not be able to extend their knee against gravity, but all have some form of knee weakness. An audible pop may have been heard at the time of injury.

B. SIGNS

Patients with a tibial tubercle fracture have focal anterior tibial tenderness. Those with an intraarticular extension of their fracture will have an associated knee effusion or hemarthrosis. Patients demonstrate weakness or complete absence of knee extension. Associated injuries may also occur. A thorough knee examination should be performed looking for associated joint line tenderness or ligamentous instability indicative of a meniscal tear or intraarticular ligament tear, respectively.

C. IMAGING STUDIES

A true lateral radiograph of the tibial tubercle is essential to accurately diagnose a tibial tubercle avulsion. Anteroposterior and oblique radiographs should also be obtained. Because the tubercle lies lateral to the midline, slight internal rotation of the knee prior to shooting the lateral film will help visualize the tibial tubercle. Although uncommon, an MRI may be obtained if suspicion exists for an associated intraarticular injury.

Treatment

The Ogden modification of the Watson–Jones classification is used to categorize these injuries and guide treatment. There are three types, each with an A and B subtype. Type I is a fracture distal to the normal junction of the ossification centers of the proximal end of the tibia and tuberosity. Type II is a fracture at the junction of the ossification centers of the proximal end of the tibia and tuberosity. Type III fractures extend into the joint. Further subtyping is used to describe the absence (subtype A) or presence (subtype B) of displacement and comminution (Figure 3–8).

Treatment goals include anatomic fracture reduction, maintenance of articular congruency, and restoration of the extensor mechanism.

A. Nonsurgical

Nondisplaced type I fractures (IA) can be successfully treated with a cylinder cast or long leg cast in extension for 4–6 weeks. Some displaced type I (IB) and IIA fractures may similarly reduce anatomically with extension in a cast.

B. Surgical

Those type IB and IIA fractures that do not reduce, as well as most type IIB and III injuries, are best treated with open reduction and internal fixation.

The approach is typically directly anterior or slightly off midline, with dissection carried down adjacent or posterior to the patellar tendon insertion. Any interposed soft tissue or periosteum is removed and an anatomic reduction is obtained. The use of intraoperative fluoroscopy is helpful. Fixation may be accomplished with the use of cannulated screws and/or a tension band construct. Grade III injuries should be evaluated for associated ligamentous or meniscal injury.

Whether operative or nonoperative treatment is chosen, a cast is typically worn for 4–6 weeks, at which time progressive knee range-of-motion exercises are started. Quadriceps strengthening is typically started at approximately 6 weeks or when full range of motion has been obtained. Patients may return to regular activities after quadriceps strength has returned to 85% of the contralateral leg. Return to full sports activities is expected by 3–6 months.

Complications & Prognosis

The prognosis for tibial tubercle avulsion fractures is very good with few complications. Genu recurvatum has not been reported, likely due to the fact that these patients are at or near skeletal maturity when their injury occurs. Loss of motion, patellar malposition, and compartment syndrome have been observed. Careful attention to anatomic alignment of the fracture and comparison to the contralateral knee is helpful to avoid patellar complications. Compartment syndrome due to laceration of a small recurrent artery is possible, and patients should be carefully observed postoperatively. The institution of an early, aggressive therapy protocol can help to obtain full knee range of motion. Nonunion is rare.

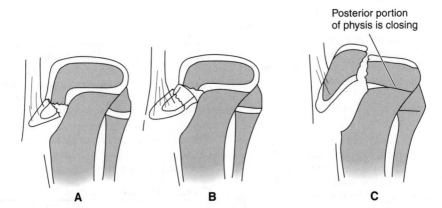

Posterior portion of physis is closing

A **B** **C**

Figure 3–8. Avulsion fractures of the tibial tubercle. ***A:*** Type I fracture across the secondary ossification center at a level with the posterior border of the inserting patellar ligament. ***B:*** Type II fracture at the junction of the primary and secondary ossification centers of the proximal tibial epiphysis. ***C:*** Type III fracture propagates upward across the primary ossification center of the proximal tibial epiphysis into the knee joint. This fracture is a variant of the Salter–Harris III separation and is analogous to the fracture of Tillaux at the ankle, because the posterior portion of the physis of the proximal tibia is closing. (Reproduced, with permission, from Odgen JA et al: Fractures of the tibial tuberosity in adolescents. *J Bone Joint Surg Am* 1980;62:205.)

McKoy BE, Stanitski CL: Acute tibial tubercle avulsion fractures. Orthop Clin North Am 2003;34(3):397.

Mosier SM, Stanitski CL: Acute tibial tubercle avulsion fractures. J Pediatr Orthop 2004;24(2):81.

Zionts LE: Fractures around the knee in children. J Am Acad Orthop Surg 2002;10:345.

■ KNEE INSTABILITY

Anatomy

Knee instability entails four primary ligaments as stabilizing structures of the knee. These ligaments include the anterior cruciate ligament (ACL), the posterior cruciate ligament (PCL), the medial collateral ligament (MCL), and the lateral collateral ligament (LCL). There are also several accessory or secondary stabilizers of the knee, including the menisci, iliotibial band, and biceps femoris. These secondary stabilizers become more important when a primary stabilizer is injured.

The MCL, the primary static medial stabilizer against valgus stress at the knee, originates from the central sulcus of the medial epicondyle (Figure 3–9). The sulcus of the C-shaped medial epicondyle is located anterior and distal to the adductor tubercle. The MCL is made up of three main static medial stabilizers of the knee: the superficial MCL, the posterior oblique ligament, and the deep capsular ligament.

The LCL, the primary static lateral stabilizer against varus stress at the knee, originates from the lateral epicondyle. This is the most prominent point of the lateral femoral condyle. The LCL insertion is on the styloid process of the fibular head, which projects superiorly from the posterolateral fibular head. The LCL joins with the arcuate ligament, the popliteus muscle, and the lateral head of the gastrocnemius to form a lateral arcuate complex that statically and dynamically controls varus angulation and external tibial torsion (Figure 3–10). The iliotibial band and biceps femoris also contribute to stability on the lateral aspect of the knee.

The ACL, the primary static stabilizer of the knee against anterior translation of the tibia with respect to the femur, originates from the posteromedial surface of the lateral femoral condyle in the intercondylar notch (Figure 3–11). It inserts on the tibial plateau just medial to the anterior horn of the lateral meniscus about 15 mm posterior to the anterior edge of the tibial articular surface. The blood supply to the ACL and PCL is the middle geniculate artery. Both the ACL and PCL are covered by a layer of synovium making these ligaments intraarticular and extrasynovial.

The PCL, the primary static stabilizer of the knee against posterior translation of the tibia with respect to the femur, originates from the posterior aspect of the lateral surface of the medial femoral condyle in the intercondylar notch (Figure 3–12). It inserts on the posterior aspect of the tibial plateau in a central depression just posterior to the articular surface. The insertion extends distally along the posterior aspect of the tibia for up to 1 cm in length. The PCL is a complex structure consisting of two major bands: the anterolateral and the posteromedial. The anterolateral band is tight in flexion and loose in extension. The posteromedial band is loose in flexion and tight in extension. The cross-sectional area of the anterolateral band is twice as large as the posteromedial band. The meniscofemoral ligaments, the ligaments of Wrisberg and Humphrey, are the third

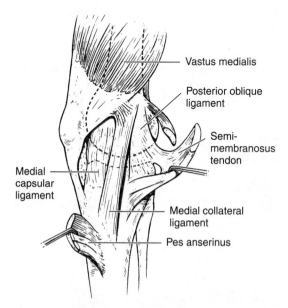

Figure 3–9. Medial capsuloligamentous complex. (Reproduced, with permission, from Feagin JA Jr: *The Crucial Ligaments.* New York: Churchill Livingstone, 1988.)

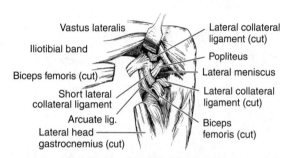

Figure 3–10. The lateral supporting portions of the knee. (Reproduced, with permission, from Rockwood CA Jr et al: *Fractures in Adults.* New York: Churchill Livingstone, 1984.)

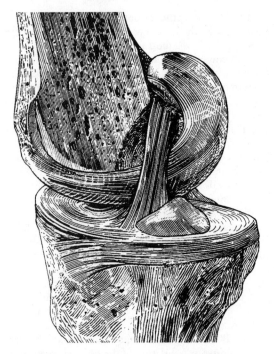

Figure 3–11. The anterior cruciate ligament with the knee in extension, showing the course of the ligament as it passes from the medial aspect of the lateral portion of the medial tibial spine. (Reproduced, with permission, from Girgis FG et al: The cruciate ligaments of the knee joint: Anatomical, functional, and experimental analysis. *Clin Orthop* 1975;106:216.)

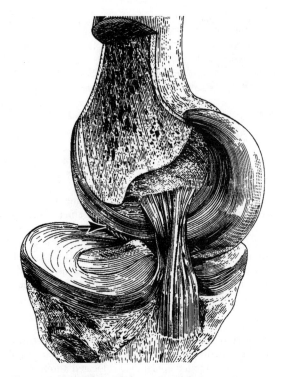

Figure 3–12. The posterior cruciate ligament showing the course of the ligament as it passes from the lateral aspect of the medial femoral condyle to the posterior surface of the tibia. (Reproduced, with permission, from Girgis FG et al: The cruciate ligaments of the knee joint: Anatomical, functional, and experimental analysis. *Clin Orthop* 1975;106:216.)

component of the PCL. The meniscofemoral ligaments travel from the posterior horn of the lateral meniscus to the posteromedial femoral condyle.

Fu FH et al: Current trends in anterior cruciate ligament reconstruction. Part 1: Biology and biomechanics of reconstruction. Am J Sports Med 1999;27:821.

DIFFERENTIAL DIAGNOSIS

The differential diagnosis of acute or chronic knee instability can involve any of the following structures: the ACL, the PCL, the MCL, the LCL, and the other structures of the posterolateral corner. Of course there are often combinations of the above ligamentous injuries in addition to injuries of secondary stabilizing structures such as the menisci that produce an unstable knee. The history and mechanism of injury are valuable pieces of information if available. Similarly, the location of pain with palpation can help to narrow the diagnosis. Clearly, however, a thorough physical examination helps to distinguish which ligaments are responsible for knee

instability. Additionally, imaging studies are often obtained to confirm clinical suspicions and to evaluate for occult injuries in the setting of a suspected multiligamentous knee injury.

MEDIAL COLLATERAL LIGAMENT INJURIES

ESSENTIALS OF DIAGNOSIS

- *The most commonly injured ligament of the knee.*
- *Mechanism: valgus stress to the knee joint.*
- *History: medial knee pain and instability.*
- *Pain and laxity with valgus stress at 30° of flexion.*
- *Primary nonoperative treatment with protected mobilization.*

Prevention

Prevention of MCL injury can be achieved by a variety of methods. Increased strength of the thigh muscles and proprioceptive training can help protect from knee injuries. Hinged knee braces may provide some protection from excessive valgus stresses.

Clinical Findings

An MCL tear typically presents with medial knee pain after either a noncontact rotational injury or a direct valgus blow to the lateral knee. Instability may or may not be present depending on the severity of the injury.

A. SYMPTOMS

How and when the patient was hurt are important parts of the history. Lower grade MCL injuries typically involve a noncontact external rotational injury whereas higher grade injuries generally involve lateral contact to the thigh or upper leg. Other important information includes the location and presence of pain, instability, timing of swelling, and sensation of a "pop" or tear. Surprisingly, grade I and II injuries are often more painful than complete (grade III) MCL injuries. Immediate swelling may indicate an associated cruciate ligament injury, fracture, and/or patellar dislocation.

A prior history of knee injuries or instability should always be sought when evaluating a new knee injury.

B. SIGNS

MCL injuries are evaluated with a complete knee examination to determine the presence of any coexisting injuries. This is especially important with ACL and PCL evaluations because an injury to either of these ligaments would significantly change the course of treatment. Given the frequency of coexisting patellar dislocations in MCL injuries, palpation of the patella and the medial parapatellar stabilizing ligaments should be performed in addition to patellar apprehension testing.

Medial joint line tenderness along the course of the MCL is typical at the location of the tear. MCL ligament sprains are graded on a scale ranging from mild (grade I) to moderate (grade II) and severe (grade III) sprains. Laxity to valgus stresses is assessed by the amount of medial joint space opening that occurs at 30° of flexion (Figure 3–13). It is important to stress the knee at 30° of flexion because with the knee in full extension the posterior capsule and PCL will stabilize the knee to valgus stress, which in full extension could lead the examiner to believe that the MCL is intact. Zero opening is considered normal, with 1–4 mm indicating a grade I injury, 5–9 mm indicating a grade II injury, and 10–15 mm indicating a complete or grade III injury. Additionally, in grades I and II, injuries

typically have a firm end point, whereas in grade III, the injury tends to have a soft end point to valgus stress.

C. IMAGING STUDIES

A series of knee radiographs should be obtained in any patient with a suspected significant knee injury. Radiographs should be inspected for acute fracture, lateral capsular avulsion (Segond's fracture—see ACL imaging), loose bodies, Pellegrini–Stieda lesion (MCL calcification) (Figure 3–14), and evidence of patellar dislocation. Stress radiographs should be obtained in patients prior to skeletal maturity to rule out an epiphyseal fracture.

MRI is most useful for confirming the site of MCL injury and identifying meniscal and other coexisting injuries to the knee. Relative indications for an MRI include an uncertain ACL status despite multiple examinations, evaluation of a suspected meniscal tear, or preoperative evaluation for a planned MCL reconstruction or repair.

D. SPECIAL TESTS

An examination under anesthesia can be valuable when a conventional physical examination is thought to be unreliable secondary to patient guarding. Diagnostic arthroscopy can also be used to evaluate for coexistent pathology. However, both of these diagnostic methods have largely been replaced by MRI as a first line diagnostic test.

Treatment

Treatment of an isolated MCL injury is generally nonoperative and involves protection against valgus stress and early motion. Classically, MCL injuries were treated with surgical repair. However, the results of nonoperative treatment paralleled operative intervention.

Grade I and grade II injuries can be treated by placing the knee in either a cast or a brace with weight bearing as tolerated. Generally, knee motion is started within the first week or two and full recovery is usually achieved more rapidly with early knee range of motion.

Treatment of grade III injuries is more controversial. Increased instability has been shown in grade III tears treated nonoperatively, although in most instances knees with multiligamentous injuries were not excluded. Comparing isolated grade III MCL tears treated with surgical reconstruction versus conservative management, the conservative treatment group enjoyed better results in both subjective scoring and earlier return to activity.

The exception to the current trend of nonoperative treatment of grade III injuries involves multiligamentous knee injury. In this group, particularly with a distal tibial avulsion of the MCL, nonoperative treatment has not fared nearly as well as in isolated MCL injuries.

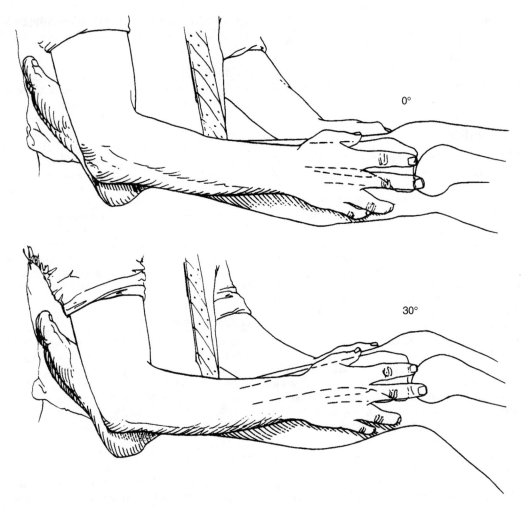

Figure 3–13. The collateral ligament being tested in extension and 30° of flexion with the foot between the examiner's elbow and hip. (Reproduced, with permission, from Feagin JA Jr: *The Crucial Ligaments.* New York: Churchill Livingstone, 1988.)

Surgical MCL repair in the acute setting can include a primary repair, with shortening if needed, of the torn ligament. Similarly, avulsion fragments are treated with reduction and fixation in the acute setting. Primary repairs can be reinforced if needed with autograft or allograft tissues if the remaining MCL is insufficient for a stand alone repair. Chronic reconstructions also often include autograft or allograft tissue reconstruction.

Traditionally, casting or operative treatment of MCL injuries significantly limited an early return to range-of-motion exercises. With the addition of functional bracing and early motion to a conservative treatment protocol, motion and strengthening of the knee can occur at an early stage while the ligament is protected from valgus stress. As knee motion improves, isotonic strengthening exercises are introduced. As the strength of the extremity improves, the intensity of functional rehabilitation increases accordingly.

Complications

With nonoperative treatment becoming the standard of care, the amount of complications associated with an MCL injury has significantly decreased. The main potential complication of nonoperative therapy is residual valgus laxity or medial knee pain. Radiographs may also show residual calcification of the MCL (Pelligrini–Steida lesion). Potential surgical complications include arthrofibrosis, infection, damage to the saphenous nerve or vein, or recurrent valgus laxity.

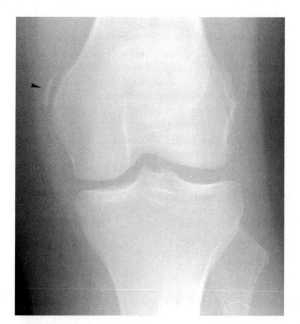

Figure 3–14. Pellegrini–Steida lesion. There is a curvilinear calcification at a site of the previous medial collateral ligament injury. (Reproduced, with permission, from Anderson J: *An Atlas of Imaging in Sports Medicine.* McGraw-Hill, 1999.)

Prognosis & Return to Play

In general, in isolated MCL injuries good outcomes can be achieved with conservative treatment and rehabilitation. A 98% return to professional football after nonoperative treatment of isolated MCL injuries has been shown.

Gardiner JC et al: Strain in the human medial collateral ligament during valgus loading of the knee. Clin Orthop Related Res 2001;391:266.

Mazzocca AD et al: Valgus medial collateral ligament rupture causes concomitant loading and damage of the anterior cruciate ligament. J Knee Surg 2003;16(3):148.

Nakamura N et al: Acute grade III medial collateral ligament injury of the knee associated with anterior cruciate ligament tear. The usefulness of magnetic resonance imaging in determining a treatment regimen. Am J Sports Med 2003;31(2):261.

Robinson JR et al: The posteromedial corner revisited. An anatomical description of the passive restraining structures of the medial aspect of the human knee. J Bone Joint Surg B 2004;86(5):674.

Sawant M et al: Valgus knee injuries: evaluation and documentation using a simple technique of stress radiography. Knee 2004;11(1):25.

Wilson TC et al: Medial collateral ligament "tibial" injuries: indication for acute repair. Orthopedics 2004;27(4):389.

LATERAL COLLATERAL LIGAMENT INJURIES

ESSENTIALS OF DIAGNOSIS

- *Much less common than an MCL injury.*
- *Rarely seen in isolation.*
- *Often overlooked in a multiligamentous knee injury.*
- *Mechanism: varus stress and external tibial torsion.*
- *Pain laterally with varus instability.*
- *Operative repair/reconstruction is the mainstay of treatment.*

Prevention

Bracing has not been shown to be effective in prevention of LCL injuries.

Clinical Findings

Because this is a relatively rare injury seen in combination with other ligamentous injuries, the clinical findings of an LCL and posterolateral corner injury can frequently go unnoticed. Subtle findings such as lateral and posterolateral pain and ecchymoses should be noted and investigated further.

A. Symptoms

The most consistent symptom of an acute LCL injury is lateral knee pain. However, the symptoms of lateral and posterolateral instability are quite variable and depend on the severity of injury, level of patient activity, overall limb alignment, and other associated knee injuries. For example, a sedentary individual with minimal laxity and overall valgus alignment will have few if any symptoms. However, if LCL laxity is combined with overall varus alignment, hyperextension, and an increased level of activity, symptoms will be quite pronounced. These patients may complain of lateral joint line pain and a varus thrust of their leg with everyday activities, often described as the knee buckling into hyperextension with normal gait.

B. Signs

Patients with an LCL and/or posterolateral corner injury often have additional ligamentous injuries to the knee. Therefore a thorough knee examination should be performed to evaluate for coexistent knee pathology. Additionally, a careful neurovascular examination should be performed as the incidence of neurovascular injury, particularly peroneal nerve injury, in posterolateral knee injuries has been reported to be 12–29%.

The integrity of the LCL is assessed with a varus stress with the knee in full extension and 30° of flexion. Baseline varus opening is widely variable and should be compared to the contralateral leg. The average baseline for varus opening is 7°. Examination findings with an isolated LCL injury should include varus laxity at 30° of flexion and no instability in full extension. This is due to the stabilizing effect that the intact cruciate ligaments provide in full extension.

It is important to note that a significant posterolateral knee injury can be present without significant varus laxity. The most useful test to evaluate for posterolateral instability is the dial test, performed by externally rotating each tibia and noting the angle subtended between the thigh and the foot. The dial test is performed at 30° and 90° of flexion with a significant difference being an angle 5° or greater than the contralateral leg.

C. Imaging Studies

A series of knee radiographs should be obtained in any patient with a suspected significant knee injury. Radiographs should be inspected for acute fractures, lateral capsular avulsion (Segond's fracture—see ACL imaging), loose bodies, fibular head avulsions (Figure 3–15), and evidence of patellar dislocation. With chronic posterolateral instability, degenerative changes of the lateral compartment are often noted. Lateral joint space narrowing with osteophytes and subchondral sclerosis can be seen.

Stress radiographs can help to quantify the amount of varus angulation present.

MRI is often a useful adjunct for diagnosing posterolateral corner and LCL injuries in the severely injured knee. As previously mentioned, this posterolateral injury can often go unnoticed during an initial evaluation and MRI findings can refocus the examination to the posterolateral structures. Pain and guarding at the time of injury can often obscure posterolateral injury and MRI can prove to be an extremely valuable adjunct in diagnosis.

D. Special Tests/Examinations

1. Reverse pivot shift test—This test involves starting with the knee flexed to 90°. With the knee extended, the leg is loaded axially with a valgus stress applied to the knee and the foot is held in external rotation. A palpable shift is noted as the tibia reduces from its posteriorly subluxed position as the knee is extended.

2. External rotation recurvatum test—This test is performed with the patient supine and the hip and knee fully extended. The leg is lifted off the bed by the toes. Hyperextension, varus instability, and external rotation of the tibial tubercle occur with adequate quadriceps relaxation in a patient with posterolateral instability.

3. Posterolateral drawer test—A standard posterior drawer test (see PCL physical examination) is performed with the tibia in internal rotation, neutral, and externally rotated positions. With posterolateral injury, the magnitude of the posterior drawer displacement will be greatest with external tibial rotation.

4. Examination under anesthesia—An examination while the patient is relaxed under a general anesthetic is extremely useful, particularly in the acute setting. If the patient with a multiligamentous knee injury is taken to the operating room, this is an excellent opportunity to examine the knee without guarding to improve the accuracy of the examination.

Treatment

A. Conservative

Isolated LCL ligament injuries, as noted above, are rare. However, in the case of an isolated LCL ligament injury with grade II or less magnitude, a period of immobilization from 2 to 4 weeks followed by a quadriceps strengthening program will usually yield good results. Grade III injuries will often not respond as well with conservative treatment. A combination of delayed diagnosis along with an uncertain natural history of posterolateral instability makes the treatment of these injuries a challenge.

B. Surgical

LCL and posterolateral ligaments, as discussed above, rarely occur in isolation. Therefore, other injuries must also be considered in the treatment plan of a multiligament knee injury. Ideally the posterolateral and LCL injury is diagnosed in the acute setting. This allows the preferred surgical treatment of a primary repair of the injured structures with augmentation as needed. Primary repair is generally feasible only in the first few weeks following the knee injury.

The knee with chronic posterolateral instability will often require ligamentous reconstruction or advancement to reconstitute a static restraint to varus stresses. The key biomechanical concept of any lateral ligamentous reconstruction is that the isometric point of the LCL lies between the fibular head and the lateral epicondyle. Therefore, regardless of the graft material used to reconstruct the lateral ligamentous complex, a portion of the graft must pass between the lateral femoral epicondyle and the fibular head.

C. Special Procedures

To improve the success rate of reconstruction of chronic lateral ligamentous instability, a proximal tibial valgus osteotomy may be performed to decrease the stress on the lateral structures of the knee.

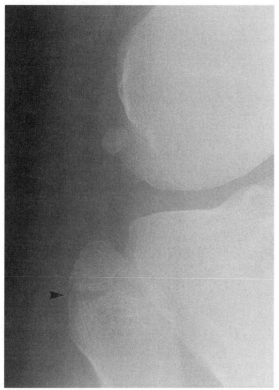

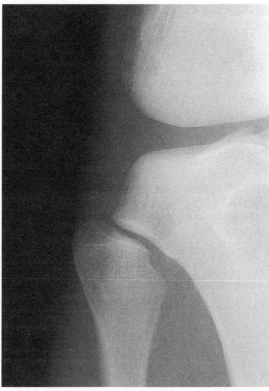

A   B

Figure 3–15. A: An oblique view of the proximal tibiofibular joint shows an avulsion fracture of the head of the fibula (***arrowhead***) due to traction by the lateral collateral ligament and/or the biceps femoris. **B:** Subluxation of the proximal tibiofibular joint, demonstrated in an oblique view. (Reproduced, with permission, from Anderson J: *An Atlas of Radiography for Sports Injuries.* McGraw-Hill, 2000.)

D. REHABILITATION

The rehabilitation of the knee after posterolateral reconstructions or repairs is largely guided by associated injuries to the ACL or posterior cruciate ligament (PCL). It is generally necessary, however, to limit weight bearing for at least 6 weeks and protect the lateral structures with a brace for at least 3 months.

Complications

The peroneal nerve runs just posterior to the fibular head. It is important to isolate the peroneal nerve prior to any lateral knee exposure to minimize the complication of a peroneal nerve injury.

Prognosis & Return to Play

If injuries to the posterolateral corner of the knee are diagnosed and repaired acutely, the results are good for restoration of varus stability and return to play. Chronic posterolateral corner injury reconstructions also do well when an isometric lateral reconstruction is achieved.

Albright J et al: Posterolateral knee instability and the reverse pivot shift. Presented at AOSSM, June 2000, Sun Valley, ID.

Buzzi R et al: Lateral collateral ligament reconstruction using a semitendinosus graft. Knee Surg Sports Traumatol Arthrosc 2004;12(1):36.

Lee MC et al: Posterolateral reconstruction using split Achilles tendon allograft. Arthroscopy 2003;19(9):1043.

Pasque C et al: The role of the popliteofibular ligament and the tendon of popliteus in providing stability in the human knee. J Bone Joint Surg B 2003;85(2):292.

Pavlovich RI, Nafarrate EB: Trivalent reconstruction for posterolateral and lateral knee instability. Arthroscopy 2002;18(1):E1.

Sugita T, Amis AA: Anatomic and biomechanical study of the lateral collateral and popliteofibular ligaments. Am J Sports Med 2001;29(4):466.

ANTERIOR COLLATERAL LIGAMENT INJURIES

ESSENTIALS OF DIAGNOSIS

- History of pain and swelling associated with an audible "pop."
- Knee instability or "giving way" with return to activity.
- Anterior laxity and acute hemarthrosis.
- Mechanism: most often twisting of the knee with the foot planted.
- Most commonly reconstructed ligamentous injury in the knee.

Prevention

Many centers are searching for improved methods and protocols to prevent ACL injury. Much of the current research centers around female athletes due to their increased incidence of ACL tears compared to their male counterparts. Strengthening, proprioceptive training, and altering the mechanics of running, jumping, and cutting are all being investigated as methods to prevent ACL injury. Unfortunately, there is no widely accepted method for prevention of ACL injury at this time.

Clinical Findings

The main clinical finding indicative of an acute or chronic ACL tear is a history of a knee injury associated with significant swelling and pain. In most patients this is often followed by symptoms of instability upon returning to athletic activities.

A. Symptoms

The mechanism of injury should be elicited in any evaluation of a knee injury. This can guide the examination to additional structures that may also be injured. ACL injury can occur from a variety of mechanisms, however, a few predominate. The most common mechanism of noncontact ACL injury involves a deceleration and rotational injury during running, cutting, or jumping activities. The most common contact injury involves either hyperextension and/or valgus forces to the knee by a direct blow.

ACL injury is often associated with a "pop" heard by the patient at the time of injury. This is not ACL specific, however. Upon return to competition the patient will often notice instability of the knee or describe the knee "giving out." Substantial knee swelling secondary to a hemarthrosis typically occurs within the first 4–12 hours following the injury.

B. Signs

With the history obtained above and a proper physical examination, it should be possible to diagnose an ACL tear without any additional tests. A complete examination of the knee should be performed to evaluate for any other associated injuries. The uninjured knee is examined first to familiarize the patient with the knee examination.

The Lachman test is the most useful test for assessing anterior laxity of the knee. It is performed with the knee in 20–30° of flexion as an anterior force is applied to the tibia with one hand while the other hand stabilizes the distal femur (Figure 3–16). The degree of anterior translation as well as the presence and character of an end point are assessed. The laxity is graded based on comparison to the uninjured contralateral knee. Grade 1 laxity is 1–5 mm of increased translation, grade 2 laxity is 6–10 mm of increased translation, and grade 3 laxity is more than 10 mm of translation as compared to the injured contralateral knee.

The anterior drawer test is also used to evaluate anterior tibial translation. This is performed with the knee in 90° of flexion as an anterior force is applied to the tibia (Figure 3–17). This test is less sensitive than the Lachman test. In the acute setting of an ACL tear there is often a window in which an accurate examination can be performed before extensive knee swelling and guarding inhibit examination. Aspiration of a hemarthrosis can help to decrease pain and improve the quality of the examination in the acute setting as well.

C. Imaging Studies

Plain radiographs of the knee should be obtained to rule out fractures. The Segond fracture (Figure 3–18), as discussed above, is an avulsion of the anterolateral capsule of the tibia. Before skeletal maturity an avulsion of the tibial insertion of the ACL can also be seen radiographically. Following radiographs, an MRI is the most useful

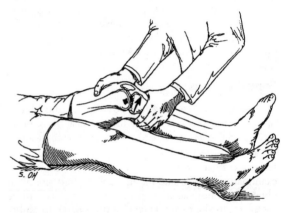

Figure 3–16. Lachman test.

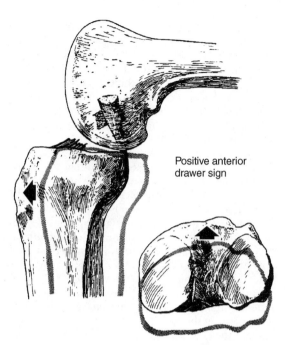

Figure 3–17. A positive anterior drawer test signifying a tear of the anterior cruciate ligament. (Reproduced, with permission, from Insall JN: *Surgery of the Knee.* New York: Churchill Livingstone, 1984.)

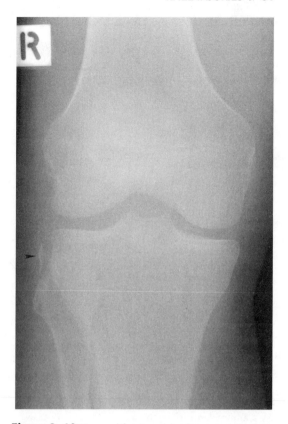

Figure 3–18. Segond fracture (also known as the lateral capsular sign) is an avulsion at the attachment of the inferior meniscal ligament and is associated with anterior cruciate ligament rupture. (Reproduced, with permission, from Anderson J: *An Atlas of Imaging in Sports Medicine.* McGraw-Hill, 1999.

method to evaluate associated injuries. Although generally not needed for diagnosis of an ACL tear, MRI can diagnose an ACL tear with 95% or better accuracy. Bone bruises of the lateral femoral condyle and lateral tibial plateau are noted in up to 80% of ACL injuries.

D. Special Examination

The pivot shift test is performed to evaluate the rotational instability associated with an ACL tear. The test is based on the lateral tibial plateau subluxing anteriorly with extension and reduction of the lateral compartment with flexion. The most effective method of achieving this result is by flexing the knee with an axial load from full extension with valgus stress at the knee and internal rotation of the tibia (Figure 3–19). The reduction of the subluxation should occur at approximately 30° of flexion. MCL injury and some meniscal tears may produce a false-negative result.

The pivot shift test is considered the most functional test to evaluate knee stability after ACL injury. An examination under anesthesia is also often useful in obtaining a more accurate pivot shift test. This can be useful in a patient with an unclear history of instability and an equivocal examination in the office.

E. Special Tests

Instrumented laxity evaluations can augment the physical examination and provide an objective baseline for future comparison. The most commonly used arthrometer, the KT-1000 (MEDmetric, San Diego, CA), utilizes a series of standard forces to measure anterior translation of the tibia with the knee in 20–30° of flexion similar to the Lachman test.

Treatment

A. Rehabilitation

Rehabilitation following an isolated ACL injury should include an effort to regain knee motion and strengthen the muscles about the knee. Returning to activities that produce episodes of instability is discouraged. Once motion and strength have been restored, a gradual return to activities can be attempted to determine the functional level that can be attained without instability.

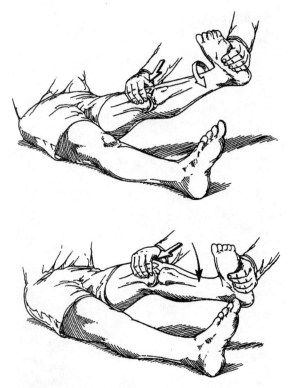

Figure 3–19. Pivot shift test.

Conservative management with rehabilitation only after an ACL injury generally yields poor results in patients that return to competitive activities. The range of clinically significant episodes of instability resulting in pain, swelling, and disability ranges from 56% to 89% in various studies following a series of conservatively managed ACL tears. These episodes of instability are thought to place the menisci and articular cartilage of the knee at risk for further injury. Fewer than 20% of athletes are able to return to strenuous competition with conservative management of ACL tears.

B. SURGICAL

The decision to surgically reconstruct an ACL tear is individualized based on the patient's desired level of continued competition, age, accompanying degenerative changes, and objective and subjective knee instability. For example, a young, active patient with both objective and subjective knee instability and with a continued desire to compete in sports involving cutting and jumping is an ideal candidate for surgical reconstruction. On the other hand, an older patient with some degenerative arthritis of the knee, minimal desire for continued competitive athletics, and no subjective instability would be much more suited to physical therapy and conservative care.

Early in the history of ACL reconstruction, it was noted that primary repairs of the ligament did not produce a good clinical result. These attempts gave way to various methods of ligament reconstruction using a variety of graft materials. Everything from synthetics to autograft and allograft tissues have been used for reconstruction of the ACL. Over time, bone–patellar tendon–bone and semitendinosis/gracilis hamstring autografts, and bone–patellar tendon–bone allograft constructs have proven to be the most commonly used grafts. All of these constructs have worked well both in the laboratory and clinically for ACL reconstructions.

The goal of ACL reconstruction is to reproduce the strength, location, and function of the intact ACL. Therefore, once a graft of adequate strength is selected, the location of placement of the graft is of utmost importance. The graft is generally passed through a bone tunnel in the tibia and a bone tunnel through the femur. The intraarticular placement of the tibial tunnel is generally in the center of the native ACL stump just in front of the PCL origin and just medial to the center of the notch in the coronal plane.

Once the graft is in place, proper tension and fixation of the graft must occur to complete a successful ACL reconstruction. Establishing proper tension in the graft is important to the function of the graft clinically. A lax ACL graft may not restore clinical stability to the knee and an overtightened graft may cause the graft to fail or limit knee range of motion. Fixation of the graft is achieved through a variety of measures. The most common method involves placing an interference screw up the bone tunnel that captures the graft in the tunnel. The graft can also be fixed via sutures tied over various devices located on the outer cortex of the tunnels.

Complications

Although ACL reconstruction usually results in a successful outcome, several potential complications can occur. One of the most common is a loss of knee motion. Efforts to minimize this include obtaining and maintaining full knee extension immediately following surgery. Knee flexion exercises are begun as soon as possible postoperatively and a goal of 90° at 1 week is set. Additionally, patellar mobilization is performed in an attempt to minimize patellofemoral scarring. Another common complication is anterior knee pain. The exact etiology of this pain is unclear, however, it is thought that patellar tendon autograft harvest may increase the incidence of patellofemoral pain. Less common complications (less than 1%) include patellar fracture, patellar tendon rupture, and quadriceps tendon rupture depending on the graft harvest site.

Prognosis & Return to Play

The goal of any rehabilitation protocol for an ACL reconstruction is to return the patient to the full desired level of activity in as short an amount of time as possible while avoiding any complications or setbacks. Because of improved surgical techniques and accelerated rehabilitation protocols, most studies have shown a 90% or better return to play and patient satisfaction. Patients generally are able to return between 4 and 6 months postoperatively with some professional athletes successfully returning to competition in 3 months. Specific criteria for a return to sports vary from institution to institution with a combination of functional testing, subjective reporting, and clinical examination contributing to the decision. In general, the criteria for return to sports include full range of motion, KT-1000 testing within 2–3 mm of the uninjured knee, ≥85% quadriceps strength and full hamstring strength, and functional testing within 85% of the contralateral leg.

An KN: Muscle force and its role in joint dynamic stability. Clin Orthop Related Res 2002;403 suppl:S37.

Bales CP et al: Anterior cruciate ligament injuries in children with open physes: evolving strategies of treatment. Am J Sports Med 2004;32(8):1978.

Beynnon BD et al: The science of anterior cruciate ligament rehabilitation. Clin Orthop Related Res 2002;402:9.

Cascio BM et al: Return to play after anterior cruciate ligament reconstruction. Clin Sports Med 2004;23(3):395.

Dunn WR et al: The effect of anterior cruciate ligament reconstruction on the risk of knee reinjury. Am J Sports Med 2004;32(8):1906.

Huston LJ et al: Anterior cruciate ligament injuries in the female athlete. Potential risk factors. Clin Orthop Related Res 2000;372:50.

McDevitt ER et al: Functional bracing after anterior cruciate ligament reconstruction: a prospective, randomized, multicenter study. Am J Sports Med 2004;32(8):1887.

Spindler KP et al: Anterior cruciate ligament reconstruction autograft choice: bone-tendon-bone versus hamstring: does it really matter? A systematic review. Am J Sports Med 2004;32(8):1986.

POSTERIOR CRUCIATE LIGAMENT INJURIES

ESSENTIALS OF DIAGNOSIS

- *Increasingly recognized knee injury.*
- *Caused by forced posterior translation of the tibia.*
- *Posterior "sag" sign on inspection.*
- *Posterior drawer test.*
- *Most commonly after a motor vehicle accident "dashboard injury" or sports injury.*
- *Posterolateral knee injury associated with 60% of PCL injuries.*

Prevention

The energy required to tear the PCL is significant. Beyond maintaining good strength in the musculature around the knee, there is no effective prevention beyond limitations in activity. A direct blow to the knee is the most common sports mechanism for PCL injury and therefore contact sports show the highest incidence.

Clinical Findings

PCL injury is associated with a significant injury to the knee. This is generally seen after a direct blow to the knee or an injury from an impact with the dashboard in a motor vehicle accident. PCL injury is associated with a large hemarthrosis and knee pain.

A. Symptoms

When evaluating a patient for a PCL injury it is important to determine the mechanism of injury, the severity of the injury, and any potential associated injuries. In contrast to an ACL tear, it is rare for patients with PCL injuries to report hearing a "pop" or report any feelings of subjective instability. More commonly patients will complain of knee pain, swelling, and stiffness.

The presentation of a patient with a subacute or chronically injured PCL can range from asymptomatic to significant instability and pain. Patients with significant varus alignment or injury to the lateral structures of the knee will often complain of feelings of instability and giving way. A few characteristic mechanisms of PCL injury differ significantly from the mechanism of ACL injuries. As above, one of the most common mechanisms of PCL injury is the "dashboard" injury during which the anterior tibia sustains a posteriorly directed force from the dashboard with the knee in 90° of flexion. Sports injuries to the PCL come from an outside force or blow in contrast to the typical deceleration twisting mechanism of an ACL injury. The most common methods of incurring a sports-related PCL injury are a direct blow to the anterior tibia or a fall onto the flexed knee with the foot in plantar flexion. The most common mechanism of incurring an isolated PCL injury in the athlete is a partial tear associated with hyperflexion of the knee. Additionally, significant knee multiligamentous injuries with PCL tears can be seen after a varus or valgus stress is applied to the hyperextended knee.

B. Signs

A thorough knee examination should accompany the evaluation of any significant knee injury. Specific cues to injury of the PCL on initial inspection include abrasions or ecchymosis around the proximal anterior tibia and ecchymosis in the popliteal fossa. Assessment for meniscal damage and associated ligamentous injury should be performed. Evaluation of ACL laxity in the presence of a PCL injury is challenging due to the lack of a stable reference point to perform a Lachman or anterior drawer test.

Examination of the PCL in the acutely injured knee can be challenging. Despite increased awareness of the injury, many PCL injuries go undiagnosed in the acute setting. The most accurate clinical test of PCL integrity is the posterior drawer test (Figure 3–20). The knee is flexed to 90° with the patient supine and a posteriorly directed force is applied to the anterior tibia. The amount of posterior translation and the presence and character of the end point are noted. The extent of translation is assessed by noting the change in the distance of the step-off between the anteromedial tibial plateau and the medial femoral condyle. The tibial plateau is approximately 1 cm anterior to the medial femoral condyle on average. However, the contralateral knee must be examined to establish a baseline.

Another test with which to examine the PCL is the posterior sag or Godfrey test (Figure 3–21). This test involves flexing the knee and hip and noting the posterior pull of gravity creating a posterior "sag" of the tibia on the femur. An adjunct to this test involves noting a reduction of this subluxation with active quadriceps contraction.

The reverse pivot shift is the analog to the pivot shift in the evaluation of an ACL injury. This is performed by placing a valgus stress on the knee with the foot externally rotated. The knee is then extended from 90° of flexion and a palpable reduction of the posterolateral tibial plateau is noted between 20° and 30° of flexion.

It is extremely important to evaluate the posterolateral structures of the knee in the setting of a suspected PCL injury. Injury to the posterolateral structures has been reported to occur in up to 60% of PCL injuries.

C. IMAGING STUDIES

Given the magnitude of the forces required to injure the PCL, plain radiographs of the knee are essential to evaluate for bony injuries, dislocation, or evidence of

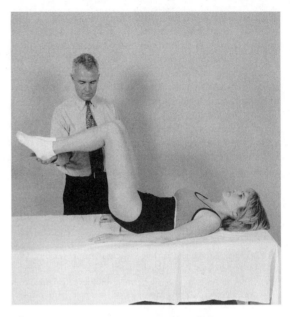

Figure 3–21. Godfrey sign. (Reproduced, with permission, from Dutton M: *Orthopaedic Examination, Evaluation, & Intervention.* McGraw-Hill, 2004.)

other associated injuries. Subtle posterior subluxation on the lateral radiograph may also indicate PCL injury. Stress posterior drawer radiographs and contralateral comparisons may also increase the sensitivity for detecting PCL injuries with plain radiographs (Figure 3–22). In the chronic setting of PCL injury, radiographs are useful to assess for patellofemoral and medial compartment degenerative changes that can occur over time.

Although plain films are necessary and useful in evaluating these injuries, MRI has become the diagnostic study of choice for the knee with a presumed PCL injury. It is reported to be 96–100% sensitive at diagnosing PCL tears. Equally or more important, MRI is extremely valuable in its ability to detect associated injuries. This is particularly important in diagnosing posterolateral corner injuries as these can often be missed on the initial clinical examination. In multiligamentous knee injuries, MRI can also be of use in assessing the ACL, as clinical examination of the ACL is challenging in the setting of a complete PCL tear.

D. SPECIAL TESTS

In the setting of a chronic isolated PCL tear, pain in the medial and patellofemoral compartments is generally evaluated with radiographs. If these are normal, some surgeons will proceed with a bone scan to evaluate for increased uptake in these areas. If these areas are under increased stress on the bone scan before signs of advanced

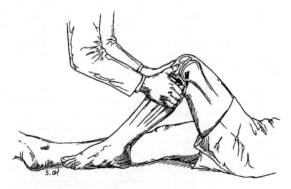

Figure 3–20. Posterior drawer test.

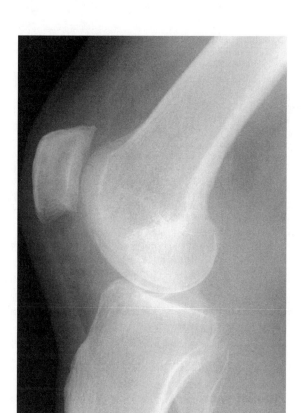

Figure 3–22. Abnormal tibiofemoral alignment. A lateral view shows posterior displacement of the tibia, indicative of posterior cruciate ligament deficiency. Also note changes of chondromalacia patellae.
(Reproduced, with permission, from Anderson J: *An Atlas of Imaging in Sports Medicine.* McGraw-Hill, 1999.)

arthritis occur, this subset of patients may benefit from a PCL reconstruction to decrease the stresses seen by these two compartments.

Treatment

There is considerable controversy regarding treatment of isolated PCL injuries. Multiple factors, including the patient's age, activity level, expectations, and associated injuries, must be evaluated in deciding how to treat a complete PCL rupture. The literature on operative versus nonoperative treatment of these injuries can be difficult to interpret, and there are no long-term follow-up studies of randomized patient groups.

A. Conservative Care and Rehabilitation

Rehabilitation of the PCL injured knee is often largely dependent on the associated injuries sustained by the knee. This is particularly true with the commonly associated posterolateral corner injury. Therefore, we will focus on the rehabilitation of the isolated PCL injured knee. Regaining motion and regaining strength are the two key objectives of a rehabilitation program. Obtaining full quadriceps strength is essential for achieving the optimal result with conservative treatment. The initial treatment is aimed at keeping the tibia reduced under the femur and minimizing tension on the injured PCL. With partial injuries (grade I and II), the prognosis is quite good and early motion with weight bearing is the usual course of therapy. In a complete PCL tear, the knee is usually immobilized in extension to protect the posterolateral structures. Early strengthening exercises focus on quadriceps strength with quadriceps sets, straight leg raises, and partial weight bearing in extension.

Overall, most patients do quite well with conservative treatment of a PCL tear. Despite objective findings of instability that are often noted on examination, most patients subjectively are satisfied with the function of the knee. Bracing is generally ineffective in controlling PCL laxity clinically.

The main subjective complaint with chronic PCL insufficiency, however, is pain rather than instability. A PCL-deficient knee with posterior tibial subluxation places significantly increased stress on the patellofemoral and medial compartments of the knee. In patients with PCL injuries followed with serial radiographs, 60% displayed some degenerative changes of the medial compartment.

B. Surgical

PCL injuries requiring surgical management include avulsion fractures, isolated acute PCL injuries, multiligament injuries, and chronic PCL insufficiency. Avulsion fractures of the PCL are rare. If nondisplaced, these injuries are treated conservatively. If significantly displaced, these fractures are generally treated with open reduction and internal fixation.

Isolated PCL injuries are usually treated with conservative care by the majority of surgeons at this time. However, nonoperative care of these injuries is not without its own consequences. Although subjectively these patients do relatively well over the short term, many continue to have objective instability and display degenerative arthritic changes over time. A follow-up of patients with PCL-deficient knees at an average of 15 years after injury found 89% had persistent pain and 50% had chronic effusions. All patients in this group showed degenerative changes when followed for 25 years. Therefore, given the risks of continued instability and an increased chance of arthritic changes, surgical reconstruction of the PCL is a reasonable choice.

Initially, surgical care of complete PCL tears consisted of a primary repair of midsubstance tears. The objective stability of these repairs was generally disappointing. Current methods of reconstruction usually involve routing either autograft or allograft tendons through bone tunnels to reconstruct the PCL in an anatomic fashion. Although there are several different methods of reconstructing the PCL, the two primary ones consist of single and double bundle repairs. Classically, reconstructions of the PCL anatomically replicated the anterolateral bundle of the native PCL with a single bundle reconstruction. As problems were noted with recurrence of posterior laxity in the postoperative period, a double bundle technique was derived to reconstruct both the anterolateral and posteromedial bundles of the native PCL. The advantages of the double bundle technique are still theoretical, and there is no long-term clinical follow-up demonstrating the superiority of a double bundle reconstruction at this time.

The severe instability noted with PCL injuries associated with multiligamentous knee injuries makes the argument for ligament reconstruction more compelling in this patient population. Many of the studies involving PCL reconstruction for these complex knee injuries have involved attempts at primary repair. Although subjective results were generally good, residual pathologic objective laxity was very common following repairs. More recently ligament reconstructions with allografts and autografts have become the dominant method of PCL reconstruction in this challenging patient population.

Complications

The most common complication following PCL reconstruction is the return of objective posterior laxity on physical examination. This does not present as subjective laxity, however, and patient satisfaction remains high despite objective laxity. Acute PCL reconstructions in the setting of a multiligamentous knee repair/reconstruction can result in arthrofibrosis with extensive postoperative scarring.

Prognosis & Return to Play

Even with conservative management of a PCL injury, the prognosis for a functional recovery and return to competition is very good. PCL laxity can be significantly compensated for by a strong quadriceps muscle and extensor mechanism. Athletes should spend a minimum of 3 months in rehabilitation before attempting a return to competition. However, a subset of patients experiences significant instability with a grade III PCL injury and cannot return to play. This group may benefit from PCL reconstruction.

On the other hand, the prognosis for a PCL tear associated with a multiligamentous knee injury is guarded with respect to return to play. Although prompt recognition of a multiligamentous injury and appropriately timed treatment, reconstruction, and rehabilitation are essential for optimal recovery, a significant percentage of patients will not be able to return to full competition.

Christel P: Basic principles for surgical reconstruction of the PCL in chronic posterior knee instability. Knee Surg Sports Traumatol Arthrosc 2003;11(5):289.

Giannoulias CS, Freedman KB: Knee dislocations: management of the multiligament-injured knee. Am J Orthop 2004;33(11):553.

Giffin JR et al: Single- versus double-bundle PCL reconstruction: a biomechanical analysis. J Knee Surg 2002;15(2):114.

Li G et al: Biomechanical consequences of PCL deficiency in the knee under simulated muscle loads—an in vitro experimental study. J Orthop Res 2002;20(4):887.

Shelbourne KD, Carr DR: Combined anterior and posterior cruciate and medial collateral ligament injury: nonsurgical and delayed surgical treatment. Instruct Course Lect 2003;52:413.

Twaddle BC et al: Knee dislocations: where are the lesions? A prospective evaluation of surgical findings in 63 cases. J Orthop Trauma 2003;17(3):198.

Wind WM Jr et al: Evaluation and treatment of posterior cruciate ligament injuries: revisited. Am J Sports Med 2004;32(7):1765.

■ KNEE PAIN

ANATOMY

Patellofemoral

The human knee is one of the most complex mechanical systems in the body. It is designed to accept and redirect very high loads with magnitudes that can be many times body weight. Some of the highest compressive and tensile loads are transmitted by the patellofemoral joint. Understanding the functional anatomy of the patellofemoral joint allows musculoskeletal specialists to better identify injuries and direct appropriate treatments. Despite its seemingly simple construction, the patellofemoral joint is one of the more complex anatomic regions of the knee. It is composed of multiple fascial layers, ligamentous attachments, bursae, and bony landmarks.

Fascial

Anatomic descriptions are most easily understood by proceeding from the most superficial subcutaneous layer to the deep capsular layer (Figure 3–1). The subcutaneous layer is the most superficial and contains relatively little fat. The skin overlying the patella is highly mobile and allows for extensive and uninhibited range of motion. As this layer progresses medially and laterally, the number of small perpendicular fascial attachments increases. These fascial attachments contain the subcutaneous prepatellar bursa in its anterior location. A more inferior subcutaneous prepatellar tendon bursa can be found immediately anterior to the patellar tendon. The bursae are highly variable in both their anatomic and their clinical location. The next deepest layer, the superficial fascial or arciform layer, is an extension of the fascia lata and is named for is transverse or "arcing" orientation over the anterior knee. This superficial fascial layer covers the iliotibial band on the lateral side, the distal quadriceps muscle on the medial side, and the patellar tendon inferiorly, and ends at the level of the tibial tubercle. This layer does not contribute to the patellar tendon, but its fibers are cut and often repaired during the patellar tendon harvest used for ACL reconstruction.

The intermediate oblique layer exists as a fascial layer anterior to the patella and is composed of fibers from the anterior portion of the rectus femoris, vastus medialis, and vastus lateralis. This layer is thicker than the arciform layer, and its fibers blend into the deeper layers just medial and lateral to the patellar margins, however, it does not contribute fibers to the patellar tendon. The potential space that lies superficial to the intermediate layer but deep to the arciform layer contains the intermediate prepatellar bursa. The deep longitudinal layer is derived from the rectus femoris and is named for the direction of its fibers as they course across over the anterior patella and become contiguous with the patellar tendon prior to inserting on the tibial tubercle. These fibers are adherent to the patella and provide the deep margin for the deep prepatellar bursa (Figure 3–5). The next deepest layer has thick fibers that are transverse in their orientation and form the medial and lateral retinaculum. These fibers provide a major static restraint to the patellofemoral articulation. The medial retinacular layer runs from the medial surface of the patella and inserts on the medial femoral condyle. The lateral retinacular layer runs from the lateral surface of the patella passing deep to the iliotibial tract and inserts on its undersurface. The deepest layer includes the capsular attachments from the medial and lateral borders of the patella as they insert on the medial and lateral meniscus (Figure 3–8).

Muscular & Ligamentous

Although the hamstrings and quadriceps are the major muscle groups that contribute to knee motion, the quadriceps muscle group also plays a critical role in patellofemoral joint structure and stabilization (Figure 3–2). The primary role of the quadriceps is deceleration through eccentric contraction during normal ambulation (Figure 3–3). At the level of the mid-thigh, the group includes the rectus femoris, vastus medialis, vastus lateralis, and vastus intermedius muscles. At the knee joint, the vastus medialis gives rise to the vastus medialis obliquus and the vastus lateralis becomes the vastus lateralis obliquus. The rectus femoris originates

on the anterior inferior iliac spine and its tendinous insertion begins on the anterior surface of the patella and continues over the anterior surface as it travels distally and becomes part of the patellar tendon. The vastus intermedius lies deep to the rectus femoris. It originates from the anterior surface of the proximal femur and has a broad fibrocartilaginous insertion on the superior pole of the patella. Its broad fibrocartilaginous insertion serves to distribute load equally across a large portion of the quadriceps tendon insertion. The articularis genus lies deep to the vastus intermedius. It originates on the distal femur and inserts on the superior capsule of the suprapatellar pouch. It serves to retract the suprapatellar pouch during knee motion and often contributes to the formation of the medial and suprapatellar plicae. The vastus medialis and vastus lateralis muscles originate from the anterior surface of the proximal femur just medial and just lateral to the vastus intermedius origin, respectively. They insert on the superior medial and superior lateral borders of the patella. The vastus medialis is usually large in size and has a more distal insertion, whereas the vastus lateralis has a long tendinous insertion on the superior lateral patella. The lateral side also receives contributions from the iliotibial tract. In addition, the vastus medialis obliquus serves an important role in medial stabilization of the patella as the knee approaches full extension.

Whereas the quadriceps musculature functions as an important dynamic patellar stabilizer, several medial ligamentous structures function as important static soft-tissue restraints to prevent lateral translation of the patella. The major medial soft tissue stabilizer, the medial patellofemoral ligament (MPFL), provides 53% of the total restraining force to lateral displacement of the patella. The patellomeniscal ligament provides 22% of the total restraining force, and the medial retinaculum ligament and medial patellotibial ligament provide lesser contributions (Figure 3–7).

Patellar Tendon

The patellar tendon has a complex organization that allows for transmission of high tensile loads from its origin on the inferior pole of the patella to its insertion on the tibial tubercle. Its fibers have a broad origin from the posterior and inferior surfaces of the patella and include anterior contributions from the rectus femoris as they progress distally to a broad insertion on the tibial tubercle. The patellar tendon is composed of densely packed collagen fibers that are primarily arranged parallel to the long axis of the tendon. Eighty-five percent of its dry weight is collagen, the majority of which is type I (90%). The tendon is surrounded by three layers: the outermost paratenon, an inner epitenon, and an innermost endotenon. The blood, nerve, and lymphatic supply to the tendon is via the endotenon, which serves to bind and bring nutrients to individual cells and collagen fibers.

Patella

The patella acts as a fulcrum and provides a mechanical advantage to the quadriceps during force transmission across the knee joint. The forces across this fulcrum are complex and include high degrees of compression and tension, with a minimal amount of friction. The patellar osseous and cartilaginous anatomy is equally complex and its design reflects its function (Figure 3–7). The anterior surface of the patella is convex and is composed of fibrous insertions from the rectus femoris and perforations for blood supply from the genicular vessels. The posterior articular surface contains thick cartilage that covers three facets. The lateral facet is the largest and extends from the superior pole to the inferior pole and articulates with the lateral femoral condyle. It is separated from the medial facet by a longitudinal central ridge that articulates with the femoral trochlear groove. The medial facet also extends from the superior to the inferior pole, but is approximately one-third smaller than the lateral facet and articulates with the medial femoral condyle. A smaller "odd" facet lies medial to the medial facet and articulates with the medial femoral condyle only during the extremes of knee flexion. The thick cartilage that covers these facets serves to increase patellofemoral congruity and dissipate compressive loads during the wide range of knee motion.

Peeler J et al: Structural parameters of the vastus medialis muscle. Clin Anat 2005;18(4):281.

Sanders TG, Miller MD: A systematic approach to magnetic resonance imaging interpretation of sports medicine injuries of the knee. Am J Sports Med 2005;33(1):131.

ANTERIOR KNEE PAIN

Patients who present with anterior knee pain are common in the practice of general orthopedics and sports medicine. The most frequent causes of anterior knee pain in the athlete include overuse injuries, patellofemoral instability, and direct trauma. Although anterior knee pain can come from many of the structures described above, in the most general sense, the cause of pain can be organized into the following categories: anterior knee pain with articular breakdown, anterior knee pain without articular breakdown, and anterior knee pain related to patellofemoral instability. Pain that is derived from the patellofemoral joint with articular breakdown often includes patients with the diagnosis of articular cartilage softening, known as chondromalacia, or frank patellofemoral chondrosis/arthrosis. Anterior knee pain without evidence of articular breakdown includes patients with the diagnosis of

patellar tilt-compression or some other form of patellar malalignment that precedes cartilage injury, patellar tendinitis or "jumper's knee," synovial plica, painful retinaculum, infrapatellar contracture syndrome, and, in children, Osgood–Schlatter disease. Anterior knee pain related to patellofemoral instability usually results from patellar tilt with or without patellar subluxation. The essentials of the diagnosis and treatment of the most common of these disorders will be described below.

Differential Diagnosis

A. SOFT-TISSUE ABNORMALITIES

1. Pathologic plica
2. Patellar tendinitis
3. Quadriceps tendinitis
4. Retinaculum
5. Infrapatellar contracture syndrome
6. Patellar tilt-compression
7. Osgood–Schlatter disease
8. Reflex sympathetic dystrophy

B. PATELLAR INSTABILITY

1. Subluxation
2. Dislocation

C. PATELLOFEMORAL CHONDROSIS/ARTHROSIS

1. Degenerative lesion
2. Direct trauma
3. Chondromalacia patella

1. Patellofemoral Chondrosis/Chondromalacia

The terms patellofemoral chondrosis or patellofemoral arthritis are reserved for describing the degenerative changes specifically observed in the patellofemoral articulation, whereas the term chondromalacia patellae is used to describe the breakdown of articular cartilage on the undersurface of the patella. Degenerative changes such as patellofemoral chondrosis or chondromalacia often cause the pain that arises from the patellofemoral joint. Because articular cartilage is not innervated, it is believed that the pain is derived from abnormal force transmission across degenerative articular cartilage to subchondral bone. Damage to the articular surface can range from localized articular softening to full-thickness lesions with exposed subchondral bone. The etiology of patellofemoral chondrosis is highly variable and includes damage to articular cartilage due to direct trauma, chondral injury following acute patellar dislocation, patellofemoral malalignment, and chronic subluxation.

ESSENTIALS OF DIAGNOSIS

- *Clinical history*
  —*Anterior knee pain with activity, for example, with stairs, running, or squatting.*
  —*History of trauma to the anterior knee or patellar dislocation.*
  —*History of effusions or crepitus from the patellofemoral joint.*
- *Physical examination*
  —*Knee effusions and crepitus are common and can be nonspecific.*
  —*Quadriceps wasting or weakness.*
  —*Pain with patellofemoral compression during knee range of motion.*
- *Imaging*
  —*Radiographs often read as normal except in end-stage arthrosis.*
  —*Abnormal patellar tilt and subluxation are often present on Merchant view or CT.*
  —*MRI can localize and quantify the extent of articular damage.*
- *Arthroscopic examination*
  —*Knee arthroscopy is the gold standard for evaluation and initial treatment.*
  —*Useful for grading, localization, and planning treatment strategies.*

Pathogenesis

During the initial history and examination it is important to ask questions about previous knee injuries, knee trauma, duration of symptoms, as well as exacerbating and remitting factors. Previous injury, surgery, and type of sport can be critical in narrowing the differential diagnosis. It is also important to distinguish symptoms of pain from those of instability. A careful history and physical examination should steer the physician to one of the three general categories listed in the differential diagnosis: anterior knee pain without evidence of articular breakdown, anterior knee pain with evidence of articular breakdown, and anterior knee pain resulting from patellofemoral instability. Plain radiographs should be obtained in all patients with possible patellofemoral pathology and should include an anteroposterior view, lateral view, tunnel view, and Merchant view. Other ancillary studies such as CT or MRI are indicated in certain cases as outlined below.

Prevention

Anterior knee pain in athletes is commonly related to overuse. The key to prevention is the identification and modification of factors that predispose the athlete to developing symptoms. Sport-specific training programs that include balanced quadriceps strengthening and patellar stabilization exercises are important elements for both the prevention of injury and long-term rehabilitation following previous injury.

Clinical Findings

A. Symptoms

Anterior symptoms related to patellofemoral chondrosis are typically described as deep and aching pain that worsens with activity or with sitting for prolonged periods with the knee in a flexed position. Symptoms are often vague and poorly localized beyond the anterior knee or patellofemoral joint. Patients with patellofemoral subluxation describe a feeling of instability localized to the anterior aspect of the knee. A history of previous patellar dislocation may be present, but more often, symptoms related to extensor mechanism imbalance are present in the history. Particular activities that increase patellofemoral contact pressures such as running, stairclimbing, and deep squats tend to exacerbate symptoms. Patients also describe intermittent knee effusions that often correlate with periods of increased activity. Popping and crepitus are common, but can be nonspecific findings present in many of the diagnoses listed above. In general, symptoms usually become worse with activity and improve with rest.

The correlation of clinical findings to articular changes is critical in both the diagnosis and treatment of anterior knee pain due to patellofemoral arthritis. Many patients may have symptoms of anterior knee pain without articular change, and previous studies have documented articular changes during arthroscopy in patients who did not have symptoms of pain. The physical examination and radiographic studies are important keys to narrowing the differential diagnosis prior to proceeding with various treatment options including knee arthroscopy.

B. Signs

All physical examinations should be performed with the athlete barefoot and wearing shorts to allow inspection and examination of the entire lower extremity. In general the athlete's attitude and cooperation with the examination may provide important clues for previous or future compliance with treatment and rehabilitation protocols. The examination should begin with an evaluation of the athlete's stance and gait, followed by careful examination of the hip, particularly in adolescents, as knee pain is often the result of hip pain until proven otherwise. Examination of the knee joint begins with inspection for overall femoral–tibial and patellofemoral alignment. Evaluation of the skin may point toward a diagnosis of reflex sympathetic dystrophy, particularly in patients with pain out of proportion to injury. Quadriceps, hamstring, and calf muscle size, definition, tone, strength, and flexibility should be assessed. Evaluation of active and passive knee range of motion focusing on knee joint stability and patellofemoral tracking throughout a full range of motion may aid in narrowing the differential diagnosis. Prone positioning is particularly helpful in evaluating quadriceps tightness and patellar tendon pathology. A careful ligamentous examination including the collaterals and cruciates should follow and may help identify other potential causes of knee pain or instability. Examination of the PCL is particularly important as chronic PCL tears have been associated with patellofemoral arthrosis. Tenderness to palpation may be present in a variety of locations and can help differentiate meniscal pathology (medial or posteromedial joint line tenderness) from the anterior retinacular pain often associated with patellofemoral pathology.

The physical examination of the athlete with ordinary patellofemoral chondrosis related to overuse is relatively nonspecific. Other causes of knee pain must be excluded by a careful history and complete physical examination. Crepitus and effusions are common, as is quadriceps wasting. Once the diagnosis of patellofemoral chondrosis or chondromalacia patellae is suspected, it is important to try and isolate the location of the articular pathology. This can be determined by applying patellofemoral compression while taking the knee through a full range of motion and documenting the point or points at which maximal pain occurs. The quadriceps angle (Q angle) should be documented with the knee in slight flexion and at 90° (Figure 3–6). An abnormal Q angle and patellar apprehension with attempts to move the patella laterally out of the trochlea may indicate chronic subluxation due to patellar malalignment or a tight lateral retinaculum. This will be discussed further in the section on patellar maltracking.

Articular degeneration within the patellofemoral joint can be classified into four types based on location and may identify potential causes and guide treatment strategies. Type I includes a distal mid-patellar lesion that is caused by chronic subluxation and/or patellar tilt. Type II lesions are subdivided into IIA and IIB: IIA lesions result from lateral patellar pressure syndrome and exhibit articular breakdown of the lateral patellar facet; IIB lesions, which include combinations of types I and IIA, also result from chronic subluxation and excessive patellar tilt. Type III lesions involve the medial patellar facet and can result from a variety of causes including a forceful reduction of acute patellar dislocation and deficient contact pressures secondary to chronic

subluxation/patellar tilt, or can follow tibial tubercle transfers with posterior displacement of the tibial tubercle. Type IV lesions include IVA lesions, which involve the proximal patella, and IVB lesions, which involve the proximal patella plus at least 80% of the whole patella. Type IV lesions are typically the result of direct trauma to the anterior aspect of the flexed knee. In general, distal lesions are more painful early in the knee flexion arc, whereas proximal lesions are more painful during deep flexion.

C. IMAGING STUDIES

Initial radiographic evaluation includes standard weight-bearing anteroposterior, lateral, and tunnel views, as well as an axial Merchant view. Although the anteroposterior and lateral views provide important clues regarding patellar alignment, particularly with regard to patellar alta and baja, the axial Merchant view may show subtle irregularities such as joint space narrowing in the lateral patellofemoral joint. It is often useful for diagnosis of patellar tilt, with and without frank patellar subluxation. The Merchant view is typically taken with the knee flexed 45° and the x-ray beam projected caudad at an angle of 30° from the plane of the femur (Figure 3–4). Radiographic evaluation is often normal, particularly in the early stages of patellofemoral chondrosis. CT scan is typically reserved for evaluation of patellar maltracking (Figure 3–9). It offers sequential axial images at any desired degree of knee flexion, and therefore allows the physician to determine the specific pattern of patellofemoral malalignment. In addition, in more advanced cases, CT allows visualization of subchondral and cystic irregularities that are often present in the lateral patellofemoral joint. MRI is perhaps the most useful imaging modality to quantify the extent and location of articular surface injury. Because it provides very clear images of chondral, osteochondral, and soft tissue lesions throughout the knee it is a useful tool in the diagnosis of patellofemoral chondrosis, but is often less helpful than plain radiographs and CT in evaluating patellofemoral malalignment.

Treatment

A. NONSURGICAL

Treatment of anterior knee pain due to patellofemoral chondrosis or chondromalacia usually begins with nonoperative management. After rest, NSAIDs, and modification of activity have decreased the acute symptoms, a well-structured rehabilitation program is ordered. The program should focus on stretching of the extensor mechanism, iliotibial tract, retinaculum, and hamstrings. Strengthening of the quadriceps, which is also important, is usually directed toward the vastus medialis obliquus (VMO) as it is the major dynamic medial patellar stabilizer. The VMO is believed to be deficient relative to the larger vastus lateralis and thus is unable to resist lateral patellar subluxation. It is important to encourage short-arc quadriceps strengthening exercises and straight leg rises to minimize the patellofemoral joint reactive force. Additional modalities include elastic knee supports, patellar taping, orthotics, and reassurance. The majority of patients with anterior knee pain due to isolated patellofemoral chondrosis will improve with nonoperative modalities. Persistent pain, effusions, and crepitus in conjunction with patellar malalignment indicate worsening articular cartilage degeneration and alternative treatment strategies should be pursued.

B. SURGICAL

A variety of surgical treatment options for patellofemoral chondrosis exist. For the athlete these include procedures directed at anatomic realignment and in some cases articular cartilage regeneration. For severe end-stage patellofemoral arthrosis, joint resurfacing and patellectomy have sometimes been advocated.

Knee arthroscopy is an important part of both the diagnostic evaluation and the potential treatment. Although diagnostic arthroscopy with lavage and debridement has been controversial, it is helpful for staging lesions and for planning future surgical treatments. In general, arthroscopic lavage relieves pain and improves function in the short term by removing debris and inflammatory proteoglycans. Because the pathology is often not addressed by this procedure, symptoms usually return. In cases involving isolated lesions, diagnostic arthroscopy allows the lesion to be graded and provides exposure for other modalities.

The grading system defined by Outerbridge is most commonly used because of its simplicity and reproducibility. This system grades lesions based on lesion depth and must be combined with documentation of the location, shape, and size of the lesion. Grade I lesions include articular surfaces that are swollen, soft, and in some cases blistered. Grade II lesions are characterized by articular fissures and clefts with diameters <1 cm. Grade III lesions include deep fissures extending to subchondral bone with diameters >1 cm. Finally, grade IV lesions include those with exposed subchondral bone.

The use of lavage and debridement for treatment of traumatic lesions has yielded better results in patients without evidence of patellar instability than in patients with degenerative or atraumatic lesions. For patients with known patellar tilt and minimal articular involvement of primarily the lateral facet, lateral release at the time of arthroscopic evaluation has been advocated. To be effective, lateral release must be reserved for patients with objective evidence of patellar tilt and without severe articular breakdown. In general, arthroscopic lavage and debridement with or without lateral release are reserved for grade and I and II lesions, as long-term

results are generally poor with grade III and IV lesions. In cases involving more advanced articular degeneration, arthroscopic chondroplasty has been advocated. The techniques of abrasion arthroplasty or microfracture chondroplasty include mechanical penetration of subchondral bone and subsequent delivery of marrow-derived mesenchymal stem cells to articular defects to induce a fibrocartilaginous healing response. Arthroscopic chondroplasty is typically reserved for patients younger than 30 years with relatively well-defined grade III lesions. It is not indicated for more advanced articular defects or damage.

Additional treatment strategies are directed toward restoration or regeneration of normal hyaline articular cartilage. These strategies include autologous chondrocyte implantation (ACI), osteochondral autograft transfer, mosaicplasty, and osteochondral allograft transplantation. Although an in-depth discussion of each of these procedures is beyond the scope of this chapter, some key points will be highlighted. ACI was developed for the treatment of significant, symptomatic, full-thickness chondral defects involving the femoral condyle. The procedure involves harvesting autologous chondrocytes, expanding the cells in culture, and reimplanting them under a periosteal flap after debridement of the articular lesion. Results have been variable, but long-term follow-up in a multicenter study has reported 79% good to excellent results. In general, ACI is indicated in younger (aged 20–50 years) active patients with isolated (2–4 cm^2) traumatic femoral condyle defects. Results in patients with trochlear or patellar defects are much less predictable. Contraindications include diffuse osteoarthritis, instability or abnormal tracking, and previous meniscectomy.

Osteochondral autograft transfer and mosaicplasty are appealing because they can use normal donor articular cartilage to replace deep lesions. Both techniques are dependent on surgical skill to match or recreate the topography of the surface being replaced. In addition, donor sites are limited and raise the potential of donor-site morbidity. Osteochondral allografts are typically reserved for larger (10 cm^2 or greater) defects of the femoral condyles and are often used after previous treatments have failed. Fresh allografts allow greater chondrocyte survivability but carry an associated risk of an immunologic response and the potential for disease transmission. Additional considerations include a technically demanding procedure and the need for the surgeon and patient to be available on relatively short notice. Although fresh-frozen allografts confer decreased immunogenicity and allow for greater flexibility with regard to timing of the procedure, chondrocyte viability is a major concern that may affect long-term graft viability. Patellectomy and patellar resurfacing are reserved for patients with extensive articular damage to the patella, significant functional limitation related to pain, and failure of previous treatments. Results of both procedures are inconsistent. Major anatomic realignment procedures such as osteotomy, tibial tubercle transfer and elevation, and others will be discussed in the section on patella maltracking.

Prognosis

Ultimately the goal of a patellofemoral rehabilitation program is to return the patient to an acceptable level of preinjury performance or activity. To achieve this goal, rehabilitation should initially be directed toward decreasing inflammation, restoring range of motion, and regaining muscle strength, endurance, power, and flexibility while maintaining the athlete's overall cardiovascular fitness. In the final stages of rehabilitation, therapy should focus on regaining proprioceptive awareness, agility, and functional skills with sport-specific exercise and activity. The rehabilitation program must therefore be individualized and should consider the athlete's age, prior level of muscular and cardiovascular performance, familiarity with exercise equipment, and degree of motivation.

Return to Play

Regardless of the treatment strategy utilized, return to athletic activities is dependent on the restoration of normal motion, stability, and strength to the involved lower extremity. A four-phase rehabilitation protocol should be complete, and patients should be able to perform sport-specific rehabilitation activities without significant pain, functional limitation, or recurrence of knee effusions. Counseling regarding continued use of sport-specific exercises and avoidance of activities that increase patellofemoral contact pressures should also be emphasized.

Aderinto J, Cobb A: Lateral release for patellofemoral arthritis. Arthroscopy 2002;18:339.

Browne JE, Branch TP: Surgical alternatives for treatment of articular cartilage lesions. J Am Acad Orthop Surg 2000;8:180.

Cartilage Repair Registry Report: Genzyme Tissue Repair, Vol 4. Cambridge, MA, February 1998.

Christoforakis JJ, Strachan RK: Internal derangements of the knee associated with patellofemoral joint degeneration. Knee Surg Sports Traumatol Arthrosc 2005;13(7):581.

Minas T, Chiu R: Autologous chondrocyte implantation. Am J Knee Surg 2000;13:41.

Steadman JR et al: Outcomes of microfracture for traumatic chondral defects of the knee: average 11-year follow-up. Arthroscopy 2003;19:477.

2. Patellar Maltracking

Patellar maltracking falls under the general category of patellar instability and includes disorders such as patellar tilt, patellar subluxation, and patellar dislocation. In general, patellar maltracking most commonly presents in the form of abnormal patellar tilt with or without lateral subluxation. Although this can be caused by a variety of factors, it is most commonly multifactorial and includes elements of a tight lateral retinaculum, VMO atrophy, and preexisting malalignment such as genu valgum or hyperlaxity.

ESSENTIALS OF DIAGNOSIS

- Clinical history
  —Feeling of anterior knee instability or anterior knee pain.
  —History of trauma to the anterior knee or previous patellar dislocation.
  —History of previous knee surgery or lateral retinacular release.
- Physical examination
  —Extensor mechanism imbalance with VMO wasting or weakness.
  —Apprehension or reverse apprehension with lateral or medial patellar displacement.
  —Patellar hypermobility, patella alta, and abnormal Q angle are hallmarks.
- Imaging
  —Abnormal patellar tilt and subluxation are often present on axial radiographs.
  —CT may reveal subtle patellar tracking abnormalities.
  —MRI is useful for evaluating soft tissue structures (ie, MPFL) as well as for articular cartilage damage.

Pathogenesis

A thorough history and a physical examination including timing of onset, duration of symptoms, mechanism of injury, and previous patellofemoral problems are critical in narrowing the differential diagnosis. In general, patients with lateral subluxation describe a feeling of anterior instability and pain in the patellofemoral joint. Occasionally, patients also note the presence of an effusion, crepitance, and catching in the anterior aspect of the knee. They also have a history of previous knee injury or prior knee surgery. In patients with lateral patellar compression syndrome or patellar tilt, the onset of symptoms is often insidious and can be associated with minor trauma. This condition is caused by a tight lateral retinaculum that causes increased contact pressures between the lateral patellar facet and the lateral femoral trochlea. Patients often complain of diffuse anterior knee pain that localizes to the lateral retinaculum during knee flexion.

Clinical Findings

A. SYMPTOMS

With patellar maltracking, the patella articulates abnormally with the femoral trochlea so that it subluxes either laterally or medially. Lateral subluxation is the more common form of malalignment and is usually the result of overall malalignment of the involved lower extremity including genu valgum or generalized hyperlaxity. In patients with this form of malalignment, the patella is usually stabilized by the femoral trochlea during knee flexion but shifts laterally from the trochlear groove as the knee approaches full extension. Patients usually complain of the knee "giving way" during these episodes, although they rarely suffer a frank patellar dislocation. The less common form of patellar instability is medial subluxation. This is usually the result of an iatrogenic injury following a lateral release that is too extensive or poorly indicated. Both types of patellar subluxation can predispose patients to patellofemoral chondrosis. The subsequent arthritis that can develop as a result was discussed in the previous section. Patellar maltracking can also predispose athletes to acute patellar dislocation, although this injury is uncommon. Two mechanisms have been proposed: a more common indirect injury and a less common direct blow. Either mechanism can result in articular damage to either the lateral condyle of the femur or the medial patellar facet, or to both.

B. SIGNS

The basic elements of the general knee examination outlined above apply here as well. The examination should begin with an evaluation of the athlete's stance and gait. Various risk factors predispose athletes to patellar instability and must be evaluated during the initial physical examination. These factors include excessive femoral anteversion, genu valgum, patellar dysplasia, femoral dysplasia, patella alta, VMO atrophy, high Q angle, pes planus, and generalized hyperlaxity. Examination of the knee joint continues with inspection of overall femoral–tibial alignment and patellofemoral alignment. On initial inspection the Q angle should be measured and documented. This angle is measured from a line connecting the anterosuperior iliac spine and the mid-patella, and a line connecting the mid-patella and the tibial tubercle (Figure 3–10). The Q angle is commonly used as a measure of the valgus moment acting on the patellofemoral joint. In general, females have larger Q angles than males, and normal includes angles up to 20° for females and 15° for males. Q angles are increased by genu valgum, a laterally displaced tibial tubercle, increased femoral anteversion, and external tibial torsion. Although a Q angle does not necessarily predict anterior knee pain or patellar subluxation, it does potentially contribute to patellofemoral malalignment as the quadriceps contracts.

Gross dynamic evaluation of patellar tracking can be evaluated by passively extending the knee while the patient is sitting. In general the patella should follow a midline course throughout the full range of motion. In some cases, a "J sign" may be seen. This refers to the path that the patella travels (upside down J) in cases in which patellar maltracking is present and the patella is pulled laterally as the knee approaches full extension. A reverse J sign can be seen in cases of medial patellar subluxation in which the patella is pulled medially as the knee approaches full extension. If the J sign is seen during open chain knee extension, it can be indicative of VMO deficiency and may thus direct further treatment strategies.

The medial and lateral retinacular structures should also be carefully evaluated. Tenderness to palpation along the medial or lateral retinacular structures is common when these tissues are overloaded in patients with patellofemoral malalignment. Tenderness specifically over the medial epicondyle, known as Bassett's sign, may represent an injury to the MPFL in patients with a history of patellar dislocation. An additional test directed specifically at detecting a tight lateral retinaculum is the patellar tilt test. This test is performed with the knee relaxed and passively extended. The medial patellar facet is stabilized as attempts are made at lifting the lateral patellar facet. In normal patients, the lateral edge of the patella should lift approximately 15° beyond the horizontal plain. If this is not possible, a tight lateral retinaculum may be the cause of anterior knee pain and a subsequent lateral release may be indicated. The patellar apprehension test is particularly useful with regard to evaluating patellar instability (Figure 3–11). A positive test occurs when pain and guarding are elicited during lateral translation of the patella. This is highly suggestive of patellar hypermobility or instability.

The medial and lateral patellar glide tests assess for the integrity of the static retinacular restraints. The lateral patellar glide test includes evaluation of the medial joint capsule, medial retinaculum, and VMO. The patella is manually translated in the lateral direction and the distance is measured as the number of quarter widths that the patella is displaced beyond its neutral position in the trochlea. A value greater than three-quarters width indicates hypermobility, whereas a value less than one-quarter width with the medial patellar glide test indicates a tight lateral retinaculum. Although this test can provide useful information regarding the retinacular structures it is highly examiner dependent.

Although the majority of the examination is performed with the patient supine, it is also important to examine the knee with the patient prone. By stabilizing the pelvis and eliminating hip flexion, prone positioning allows accurate assessment of extensor mechanism flexibility. In addition, excessive femoral anteversion and tibial torsion can be easily assessed. Decreased internal rotation may be indicative of early hip osteoarthritis and pain that may be referred to the knee.

C. IMAGING STUDIES

The initial radiographic evaluation of the patellofemoral joint should include standard weight-bearing antero-posterior and lateral views, as well as an axial view (Figure 3–12). The anteroposterior view is useful for evaluating gross subluxation, fracture, or deformity of the patella. A true anteroposterior view must be verified before any determinations about patellar subluxation are made. The lateral view allows several important assessments. First, it provides valuable information about trochlear depth and morphology. The center of the trochlea will be seen as the most posterior line, and the medial and lateral trochlear facets can also be visualized separately. Using these landmarks allows the measurement of the appropriate trochlear depth and the assessment of potential facet dysplasia. Additional information regarding patella alta or baja can be determined from the lateral radiograph by calculating the ratio of the patellar tendon length to the greatest diagonal length of the patella. Values for normal ratios are between 0.8 and 1.0, whereas values greater than 1.0 indicate patella alta and lower values indicate patella baja.

The axial radiograph provides additional valuable information about patellar tracking. The Laurin axial radiograph is obtained with the knee flexed to 20°, whereas the Merchant view is obtained with the knee flexed to 40°. Either one of these views is acceptable and will minimize radiation exposure. The axial radiograph is the most helpful in evaluating patellofemoral alignment and diagnosing patellar tilt or patellar subluxation. Two angles are measured using this radiograph, the Laurin lateral patellofemoral angle and the Merchant congruence angle. The Laurin lateral patellofemoral angle is measured between a line drawn across the femoral condyles and a line drawn along the lateral patellar facet. Normally, this angle opens laterally, however, in cases in which the angle is parallel or opens medially, patellar tilt is likely. The Merchant congruence angle is used to assess patellar subluxation. It is measured by bisecting the femoral sulcus angle and measuring the angle between this bisector and the line drawn from the lowest point in the sulcus to the median patellar ridge. Normal congruence is −6 ± 11° with the knee at 45° of flexion. The patella should be centered within the trochlea at this angle of knee flexion and abnormal congruence indicates the potential for patellar subluxation.

CT confers several advantages over axial radiographs in the evaluation of patellar maltracking. Although many of the same measurements can be made as on axial radiographs, axial CT images offer little distortion and no image overlap. In addition, CT images can be obtained at any angle of knee flexion. This is particularly useful in assessing patellar maltracking as the knee approaches terminal extension and the patella is no longer stabilized by the lateral femoral condyle (Figure 3–13). An additional advantage of CT versus axial radiographs is the ability to evaluate lateralization of the tibial tubercle. This is assessed by measuring the distance between the tibial tubercle and trochlear sulcus when two appropriate axial images are superimposed. A value greater than 9 mm has been shown to identify patients with abnormal patellofemoral alignment with 95% specificity and 85% sensitivity. Although MRI can be used to verify the osseus findings on plain radiographs and CT, it is most useful for visualization of soft tissues and evaluation of articular cartilage damage. MRI has also been found useful in the identification of findings associated with patellar dislocation. These include tearing of the MPFL from the femoral insertion, the less common avulsion of the MPFL from the medial patellar facet, joint effusion, increased signal intensity and injury to the VMO, and bone bruises in the lateral femoral condyle and medial patellar facet.

Treatment

A. NONSURGICAL

As dynamic patellar instability is the most common cause of anterior knee pain resulting from patellar maltracking, nonoperative treatments provide the mainstay of therapy. After careful evaluation of quadriceps strength using isokinetic testing, an appropriate rehabilitation protocol can be developed. Again, the goal of any patellofemoral rehabilitation program is to return to an acceptable level of athletic performance by decreasing inflammation, restoring range of motion, and regaining muscle strength, endurance, power, and flexibility. Quadriceps strength, power, and endurance are most effectively improved with short-arc isotonic quadriceps extension exercises in the range of 0–30° of knee flexion where patellofemoral contact pressures are the lowest. Exercises should focus on restoring a balanced extensor mechanism with particular attention directed toward the VMO. The symptoms of patellofemoral instability can often be improved with patellar stabilization braces or patellar taping, both of which require patient compliance. Orthotics have also been shown to improve alignment of the lower extremity, particularly in patients who have valgus thrust that may contribute to patellar instability. Although most patients with patellar instability will improve with a well structured nonoperative treatment program, patients with persistent and disabling symptoms often require surgical treatment.

B. SURGICAL

As is true for most patellofemoral disorders causing anterior knee pain, surgical treatment begins with a complete arthroscopic examination. The examination should then use the superomedial portal to focus on the patellofemoral joint throughout the full knee range of motion. Patellar tilt can be evaluated as the knee approaches extension. In addition, passive patellar tracking is assessed as the knee is taken through a full range of motion. Normal tracking is present when the lateral facet aligns with the trochlea at approximately 20–25° of knee flexion and the mid-patellar ridge by 35–40° of flexion. Lateral overhang of the lateral patellar facet should be noted as the patella engages the trochlea. When used in combination with objective clinical or radiographic evidence of patellar subluxation, this can direct additional surgical realignment procedures.

Arthroscopic lateral release is indicated in patients with patellar tilt but without abnormal medial or lateral patellar glide. An adequate release includes the entire lateral retinaculum, vastus lateralis obliquus, and distal patellotibial band. Complete vastus lateralis release has been reported, but should be avoided to prevent retraction and atrophy with subsequent quadriceps imbalance. Lateral release should not be performed in patients without objective evidence of patellar tilt as iatrogenic medial subluxation can result. The most common complication following lateral release is hemarthrosis and delayed rehabilitation. This can be avoided by evaluation of the release with the tourniquet deflated prior to closure.

In patients who have failed nonoperative treatment and who have objective evidence of patellar subluxation, surgical treatment is often indicated. Multiple realignment procedures have been described, and the surgical procedure is determined by the type of patellar subluxation. Both proximal and distal realignment procedures exist. Proximal realignment procedures are directed at the dynamic elements of the extensor mechanism and include medial capsular imbrication, advancement of the vastus medialis, and advancement of the VMO. All procedures are aimed at centralizing the patella within the femoral sulcus and improving patellofemoral congruency through a full range of motion. For many patients with lateral subluxation due to patellofemoral malalignment, a distal realignment procedure such as an anteromedial tibial tubercle transfer usually produces satisfactory results. Medialization of the tibial tubercle typically corrects the abnormal Q angle, whereas moving the tubercle anteriorly unloads the patellofemoral joint and helps prevent the degenerative changes observed with direct medial tibial tubercle transfer. Arthroscopic evaluation should be used to verify alignment during these procedures to prevent over- or undercorrection.

The surgical treatment of patellar dislocations is controversial. Although surgical treatment is usually indicated only after patients have failed a comprehensive nonoperative treatment program, the chance of redislocation ranges anywhere from 15–44%. Recent studies have revealed markedly decreased rates of redislocation with surgical treatment in young athletic patients with acute patellar dislocation. The surgical procedure is aimed at open repair of the MPFL injury and may require additional realignment procedures. Again, arthroscopy is required both for the evaluation of patellofemoral tracking and for the evaluation of osteochondral lesions that are often associated with acute patellar dislocations. Chronic patellar dislocations are treated with the realignment procedures previously described.

Prognosis & Return to Play

Most patients with instability related to patellar tilt and/or patellar subluxation do well. Regardless of the treatment strategy utilized, return to athletic activities is dependent on the restoration of normal motion, stability, and strength to the involved lower extremity. Return to activity should be gradual. Therapy should be adjusted according to the procedure performed and allow adequate time for healing of skin, soft tissues, and bone. Ultimately, a four-phase rehabilitation protocol should be complete, and patients should be able to perform sport-specific rehabilitation activities without significant pain, functional limitation, or recurrence of symptoms.

Atkins DM et al: Characteristics of patients with primary acute lateral patellar dislocation and their recovery within the first 6 months of injury. Am J Sports Med 2000;28:472.

Katchburian MV et al: Measurement of patellar tracking: assessment and analysis of the literature. Clin Orthop Relat Res 2003;412:241.

Palmer SH et al: Surgical reconstruction of severe patellofemoral maltracking. Clin Orthop Relat Res 2004;419:144.

3. Patellar Tendinitis

Historically, the term patellar tendinopathy referred to both quadriceps and patellar tendinitis. Patellar tendinitis, commonly referred to as "Jumper's knee," is a common problem in the athletic population, and today refers to the tendinitis that affects the patellar tendon. Patellar tendinitis typically affects athletes who participate in sports that involve running and frequent jumping with eccentric loading of the patellar tendon. Although there is a predilection by sport, it can affect athletes of almost any age. The specific etiology of the tendinopathy varies depending on the particular activity and on the age of the athlete. Chronic tendon problems can result from a variety of causes including overuse injury, cumulative trauma, repetitive strain due to mechanical overload, and age-related degeneration and decreased vascular supply. The term tendinitis is a histopathologic diagnosis and implies the presence of inflammatory cells. The term tendinosis is used to describe the histopathologic alterations to cells that result from chronic tendinitis and tendon overload.

ESSENTIALS OF DIAGNOSIS

- *Clinical history*
  - —*Athletes involved in sports that require quick accelerations and jumping, for example, running, track, tennis, volleyball, basketball, and soccer.*
  - —*Anterior knee pain localized to the inferior pole of the patella or the tibial tubercle.*
  - —*Pain before, during, and/or after activity depending on injury severity.*
- *Physical examination*
  - —*Extensor mechanism tightness and/or weakness.*
  - —*Tenderness to palpation along the inferior pole of the patella or tibial tubercle.*
  - —*Pain symptoms reproduced with resisted knee extension.*
- *Imaging*
  - —*Plain radiographs are often normal, but useful for the evaluation of potential stress fractures or intratendinous calcifications.*
  - —*MRI is useful for the evaluation of the integrity of the tendon and surrounding structures.*
  - —*Ultrasound by an experienced ultrasonographer can be helpful for diagnosis.*

Clinical Findings

A. Symptoms

The histories of patients with patellar tendinitis can be variable due to the wide range of etiologic factors that cause tendon problems. In younger athletes, the most common etiology includes repetitive and/or intense mechanical overload. Athletes should be specifically questioned regarding changes in duration, intensity, and method of training programs. The use of appropriate shoes and protective equipment should be explored. In older patients, age-related changes such as altered vascular supply predispose tendons to weaken and degenerate. In these cases, the degenerative tendinopathy appears to be prevalent at the bony origin or insertion rather than the midsubstance of the tendon.

Patients with patellar tendinitis typically complain of pain localized to the inferior pole of the patella along the origin of the patellar tendon. Patients can also complain of pain localized to the patellar tendon insertion on the tibial tubercle, although this is less common. During the early stages of the injury, pain typically occurs after activity. As the injury worsens and becomes more chronic, pain can occur during and prior to activity. Patients typically describe the pain as a dull ache located within the tendon. Periods of more intense pain localized to the tendinous origin can occur during activity as symptoms

worsen. Patellar tendinitis can be classified into four stages based on symptoms. This classification can be helpful in guiding treatment and predicting outcome. Stage I includes pain after sports activities; stage II includes pain before and after, but not during sports activities; stage III includes patients with constant pain that prevents participation in sports activities; and stage IV includes complete tendon rupture.

B. Signs

Because of the superficial location of the entire patellar tendon, including its origin and insertion, the physical examination is relatively straightforward. As in all cases of anterior knee pain, a complete knee examination, as outlined in the sections above, should be performed. The pertinent examination findings in patients with patellar tendinitis include the following features. Patients typically have tenderness to palpation at the patellar tendon origin along the inferior pole of the patella. The undersurface, or joint surface, of the tendon is often involved and may require deep palpation to elicit symptoms. Occasionally, patients will have tenderness and swelling along the entire tendon indicating peritendinitis and/or tenosynovitis. Symptoms of pain can usually be reproduced with resisted knee extension and palpation of the tendon. Continuity of the quadriceps and patellar tendons should be evaluated to rule out partial or complete tendon ruptures. The straight leg raise with the knee in full extension allows tendon integrity and quadriceps strength to be determined. Finally, younger patients must be evaluated for apophysis traction injuries that affect the inferior pole of the patella (Sinding–Larsen–Johansson disease) or the tibial tubercle (Osgood–Schlatter disease) (Figures 3–14 and 3–15).

C. Imaging Studies

Routine radiographs are obtained during the initial evaluation. At a minimum, these should include anteroposterior and lateral views to identify stress or avulsion fractures and calcifications within the patellar tendon. CT scans are generally not indicated if the diagnosis of tendinopathy is reasonably certain. MRI can be helpful in evaluating the tendon itself, as well as the surrounding soft-tissue structures. Although it is common to see increased signal at the inferior pole of the patella and within the substance of the tendon, MRI does not always correlate with the degree of clinical symptoms. Because of its superficial location, the tendon can also be imaged with ultrasound. Experienced musculoskeletal ultrasonographers are able to evaluate for tendon enlargement, degenerative lesions, as well as partial and complete tears.

Treatment

A. Nonsurgical

The treatment of patellar tendinitis depends on the stage of presentation. Stages I and II can usually be successfully treated with nonoperative modalities. These include modification of activity, ice, and a short course of NSAIDs. Although NSAIDs can provide symptomatic relief, there are no data to support the contention that these medications alter the natural history of patellar tendinopathy. Antiinflammatory medications should be used with caution in older patients and should not be used in patients with known stomach or gastrointestinal problems. Local injection of corticosteroids is not indicated because of the possibility of steroid atrophy and the associated risk of tendon rupture. Patients should be encouraged to avoid eccentric loading, quick accelerations, and jumping. A comprehensive quadriceps stretching and strengthening program often allows gradual return to athletic activity; however, this can take as little as a few weeks to as long as several months. The initial treatment of stage III injuries follows the same course as that outlined for stages I and II.

B. SURGICAL

In persistent cases that fail nonoperative treatment, surgery may be indicated. The surgical treatment of patellar tendinopathy includes arthroscopic or open debridement of the degenerative tendon usually at the inferior pole of the patella. Surgery is often performed through a tendon splitting approach with the goal of removing the affected tissue. In some cases, curettage of the inferior pole of the patella has been advocated to stimulate an inflammatory and subsequent healing response. Additional surgical approaches have included partial tendon excision, wide excision with reattachment of the remaining tendon, and multiple longitudinal tenotomies. All of these procedures carry the risk of postoperative patellar tendon rupture. A stage IV injury requires operative repair. Primary repair in a timely fashion usually allows patients to regain quadriceps strength and full knee range of motion, and to return to previous levels of activity.

Prognosis & Return to Play

Regardless of the treatment strategy, proper rehabilitation is critical in allowing athletes to return to sport and prevent reinjury. After appropriate rest and modification of activity, rehabilitation is directed at improving quadriceps tightness. A four-stage rehabilitation program includes static stretching of the hamstrings, static stretching of the quadriceps, eccentric strengthening exercises, and ice packs after additional stretching. Sport-specific exercises are gradually introduced and quadriceps strength and elasticity improve. Ultimately, athletes are allowed to return to sport when they have full range of motion, when isokinetic quadriceps strength is equal to at least 90% of the normal side, and when they no longer have tenderness or pain with activity.

Panni AS et al: Patellar tendinopathy in athletes: outcome of operative and nonoperative management. Am J Sports Med 2000;28:392.

Peers KH et al: Cross-sectional outcome analysis of athletes with chronic patellar tendinopathy treated surgically and by extracorporeal shock wave therapy. Clin J Sport Med 2003;13:79.

Warden SJ, Brukner P: Patellar tendinopathy. Clin J Sport Med 2003;22(4):743.

LATERAL KNEE PAIN

Differential Diagnosis

1. Meniscal lesions
2. Bursitis
3. Stress fracture
4. Osteoarthritis
5. Iliotibial band syndrome
6. Popliteal tenosynovitis
7. Ligamentous instability

Iliotibial Band Syndrome

Iliotibial band syndrome is the most common cause of lateral knee pain in distance runners. It is not restricted to runners, however, and has been known to affect other athletes involved in knee flexion activities including cycling, soccer, tennis, football, and skiing. It is caused by a combination of intrinsic and extrinsic factors. Intrinsic factors are related to an athlete's anatomic alignment, whereas extrinsic factors include training techniques and sport-specific activities.

ESSENTIALS OF DIAGNOSIS

- *Clinical history*
  —*Athletes involved in sports that require running down hills.*
  —*Aching lateral knee pain just proximal to the joint line.*
  —*Symptoms are present during running, but usually are absent before and after.*
- *Physical examination*
  —*Point tenderness in the area overlying the lateral epicondyle.*
  —*Positive Ober's test indicating iliotibial band tightness.*
- *Imaging*
  —*Plain radiographs are often normal, but are useful in evaluating other potential conditions.*
  —*CT and MRI are also not helpful in the diagnosis but may be helpful in evaluating other pathology.*

Pathogenesis

Iliotibial band syndrome is common in runners and other athletes who use running as a training tool. Specific questions about timing of onset, duration, and changes in length or intensity of the athlete's training program should be entertained. The syndrome is typically brought on by downhill running. Running downhill significantly reduces knee flexion at foot strike and increases friction between the iliotibial band and the lateral epicondyle of the femur. Friction is typically highest at 30° of knee flexion.

Clinical Findings

A. SYMPTOMS

Patients are usually asymptomatic both before and after activity. Symptoms usually begin shortly after the onset of running and continue throughout activity. They usually resolve with rest, but return when activity is resumed. Symptoms usually correlate with the intensity and length of training.

B. SIGNS

As has been mentioned previously, a comprehensive knee examination should be performed to evaluate for potential confounding injuries. A careful physical examination provides clues that are important for making the diagnosis of iliotibial band syndrome. It is important to evaluate for the presence of potential intrinsic anatomic factors that may predispose the athlete toward developing iliotibial band syndrome, such as genu varum, tibia vara, heel varus, forefoot supination, and compensatory foot pronation. Pertinent findings on physical examination include tenderness to palpation located 2–3 cm proximal to the lateral joint line in the area of the later epicondyle of the femur. Patients will also exhibit a tight iliotibial band with the Ober test. This test is performed by having the patient lie in a lateral position on the examining table with the involved knee up. The unaffected hip and knee are flexed. The involved knee is then flexed to 90° and the ipsilateral hip is abducted and hyperextended. A tight iliotibial band will prevent the involved extremity from dropping below horizontal. A provocative test, called the Noble test, allows confirmation of the diagnosis. This test is performed with the patient lying supine and with the involved knee flexed. Pressure is applied to the lateral epicondyle and the knee is extended. This test is positive when pain is reproduced when the knee is at 30–40º of flexion. Finally, functional tests, such as asking the patient to hop on the involved extremity with the knee flexed, may reproduce lateral knee pain and confirm the diagnosis.

C. IMAGING STUDIES

Plain radiographs, CT, and MRI are usually normal in patients with iliotibial band syndrome. They can be helpful in ruling out other potential causes of lateral knee pain that are included in the differential diagnosis.

Treatment

A. NONSURGICAL

Nonoperative therapy is the mainstay of treatment. Treatment is usually aimed at modification of intrinsic abnormalities and elimination of extrinsic factors. During the initial stages of treatment, the inflammatory process should be controlled with rest, ice, NSAIDs, and ultrasound or phonophoresis. Once the acute symptoms have improved, therapy can be initiated. The entire involved lower extremity should be addressed. In addition to stretching the iliotibial band, tensor fascia lata, and hip external rotators, hip abductor tightness and weakness must be improved. Modification of extrinsic factors involves altering the athlete's training program. For runners, this includes avoidance of hills, changing the duration and intensity of training, and running on the opposite side of the road or reversing the direction on a curved track. Cyclists can alter their seat height or the position of their foot within clipless pedals. In patients who have excessive foot pronation, a rigid lateral heel wedge or custom orthotic may help modify intrinsic factors.

B. SURGICAL

Although surgical treatments have been described, they are not a mainstay of treatment. They include procedures that remove a small portion of the iliotibial band that is located directly over the lateral epicondyle when the knee is flexed to 30°. Success has been reported in athletes who have failed nonoperative treatments and continue to have significant symptoms.

Prognosis & Return to Play

Ultimately, a four-phase rehabilitation protocol should be complete, and patients should be able to perform sport-specific rehabilitation activities without significant pain, functional limitation, or recurrence of symptoms. When this program is complete, patients may return to play.

Farrell KC et al: Force and repetition in cycling: possible implications for iliotibial band friction syndrome. The Knee 2003;10(1):103.

Frederickson M, Wolf C: Iliotibial band syndrome in runners: innovations in treatment. Sports Med 2005;35(6):451.

Kirk LK et al: Iliotibial band friction syndrome. Orthopedics 2000;23(11):1209.

Lower Leg, Ankle, & Foot Injuries

4

Christian Lattermann, MD, Derek Armfield, MD, & Dane K. Wukich, MD

■ LOWER LEG PAIN

Athletes performing any sport expose themselves to a particular subset of sports-specific injuries including injury to the foot and ankle. Approximately 25% of all sports injuries involve the foot and ankle and about 45% of these are simple lateral ankle sprains. In cutting sports such as football, baseball, volleyball, and soccer these injuries account for up to 25% of lost playing time. Some sports have a low incidence of foot injuries. Swimming, for example, has a very low incidence of ankle injuries. Basketball and figure skating have the highest incidence. With respect to foot injuries, football and weight lifting are the lowest risk sports. Hiking and high-speed motor sports have a higher incidence (>50%).

Overall, every sport poses a specific threat to the athletes' foot and ankle as a result of the activity and the equipment that is used. These injuries may not be benign. Approximately 40% of all simple ankle sprains lead to chronic disabilities that may end the athlete's career.

In this chapter the diagnosis and treatment of common injuries and conditions of the lower leg and foot that frequently occur in athletes will be discussed. Anatomic, biomechanical, and functional principles of the foot and ankle will be described. We will discuss conservative as well as operative treatments.

MUSCLE STRAINS

ESSENTIALS OF DIAGNOSIS

- Immediate sharp pain in the calf.
- Hear or feel a "pop" or a "snap."
- Feeling as if someone "kicked you in the calf."
- Inability to raise the calf or pain with calf raise.
- Swelling and bruising to the calf.
- Palpable gap in the medial or lateral gastrocnemius–soleus (gastrocsoleus) muscles.

Pathogenesis

Muscle strains of the gastrocsoleus complex are the most frequent injuries in athletes who jump or sprint. Muscle injuries account for up to 30% of all injuries sustained in sports events. These injuries pose a significant challenge to every sports medicine clinician. The majority of these muscle injuries are caused by contusion or excessive strain of the muscle and they can sideline athletes for a long time.

Athletes with a prior history of muscle strains have increased risk of further injury. The closer the reinjury is to the previous calf strain the higher the risk for recurrence. There also seems to be a relationship with age, with older athletes predisposed to a higher risk for calf strains.

Prevention

Fatigue may play a key role in the incidence of calf strains since muscle strain injuries seem to occur late in either training sessions or competitive settings. It was shown that the energy absorbed before failure was significantly less in fatigued than in control muscles. Therefore, proper conditioning to reduce or delay fatigue should be part of the prevention strategy.

Calf stretching and warm-up should be an integral part of the athletes' preparation. The musculotendinous unit has specific viscoelastic properties that can be influenced by warm-up and cyclic stretching. Cyclic stretching up to 50% of the maximum stretch to failure has a beneficial effect on the amount of energy that a muscle can absorb before failure. Stretching past 50% of the maximum stretch reduces the maximal amount of energy that the muscle can absorb. Therefore, the recommendation is to perform light stretching exercises before sports activities. Viscoelasticity is temperature dependent. Therefore, the warm-up exercises help to increase the viscoelastic properties of the musculotendinous unit before athletic activity.

Clinical Findings

A. Symptoms

Calf muscle strains can occur in cutting and jumping sports such as basketball, football, soccer, tennis, and racquetball. The athlete is usually not able to return to play after a significant calf muscle strain. It is important to know if the athlete had a prior, recent, minor injury to the affected calf because a muscle reinjury is likely to be more severe. Patients report immediate pain in the back of their calf. They may have felt a sudden pop or snap. Feeling "as if someone hit them in back of the calf" is often mentioned.

B. Signs

It is important to do a thorough physical examination to determine if the injury is in the muscular portion of the medial or lateral head of the gastrocnemius or at the musculotendinous junction of the gastrocsoleus complex. A muscle strain may be palpable as a swelling of the calf. Alternatively, if a disruption of the muscle fibers has occurred a gap may be felt by physical examination before swelling occurred or after it subsided. The gap and swelling are usually felt in the muscle substance. A rupture of the medial head of the gastrocnemius is more frequent than a rupture of the lateral head. The gap is therefore palpable medial or lateral to the midline. The most important differential diagnosis of a calf strain is the rupture of the Achilles tendon. Therefore, if the gap is palpable directly in the midline and distal to the musculotendinous junction, a rupture of the Achilles tendon rather than a muscle strain should be suspected. The Thompson test or calf squeeze test is helpful in making the differential diagnosis. To perform the Thompson test the patient is positioned prone with the foot hanging over the edge of a table. The examiner squeezes the calf muscle and watches for plantar flexion of the foot. If there is plantar flexion the test is negative and identifies an intact musculotendon complex. If there is no plantar flexion, either the gastrocsoleus complex is torn at the myotendinous junction or the Achilles tendon is torn.

C. Imaging Studies

The need for imaging of the calf after a calf muscle strain depends on the severity of the injury. If the physical examination suggests a large or complete tear of the medial or lateral gastrocnemius, magnetic resonance imaging (MRI) may be used to evaluate the extent of the injury. This also aids in surgical planning. MRI may also be used to monitor the healing of a muscle strain (Figure 4–1).

Calf muscle strains can also occur in combination with other injuries such as ankle sprains, fractures of the fibula, or neurovascular injuries, in which case the associated injuries dictate the need for imaging modalities.

Treatment

Treatment for calf muscle strains begins immediately at the sideline according to the RICE (rest, ice, compression,

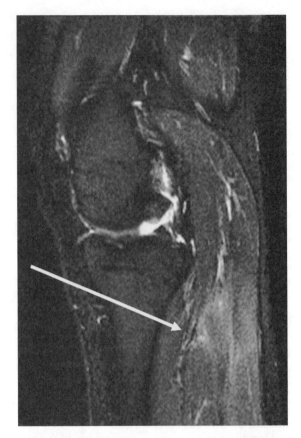

Figure 4–1. T2-weighted MRI showing edema in the medial gastrocnemius (***white arrow***). This edema is the response to the muscle strain.

elevation) principle. This initial treatment regimen is designed to avoid the formation of a large hematoma, which may affect the size of the scar tissue formed during the recovery. Initial treatment can continue for 24–48 hours.

After the initial treatment the subacute treatment protocol calls for rehabilitation as well pain control with nonsteroidal antiinflammatory drugs (NSAIDs). NSAIDs do not adversely affect healing in the initial phase of recovery from muscle strain; however, they should not be given long term (more than 7–10 days) as they may interfere with muscle healing at a later stage. A mainstay for the treatment of muscle strains is rehabilitation. Light stretching and strengthening as well as ultrasound therapy provide significant pain relief and begin to recondition the muscle fibers and help the scar tissue heal. The key is not to disrupt healing of the soft tissue. Treatment should be started after a few days of rest. Light stretching exercises such as towel stretches, standing calf stretches, and progressive resistive exercises can be performed very early. The exercise should be performed within the pain-free range of motion (ROM). After 7–10 days, light strengthening exercises can be performed using standing heel raises, single leg exercises such as hops, and gradual return to sports-specific exercises involving running, cutting, and jumping.

SURGICAL TREATMENT

Injury resulting in tears of the entire muscle mass are more frequent in the abdominal, hamstring, or rectus muscles but also occur in the calf. These injuries usually involve a very large palpable gap and result in significant loss of function. Conservative treatment of massive muscle tears results in very large amounts of scar tissue that may preclude return to sport. Primary muscle repair in complete disruptions of the muscle belly may lead to smaller scar formation and better functional recovery.

Return to Play

Generally, the severity of the muscle strain will determine the time to return to play. It is important to keep in mind that a previous calf strain predisposes the athlete to a more severe calf strain. It may therefore be prudent to let the strain heal fully before the athlete returns to play. Depending on the severity of the strain recovery time may range from 1 to 4 weeks. An important criterion for return to play is an isometric muscle strength that is within 90% of the opposite side or the preinjury value. The athlete has to be able to perform all of the cutting and specialty maneuvers required for the sport without having pain.

Leadbetter WB: Soft tissue athletic injury. In: *Sports Injuries: Mechanism, Prevention, Treatment.* Fu FH, Stone DA (editors). Lippincott Williams & Wilkins, 2001.

Noonan TJ, Garrett WE Jr: Muscle strain injury: diagnosis and treatment. J Am Acad Orthop Surg 1999;7(4):262.

STRESS FRACTURES & STRESS REACTION

ESSENTIALS OF DIAGNOSIS

- *Pain with activity.*
- *Insidious onset.*
- *Point tenderness over the fracture site.*
- *Radiographs initially are not diagnostic but may show sclerosis.*

Pathogenesis

Stress fractures of the tibia can commonly be seen in dancers and runners. There is a higher occurrence of tibial stress fractures in female athletes. Stress fractures around the foot and ankle most often occur in the metatarsal bones. The second or third metatarsals are the most common locations followed by the fifth metatarsal and the navicular. Other sites for stress fractures are the calcaneus and the cuboid.

In general, stress fractures are the result of chronic overload. This chronic overload can be due to anatomic predisposition (eg, anterior bow of the tibia in dancers) or to participation in sports that elicit extreme deceleration or chronic deceleration forces in the tibia such as the bravura technique in ballet dancers. Stress fractures in the foot are often due to overly heavy gear (eg, third metatarsal "marching fracture"), faulty training routines, or atypical foot alignment (eg, short first ray), which may predispose the metatarsals to overload. Alterations in footwear, previous injuries and fractures, as well as underlying health problems such as osteopenia, osteoporosis, and metabolic disorders can lead to the occurrence of stress fractures around the foot. As preventive measures, the athlete should not overtrain and should use appropriate training techniques. In ballet dancers the "Balanchine" technique, which requires more fluid motion and very few jumps into "pose," puts the dancer at much less risk than the "bravura" technique.

The best footwear for the sporting activity should be used and may need to be customized in case of anatomic variation (eg, high arch, flat foot, short first ray). In case of suspected osteopenia or osteoporosis, a bone densitometry analysis should be performed.

Clinical Findings

A. SYMPTOMS

Athletes will have pain at the site of the stress fracture after exercise. Most commonly this is at the junction of the middle and distal third of the tibia on its medial side. If the stress fracture is in the foot, the athlete may notice swelling after exercise and some local point tenderness. For example, for a navicular stress fracture the "N" spot should be palpated. The pain typically appears during exercise. Often athletes will not experience tenderness after initial activity but after a certain amount of exercise, the pain will set in. In fact, the pain may occur after a repeatable distance or time after exercise begins. Athletes are often able to continue with their activity, although with pain at the site of fracture.

Signs

It is crucial to do a full physical examination of the tibia and the foot. The tender spots need to be palpated to define the anatomic location of the injury. Navicular

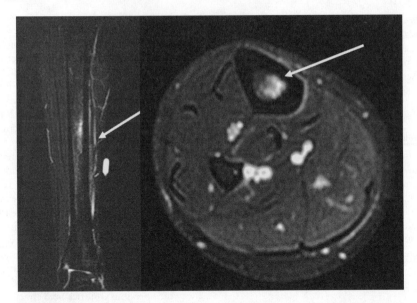

Figure 4–2. T2-weighted MRI image showing edema in the tibia. The coronal section shows the typical medial location of the stress fracture (***left arrow***). The axial cut shows the marrow edema that accompanies the fracture and healing response (***right arrow***).

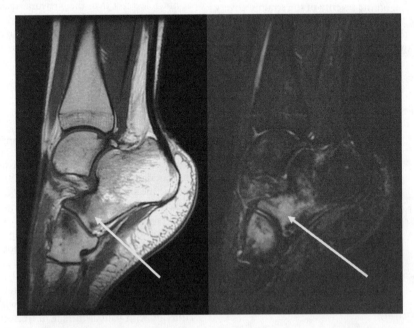

Figure 4–3. T1- and T2-weighted MRI image of the midfoot showing a stress fracture of the anterior process of the calcaneus and the cuboid. The left image is the T1-weighted image that shows some blood and cortical irregularity in the anterior calcaneus (***arrow***). The right image shows the typical edema that accompanies stress fractures in the anterior calcaneus and the cuboid.

stress fractures, for example, typically hurt in the midportion of the navicular very close to the insertion of the tibialis anterior. To differentiate tibialis anterior tendinitis from a navicular stress fracture it is important to examine the tibialis tendon and its function and to directly palpate the outline of the navicular. For metatarsal stress fractures, it is important to inspect the plantar aspect of the foot for plantar calluses that may provide a clue about improper force distribution in the forefoot.

C. IMAGING STUDIES

A stress fracture is usually diagnosed based upon clinical suspicion. Very often, the initial radiographs are negative. A stress fracture will be detectable on radiographs once the healing response and sclerosis at the fracture site have begun. This usually occurs 2–3 weeks after the onset of the symptoms. Radiographic changes are very subtle and consist of cortical thickening, trabecular sclerosis, and possibly cortical defects. In the tibia the dreaded "black line" can be identified at a later stage, once the stress fracture has essentially become a nonunion. For further imaging, usually an MRI or a bone scan is required. We believe that a bone scan is the most sensitive test. It will show a hot spot right at the fracture site. The advantage is that it will also assess surrounding bones and indicate other bones that are in danger. An MRI scan is an excellent tool with which to evaluate the surrounding soft tissues as well as the involved bone. Typically, a stress fracture leads to edema at the fracture site, which can easily be visualized by MRI (Figure 4–2). Edema typically shows up as a very low signal on the T1 sequences and as a high-density area on the T2 sequences. Inversion recovery images can be utilized to display more subtle stress reactions in smaller bones such as the anterior process of the calcaneus or the navicular (Figures 4–3 and 4–4).

Complications

The most serious complications of a stress fracture result from ignoring the telltale signs and not being responsive to the athlete's complaint. Nonoperative treatment has certain risks that are associated with the casting treatment including deep vein thrombosis and skin injuries. It is important to arrange periodic follow-up after cast treatment to inspect the soft tissues. Operative treatment has surgical risks and may result in painful hardware that may have to be removed once the fracture is healed.

Treatment

The treatment of stress fractures around the foot is largely nonoperative. Stress fractures generally require immobilization in a hard-soled shoe or cast for 6–8 weeks. Stress fractures of the forefoot (ie, metatarsal fractures)

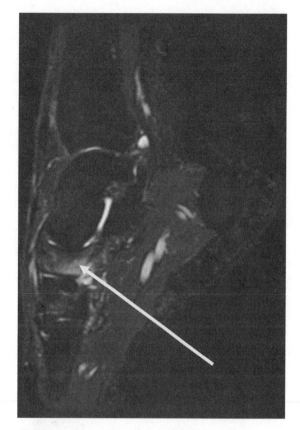

Figure 4–4. Inversion recovery MRI image of a navicular stress fracture. This may be a subtle finding on a T2-weighted image so special MRI techniques such as inversion recovery may be required.

can be treated in a hard soled shoe (eg, cast shoe) or a removable boot with a rocking sole. Stress fractures of the tarsal bones usually need to be protected or non-weight bearing for 6–8 weeks. Once the fracture has healed, a gradual return to activities can be allowed. Precautions should be taken to avoid the training errors or activities that led to the initial stress fracture. Very rarely a stress fracture will advance to a nonunion, the most notorious involving the base of the fifth metatarsal fracture, known as the "Jones fracture." This stress fracture occurs in athletes who jump a lot such as basketball, football, or volleyball players. In high-level athletes with fifth metatarsal stress fractures, an intramedullary screw allows faster return to play. In the average recreational athlete, however, the treatment of choice is modification of activity and cast or boot treatment for 4–6 weeks.

For a stress fracture that proceeds to become a nonunion or a malunion the same rules apply as for acute fractures. Any rotational misalignment needs to be corrected. A painful nonunion needs to be taken down operatively and bone grafted. Rigid fixation with an intramedullary nail, screws, or plates is then necessary.

Verma RB, Sherman O: Athletic stress fractures: part II. The lower body. Part III. The upper body with a section on the female athlete. Am J Orthop 2001;30(12):848.

Wilder RP, Sethi S: Overuse injuries: tendinopathies, stress fractures, compartment syndrome, and shin splints. Clin Sports Med 2004;23(1):55.

EXERTIONAL COMPARTMENT SYNDROME

ESSENTIALS OF DIAGNOSIS

- *Dull ache in a tibial muscle compartment (usually anterolateral).*
- *Insidious onset with activity followed by relief once activity is halted.*
- *No history of acute trauma.*
- *Reproducible onset of pain after a specific duration or intensity of exercise.*
- *Pain with passive stretch, numbness, weakness.*
- *Measurement of compartment pressures.*

Pathogenesis

Although athletes, and especially runners, are predisposed to overuse injuries, exertional compartment syndrome must be differentiated from two other conditions. The first of these and the most common is the medial tibial stress syndrome. Typically, the athlete has distinct pain along the posteromedial border of the middle to distal third tibia. There are no sensory, motor, or vascular anomalies. The distal one-third of the tibia is tender posteromedially and the pain can be elicited with a forced plantar flexion against resistance. This syndrome was previously referred to as classic "shin splints." Prevention of and therapy for this problem involve careful cross-training, light stretching, and a combination of initial rest and subsequent careful strengthening of the weak muscle groups.

The second condition that needs to be ruled out before a diagnosis of exertional compartment syndrome is made is a muscle strain in the medial gastrosoleus. Discussed earlier in this chapter, it may present in a fashion similar to the medial tibial stress syndrome.

Exertional compartment syndrome results from overcompression of the calf muscles during strenuous physical exercise. There are four major muscle compartments within the calf: anterior, lateral, posterior, and deep posterior. Others separate the calf into as many as seven compartments. During exercise, the muscle compartment can undergo a normal volume increase of up to 20%. Most often, the involved compartment is the anterior compartment followed in frequency by the deep posterior compartment. Fascial membranes make up the compartment and provide the anatomic casing for the muscles lying within its confines. As the muscle volume increases with exercise, it expands against the fascia, yet the fascia does not yield. Henceforth the intramuscular (intracompartmental) pressure will rise. As long as this pressure remains below a threshold that will not compromise blood flow and soft tissue integrity, the muscle functions within its physiologic capabilities and can recover. If the pressure rises above this physiologic threshold, the soft tissues are compromised. There is no preventive program.

Clinical Findings

A. SYMPTOMS

Exertional compartment syndrome typically presents as a dull ache or pain in the involved compartment. Patients usually indicate that the onset follows a very specific duration or type of exercise. This onset is so reproducible that it has been given the eponym "third lap syndrome." In 75–90% of patients, symptoms are bilateral, usually with one leg being worse than the other. The dull ache and discomfort typically remain for a certain duration after the exercise (minutes to hours) and then dissipate. In some patients, this may be accompanied by weakness, numbness, or paresthesias.

B. SIGNS

Immediately after exercise, the affected compartment may be tender or may feel significantly swollen. This, however, is usually helpful only if just one side is affected. In some patients muscle herniations can occur and be palpated. The presence of these herniations, although frequently found in patients with compartment syndrome, is usually incidental and has no diagnostic value.

C. IMAGING STUDIES

Imaging modalities can aid in ruling out the diagnoses of medial tibial stress syndrome, medial gastrocnemius rupture, and stress fracture of the tibia. Radiographs in two orthogonal planes (ie, anteroposterior and lateral) will usually show the periosteal stress reaction in posteromedial stress syndrome. It may or may not show a stress fracture. MRI scanning is very sensitive in evaluating edema around the calf. In case of a muscle injury, it will show a significant signal change with a high intensity in the T2-weighted image. A chronic compartment syndrome may show chronic scarring in the affected compartment. A bone scan cannot be used to diagnose chronic exertional compartment syndrome but it may rule out a stress reaction or stress fracture.

D. Compartment Pressure Measurements

The most helpful tool for the diagnosis of chronic exertional compartment syndrome is the direct measurement of compartment pressures immediately after exercise in combination with the clinical findings. There are multiple different techniques to measure compartment pressures ranging from a handheld pressure measurement device to the utilization of an arterial line and arterial pressure monitor.

Chronic exertional compartment syndrome is diagnosed if any one of the following three criteria are met:

1. A preexercise compartment pressure that is equal to or higher than 15 mm Hg.
2. One-minute after-exercise pressures that are above 50 mm Hg.
3. Five-minute postexercise pressures that are above 15 mm Hg.

These measurements are not affected by age but may be affected by position. The correct position during the test involves having the patient supine and the foot vertical.

Treatment

Conservative treatment of a chronic exertional compartment syndrome is generally unsatisfactory. Attempts can be made with the use of NSAIDs and rest, but usually the symptoms will improve only if the athlete is willing to completely stop the activity that brings on the symptoms. If the athlete wishes to continue the activity, operative intervention is the treatment of choice.

A. Surgical Compartment Release

All involved compartments need to be surgically released with great care and adequate homeostasis. Multiple different techniques have been described from a single incision to a two-incision technique. Care must be taken to identify the peroneal and saphenous nerves as well as the saphenous vein.

The results of operative compartment release have been consistently good; 90% of patients have a complete recovery with no residual symptoms.

B. Surgical Complications

Correctly diagnosing exertional compartment syndrome in an athlete with lower leg pain can be difficult. Successful treatment, of course, depends on the correct diagnosis. Failure of treatment largely results from excessive scarring or incomplete compartment release, especially of the deep compartment. This may happen when the surgeon, for cosmetic reasons, makes the skin incisions too small. Patients must realize that this is not a cosmetically pleasant procedure and it cannot be done through small incisions. Five to 10% of patients have residual symptoms after surgery. Failure can also result in infection, scarring, nerve and vessel damage, as well as recurrence of symptoms despite adequate compartment release.

Return to Play

After surgical treatment, the patient can start gradual strengthening and aerobic training as soon as the incisions have healed. The athlete should be able to return to a full exercise program 8–12 weeks after surgery.

Linz JC et al: Foot and ankle injuries. In: *Sports Injuries: Mechanism, Prevention, Treatment.* Fu FH, Stone DA (editors). Lippincott Williams & Wilkins, 2001.

Shah SN et al: Chronic exertional compartment syndrome. Am J Orthop 2004;33(7):335.

ANKLE PAIN

Ankle injuries are among the most common injuries in athletes. Soft tissue sprains and strains as well as ligament ruptures make up the vast majority of all ankle injuries. Ankle sprains and ligament tears can usually be treated successfully with nonoperative management and athletes recover quickly from these injuries. Some pathologic conditions, however, can lead to chronic irritation and inflammation of the ankle and pose substantial problems over a prolonged period.

POSTERIOR TIBIAL TENDONITIS

ESSENTIALS OF DIAGNOSIS

- *Pain of the medial aspect of the ankle.*
- *Pain with weight-bearing exercise.*
- *Usually follows an injury to the medial side of the ankle.*
- *Pain is exacerbated with active inversion and eversion of the subtalar joint.*
- *Often associated with a flat foot deformity.*

Pathogenesis

Posterior tibial tendinitis is a very rare occurrence in athletes under the age of 30 years. The majority of posterior tibial tendon problems occur in middle-aged athletes and particularly in women. Posterior tibial tendon injuries rarely develop acutely. There is usually a precipitating incident and subsequent slowly developing pain along the course of the posterior tibial tendon. This makes the tendinitis and subsequent rupture of the posterior tibial tendon a chronic disease process. Although it is a rather rare problem for athletes it is devastating should the tendon rupture since the therapeutic options are not ideal and usually lead to a dysfunction.

The posterior tibial tendon is predisposed to injury due to its critical zone of local hypovascularity combined with great mechanical stress acting on the tendon. The large distance between the posterior tibial tendon insertion and the axis of the subtalar joint provides a large lever arm that magnifies the stress on the tendon. Rapid changes in direction (ie, cutting) and jumping activities place the greatest stress on the tendon. Sports such as basketball, tennis, ice hockey, and soccer predispose the athlete to posterior tibial tendon injuries.

Clinical Findings

A. SYMPTOMS

Athletes complain of medial-sided ankle pain, worse with activity. Night or morning pain indicates more severe injury.

B. SIGNS

Physical examination reveals medial-sided point tenderness just inferior and posterior to the medial malleolus. This pain is usually exacerbated by forced inversion or eversion against resistance. A single leg toe raise is usually not possible. Commonly, the athlete will have a flat foot. Athletes usually show up early in the course of this disease because it is debilitating and usually not well tolerated for longer periods of athletic activity.

Imaging Studies

Posterior tibial tendinitis is a clinical diagnosis and does not require imaging. However, it is useful to obtain an MRI for the purpose of documentation and to evaluate the integrity of the tendon and the success of treatment (Figure 4–5). X-Rays of the foot and ankle are utilized to rule out other pathologic entities such as an accessory navicular stress fracture, degenerative joint disease, or anterior tibiotalar impingement.

Ultrasonography is equally accurate in diagnosing tendinitis as well as a rupture of the tibialis posterior tendon and can be easily done in an office setting.

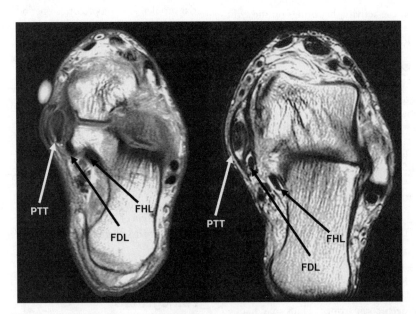

Figure 4–5. T1-weighted MRI images of the hindfoot. The left image shows a normal hindfoot with the posterior tibial tendon (PTT), the flexor digitorum longus (FDL), and the flexor hallucis longus (FHL). The tendons appear dark and do not show fraying or degeneration. On the right, there is significant fraying and even a tear in the posterior tibial tendon (***arrow***). The FDL and FHL look normal but there is some fatty degeneration inside the tendon sheaths (white areas within the tendon sheath).

Treatment

Nonoperative treatment is successful in the majority of patients with posterior tibial tendinitis. The initial treatment follows the earlier described RICE principle. A reduction in the current training program combined with NSAIDs is usually successful. In some athletes, a medial arch support may be helpful, particularly if they have a pronounced flat foot deformity. This treatment should be tried for 6 weeks. If this is not successful then immobilization in a cast or cast-boot should be tried for 4–6 weeks.

If no improvement of symptoms is obtained by 4–6 months surgical treatment options should to be considered.

SURGICAL TREATMENT

Operative treatment for posterior tibial tendinitis includes tendon inspection and a tenosynovectomy. The adjacent structures such as the anterior deltoid ligament and the immediately adjacent spring ligament need to be inspected for fraying and tears. If torn, they should be repaired. For more severe injuries, a tendon reconstruction using the flexor hallucis longus or the flexor digitorum longus tendons may be necessary. For severe and chronic injuries with a flexible hind foot, a medial slide osteotomy of the calcaneus may be needed in addition to tendon reconstruction to rebuild the medial arch; however, this is rare in athletes.

Return to Play

Return to play after nonoperative treatment is guided by the absence of pain. The process usually takes 2–4 months before full athletic activity can be resumed. Postoperatively a full ROM needs to be achieved and the return to 80% or more inversion strength and toe raise strength should be obtained before return to full activities. This takes between 4 and 12 months depending on the magnitude of surgery done.

ANTERIOR TIBIOTALAR IMPINGEMENT

ESSENTIALS OF DIAGNOSIS

- *Differentiate between anterior and anterolateral tibiotalar impingement.*
- *Usually insidious onset anterior ankle pain.*
- *Pain with forced dorsiflexion.*
- *Usually present only with activity; no pain with rest.*
- *Local tenderness over the anterior or anterolateral ankle.*

Pathogenesis

True anterior tibiotalar impingement was first described in 1943 as the "athlete's ankle" and was subsequently described as the "footballer's ankle" in 1950 and as "impingement exostosis of the tibia and talus" in 1954. Athletes who perform sports requiring repetitive forced dorsiflexion of the ankle (ie, soccer, football, dance, and gymnastics) report repetitive small sprains to the anterior ankle that they sustain in full dorsiflexion of their foot. These repetitive injuries lead to chronic sprains of the anterior ankle capsule and microtrauma to the anterior cartilage cap of the distal tibia. These microinjuries lead to a continuous cycle of microtrauma, inflammation, scarring of the capsule, subsequent calcification, and finally formation of bone spurs. Once the bone spurs grow large, they can directly impinge on each other and cause limited dorsiflexion. They may also fracture resulting in the formation of loose bodies in the ankle.

Prevention

Both anterior and anterolateral tibiotalar impingement are chronic conditions that are the result of repetitive microtrauma and therefore are very difficult to prevent. Anterior shin guards extending over the span of the ankle have been tried on soccer players; however, acceptance has been very low since these guards tend to interfere with the soft touch that these athletes require while handling the ball. Taping the ankle against maximally forced dorsiflexion as well as stretching and strengthening exercises should be routine measures for any competitive athlete. The athlete may use local antiinflammatory measures such as cryotherapy if the ankle is sore or after a minor ankle sprain. This may prevent the vicious cycle of chronic inflammation and scar formation early in the process.

Clinical Findings

A. SYMPTOMS

Patients most often present with a history of anterior ankle or midfoot pain radiating toward the lateral aspect of the ankle joint or the fibula. Initially this pain occurs after vigorous activity and dissipates soon after the activity is stopped. Gradually these symptoms may appear with light or even daily activity and may not dissipate after the activity is stopped. Patients typically report difficulties with climbing stairs and squatting as well as stiffness of the ankle.

B. SIGNS

Physical examination may reveal marked tenderness over the anterior border of the tibia and sometimes over the dorsum of the talus when the foot is plantar flexed. A ridge may be palpable over the dorsum of the talus. Patients usually display reduced dorsiflexion and a tight heel chord. A ligamentous examination of the ankle is usually within normal limits and does not show ligamentous injury.

C. IMAGING STUDIES

Radiographs of the ankle show that the anterior margin of the tibia has lost its round contour. Sometimes a bone spur can be seen on the dorsal surface of the neck of the talus. These spurs may be fragmented and can be a source of loose bodies.

Treatment

The initial treatment is nonoperative and involves rest and the use of NSAIDs. If this fails immobilization in a cast or cast-boot for 4–6 weeks should be tried. If the symptoms do not dissipate with modified activities and conservative treatment then an operative procedure should be considered.

Operative treatment addresses the bone spurs and involves removing the anterior osteophyte on the tibia as well as the dorsal bone spur on the neck of the talus. This can be done with an arthroscopic or a miniopen technique. The arthroscopic technique may result in a faster return to activities and enables the surgeon to inspect the ankle joint and thus recognize concomitant pathologies such as osteochondral defects, loose bodies, or formation of scar tissue. For anterolateral impingement the arthroscopic technique is preferred.

Postsurgical rehabilitation aims at restoration of motion and muscle strengthening. Once the surgical incisions have healed a gradual return to activities can be started.

Return to Play

Full ROM of the ankle and 80–100% of inversion/eversion and plantar flexion dorsiflexion strengths should be regained before return to competitive athletic activity.

ANTEROLATERAL TIBIOTALAR IMPINGEMENT

Pathogenesis

Anterolateral tibiotalar impingement has a different underlying pathology. Diagnosed much less frequently, it follows repetitive ankle sprains or chronic overuse in sports that involve pivoting. Anterolateral tibiotalar impingement can also follow nondisplaced fibula fractures or ligamentous avulsions of the fibula. The underlying pathology is believed to be a chronic synovitis and thickening of the distal most portion of the anterior inferior tibiofibular ligament complex (eg, anterior syndesmotic band) as a result of repetitive inversion injuries to the ankle. This scar formation was first described as a

"meniscoid band" in 1950. Subsequently, a separate band was described as being within the distal aspect of the anteroinferior tibiofibular ligament that is separated, through a fatty-fibrous layer, from the rest of the ligament and can impinge on the talar dome in maximal dorsiflexion of the ankle.

Prevention

Prevention of anterolateral tibiotalar impingement should follow the general principles of preventing ankle sprains, particularly inversion trauma to the ankle. Taping as well as off-the-shelf or custom lace-up braces to provide restraints against forced inversion of the ankle as well as proper strengthening and stretching exercises are the best preventive measures for chronic ankle sprains. High-top athletic shoe-wear, particularly for basketball players, is another means of trying to protect the ankle against inversion injury.

Clinical Findings

A. SYMPTOMS

Anterolateral tibiotalar impingement is a chronic condition that needs to be considered in patients who have severe anterolateral point tenderness and soreness for a prolonged period of time. Most importantly, it needs to be differentiated from symptoms of chronic instability. It is usually a diagnosis of exclusion and should not be made before all nonoperative treatment options such as NSAIDs, rest, ice, rehabilitation, and modalities have been exhausted.

B. SIGNS

Patients typically have anterolateral pain with dorsiflexion and sometimes clicking with motion of the ankle. Anterolateral impingement does not cause ankle instability.

C. IMAGING STUDIES

Radiographs need to be obtained to rule out stress fractures or fracture of the lateral process of the talus. An MRI can be helpful in identifying the thickened synovial band in the anterolateral recess of the ankle joint. MRI can be helpful in differentiating anterolateral impingement from chronic ruptures of the anterior talofibular ligament (ATFL). The "gold standard" for this diagnosis is ankle arthroscopy, characterized by a thickening of the anterolateral inferior band of the syndesmosis and a synovial fold in the anterolateral recess. Sometimes a small meniscus can cause the symptoms.

Treatment

The initial nonoperative treatment is identical to the treatment of anterior tibiotalar impingement. Operative treatment is an arthroscopic debridement of the synovial fold and the inferior anterior band of the syndesmosis. Once this is resected patients usually have a substantial reduction in pain.

Return to Play

Ambulation should be allowed immediately after surgery. Most importantly these patients need to undergo a vigorous rehabilitation program to regain their ROM. Because many of these patients have been deconditioned for a long period of time the coordination and strength of the ankle flexors and extendors as well as pronators and supinators need to be regained and proprioceptive exercises should be part of the rehabilitation process. Return to play should be possible after a 6-week rehabilitation period.

Mosier SM et al: Pathoanatomy and etiology of posterior tibial tendon dysfunction. Clin Orthop Relat Res 1999;(365):12.

Urguden M et al: Arthroscopic treatment of anterolateral soft tissue impingement of the ankle: evaluation of factors affecting outcome. Arthroscopy 2005;21(3):317.

ANKLE INSTABILITY

Injuries to the ankle are among the most common lower extremity injuries in sports. Overall there are as many as 23,000 ankle sprains in the United States each day. Women have a slightly higher risk of suffering a grade 1 ankle sprain than men on a collegiate level. The recurrence rate after a lateral ankle sprain is high. In high-demand sports such as basketball, the rate of recurrence may be as high as 70%.

Pathogenesis

Lateral ankle sprains most commonly occur due to excessive supination of the rear foot about an externally rotated lower leg soon after initial contact of the rear foot during gait or landing from a jump. Excessive inversion and internal rotation of the rear foot, coupled with external rotation of the lower leg, result in strain to the lateral ankle ligaments. If the strain in any of the ligaments exceeds the tensile strength of the tissues, ligamentous damage occurs. Increased plantar flexion at initial contact appears to increase the likelihood of suffering a lateral ankle sprain.

The ATFL is the first ligament to be damaged during a lateral ankle sprain, followed most often by the calcanofibular ligament (CFL). After the ATFL is ruptured, the amount of transverse-plane motion (internal rotation) of the rear foot increases substantially, thus further stressing the remaining intact ligaments. This phenomenon, described as "rotational instability" of the ankle, is often overlooked when considering laxity patterns in the sprained ankle. Concurrent damage to the talocrural joint capsule and the ligamentous stabilizers

of the subtalar joint is also common with lateral ankle sprains. The incidence of subtalar joint injury may be as high as 80% among patients suffering acute lateral ankle sprains.

The cause of lateral ankle sprain may be an increased supination moment at the subtalar joint. An increased supination moment about the ankle moment could thus cause excessive inversion and internal rotation of the rear foot in the closed kinetic chain and potentially lead to injury of the lateral ligaments. Individuals with a rigid supinated foot would be expected to have a more laterally deviated subtalar axis of rotation and a calcaneal varus (inverted rear foot) malalignment, which could predispose those with a rigid supinated foot to lateral ankle sprains.

Whether the peroneal muscles are able to respond quickly enough to protect the lateral ligaments from being injured once the ankle begins rapid inversion has been questioned. The peroneal muscles are active before initial foot contact during stair descent and when landing after a jump. This preparatory activity, along with similar activity in the other muscle groups that cross the ankle, is likely to create stiffness in tendons before initial foot contact with the ground. If the peroneal muscles are to protect against unexpected inversion of the rear foot, preparatory muscle activation before foot contact with the ground is necessary.

Structural predispositions to first-time ankle sprains include increased tibial varum and nonpathologic talar tilt, whereas functional predispositions include poor postural-control performance, impaired proprioception, and higher eversion-to-inversion and plantar flexion-to-dorsiflexion strength ratios. Further research into prevention programs based on these predisposing factors is clearly warranted.

Clinical Findings

A. SYMPTOMS

Typically an inversion injury has occurred that can be associated with an audible "pop" or a click. The ankle typically becomes swollen, tender, and painful with movement and full weight bearing.

B. SIGNS

The examiner must delineate the extent of the injury to determine if the patient injured one or multiple ligaments, tendons, bone, or even nerves. Systematically the examiner should palpate the ATFL, the CFL, and the posterior tibiofibular ligament (PTFL). The syndesmosis needs to be examined as well as the medial aspect of the ankle, the deltoid ligament, and the medial malleolus. The lateral malleolus should be palpated at its posterior border and tested for tenderness. Peroneal tendons and the base of the fifth metatarsal also need to be palpated. The clinician should stress the ATFL by performing an anterior drawer test. This may or may not be possible in the acute setting depending on the level of pain. The test is performed with the patient sitting and the lower leg hanging freely. The examiner holds the heel and positions the foot in slight plantar flexion. Then the heel is directed anterior while the other hand pushes the tibia posterior. This test is compared to results from the uninjured side. A difference is positive and is considered pathologic. The ankle inversion test can be used to differentiate between the ATFL and the CFL. A forced ankle inversion is performed and any difference from the opposite side is recorded. The inversion tested in plantar flexion evaluates the ATFL. The CFL is tested in dorsiflexion.

To examine the syndesmosis either the Hopkinson's syndesmotic squeeze test or a forced external rotation of the tibia can be performed. Pain when squeezing the fibula and tibia together approximately 10 cm above the joint and pain with forced external rotation of the tibia versus the talus (Keigler test) is suspicious. Tenderness at the inferior syndesmotic band in any of these tests is to be regarded as evidence of a syndesmotic injury until proven otherwise.

C. IMAGING STUDIES

Radiographs are used to rule out a fibular fracture, anterior process of the calcaneus fracture, lateral or posterior process of the talus fractures, midtarsal fractures, osteochondral lesions of the talus, and disruptions of the ankle mortise indicating a syndesmotic injury ("high ankle sprain"). MRI can be useful in determining the presence of bone contusions and ligament injuries (Figure 4–6).

Treatment

The initial treatment of an ankle sprain consists of the RICE principle. Additional modalities such as electrical stimulation or iontophoresis may be helpful adjuncts to reduce pain and swelling. Provided the injury does not involve the syndesmosis and there is no fracture, rehabilitation of the ankle sprain should be started as soon as pain control has been achieved. The rehabilitation process has to address ROM, strength, and proprioception. Once this phase has been completed and the athlete is pain free with exercises the third phase, designed to bring the athlete back to sports-specific drills and maneuvers such as cutting, jumping, and running, can begin. When the patient returns to athletic activities a protective, lace-up ankle brace should be worn to reduce recurrence of the injury.

If patients report recurrent sprains, continue to experience pain for a long period of time, and continue to have swelling and instability, surgical treatment options may need to be considered.

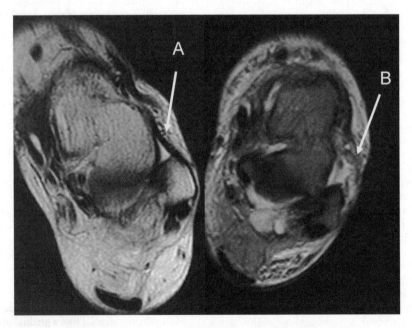

Figure 4–6. Inversion recovery MRI image of the anterior talofibular ligament (ATFL). On the left, the ATFL (***arrow A***) is intact. It is visible as a strong dark band. On the right (***arrow B***), it is disrupted, disorganized, and not visible as a collagenous dark structure.

A. SURGICAL TREATMENT

A myriad of different techniques have been described for the repair of the ATFL and CFL. The most common operative technique today is probably the Gould modification of the Brostrom technique. This technique essentially repairs the ATFL and CFL directly and imbricates the extensor retinaculum over the top of the direct ligament repair thus serving as a reinforcement of the ATFL and CFL repair. This technique has led to excellent results in high-level athletes and dancers. Using this technique there is no need to harvest any other tendon around the ankle as is required for many of the other ATFL and CFL reconstruction techniques. After a modified Brostrom procedure the athlete must wear a cast or cast-boot for about 6 weeks followed by ROM exercises and the formal rehabilitation program outlined above.

B. SYNDESMOTIC INJURY

If a syndesmotic injury is suspected, it is imperative that the integrity of the syndesmosis (ie, ankle mortise) is scrutinized. Any increase in medial joint space, disruption of the mortise, or widened gap between the fibula and the tibia may indicate a syndesmotic injury. These "high" ankle sprains are not uncommon. Up to 10% of all ankle sprains also involve the syndesmosis. They occur more frequently in high-energy collision sports such as ice hockey, football, and soccer.

If the athlete suffered a syndesmotic sprain the initial treatment is a cast or cast-boot for a minimum of 2–4 weeks followed by a reexamination. If the tenderness at the anterior syndesmotic band persists, the cast treatment needs to be continued for an additional 2 weeks. Once the anterior syndesmotic tenderness has subsided, the rehabilitation protocol can begin. It is important to know that athletes with a "high" ankle sprain will be sidelined significantly longer than athletes with a simple ankle sprain. If the syndesmosis is disrupted surgical repair with insertion of a syndesmotic screw needs to be performed. This will require wearing a cast and cast-boot for 6–9 weeks followed by rehabilitation.

Return to Play

Patients with simple ankle sprains can be treated with RICE and can return to play as soon as they experience no pain with their sports-specific activities. Those with ATFL tears should undergo formal rehabilitation and can return to play after the third phase of the rehabilitation has been concluded successfully. This usually takes 3–6 weeks. Patients with "high" ankle sprains will be sidelined for 4–12 weeks depending on the treatment necessary.

Osborne MD, Rizzo TD Jr: Prevention and treatment of ankle sprain in athletes. Sports Med 2003;33(15):1145.

Zoch C et al: Rehabilitation of ligamentous ankle injuries: a review of recent studies. Br J Sports Med 2003;37(4):291.

■ FOOT PAIN

ACHILLES TENDONITIS

ESSENTIALS OF DIAGNOSIS

- *Onset of tenderness and swelling approximately 2–6 cm above the insertion of the tendo Achilles (TA).*
- *Initial pain after activity followed in later stages by onset of pain during activity.*
- *Diffuse pain with palpation of the TA.*
- *Pain over the insertion of the TA with pressure and during the night (insertional tendinitis).*
- *Decreased dorsiflexion of the ankle with tight heel chord.*

Pathogenesis

There are three different inflammatory entities of the TA that are closely related and require the same initial treatment regime:

1. Achilles peritendinitis: inflammation of the paratenon with or without degeneration of the TA.
2. Achilles tendinosis: inflammation and degeneration of the TA without involvement of the paratenon.
3. Insertional Achilles tendinitis: inflammation and degeneration at the TA insertion with or without calcifications and bone spur formation.

A predominantly sedentary life-style followed by a sudden increase in physical activity involving walking, jogging, and running in the mid ages (40–60 years of age) in combination with tight heel chords and decreased ROM of the ankle leads to TA injury. As a general precaution stretching of the TA combined with a gradual increase in activity for elder athletes helps to avoid TA injury. Achilles tendinitis in high-level athletes is usually a sign of faulty training, improper running techniques, or overuse.

Clinical Findings

A. SYMPTOMS

Most patients complain of a gradual onset of pain in the posterior calf approximately 2–6 cm above the insertion of the TA. Often this pain is accompanied by swelling. Initially the pain will appear after physical activity. This can change and the athlete may experience pain during physical activity, usually indicating a worsening of the pathology. Insertional TA tendinitis presents similarly with the exception that it often appears as night pain when the athlete rests the foot on the back of the heel while sleeping.

B. Signs

The diagnosis of Achilles peritendinitis versus tendinosis can theoretically be made by evaluating the location of the point of maximal tenderness. In peritendinitis the entire paratenon is inflamed and therefore will not be affected by ankle ROM during the examination. TA tendinosis is a localized inflammation, in which case ROM will lead to a migration of the point of maximal tenderness throughout the examination. It is important to rule out a tear of the Achilles tendon, which can be done with the Thompson test as described in the section on muscle strains.

C. Imaging Studies

Standard radiographs of the ankle may show some calcification along the TA. There may be a thickened soft tissue shadow visible. In case of an insertional tendinitis there may be calcifications anterior to the insertion of the TA (Figure 4–7). An MRI may be helpful in differentiating tendinitis from tendinosis. In tendinitis there is significant fluid retention within the tendon without hypertrophy of the tendinous tissue. This is an acute finding and can usually be successfully treated with antiinflammatory medication and RICE. Significant hypertrophy of the tendon indicates replacement of tendon tissue with a fibrous scar (Figure 4–8). This tendinosis can predispose the patient to a rupture of the TA.

Treatment

All three injuries of the Achilles tendon initially receive the same treatment. This consists of nonoperative management including NSAIDs and rehabilitation exercises such as stretching and strengthening of the TA and strengthening of the gastrocsoleus complex. If the patient has significant hindfoot varus or valgus a correcting orthosis may need to be issued. Modalities such as iontophoresis and electrotherapy do not have proven

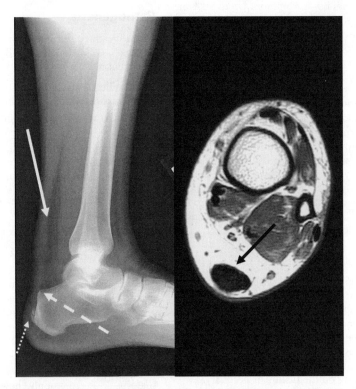

Figure 4–7. The left image shows a plain radiograph with an increased widened soft tissue shadow along the tendo Achilles (TA) (***fat arrow***). In addition, this patient has calcifications on the TA insertion (***dotted arrow***) and a Haglund's deformity (***dashed arrow***). On the T1-weighted axial MRI image there is an easily appreciated very thick inhomogeneous TA (***arrow***).

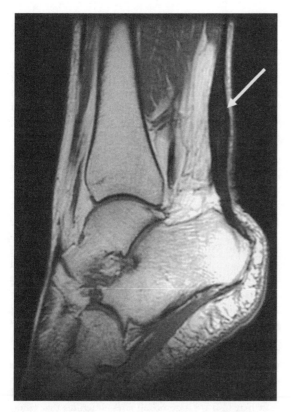

Figure 4–8. This T1-weighted image of the ankle shows a sagittal view of Achilles tendonopathy. The **arrow** marks the area of hypertrophic scarring.

efficacy but may be employed if pain relief can be obtained. It is usually not necessary to treat patients immobilized in a cast, although in rare cases this may be necessary for recalcitrant pain.

Steroid injections should not be given into the tendon or the tendon insertion as these can lead to an early rupture of the tendon making a primary repair difficult, if not impossible, secondary to the degeneration that the tendon undergoes in response to the steroid injection.

SURGICAL TREATMENT

Recalcitrant cases that have not responded to treatment in over 6 months may require surgical debridement of the paratenon and the tendinosis. Using a slightly medially based skin incision the paratenon is incised and debrided and the thickened tendon is thoroughly debrided. If more than 50% of the tendon is involved the plantaris tendon may be woven into the defect to strengthen the repair. The tendon is repaired as well as the paratenon. To ensure that the paratenon is not tightened too much, it can be released carefully on its anterior aspect thus allowing posterior closure without

undue tension. A lateral approach is used for insertional tendinitis and the calcaneal bursa is excised. In some cases there is a prominent bony ridge of the posterior calcaneus (ie, "Haglund's deformity") that may abut the tendon insertion. This bony ridge needs to be removed with an osteotome. Postoperatively the patient is put into a cast or cast-boot for 4–6 weeks. Weight bearing is usually allowed between 2 and 4 weeks and is followed by rehabilitation for 6 weeks.

Return to Play

Once the symptoms have subsided a gradual return to former activities can be allowed. If symptoms return, the eliciting activity should be stopped immediately and a more gradual return should be tried. After operative treatment the rehabilitation protocol is similar after the initial postoperative casting period.

Linz JC et al: Foot and ankle injuries. In: *Sports Injuries: Mechanism, Prevention, Treatment.* Fu FH, Stone DA (editors). Lippincott Williams & Wilkins, 2001.

Mizel MS et al: Evaluation and treatment of chronic ankle pain. Instr Course Lect 2004;53:311.

HEEL PAIN

ESSENTIALS OF DIAGNOSIS

- *Very common in runners and overweight athletes.*
- *Usually stabbing pain in the morning for the first few steps.*
- *Medial calcaneal pain.*
- *Often associated with tight heel chords.*
- *Takes 1–2 years to resolve completely.*

Pathogenesis

Plantar heel pain has many medical names such as plantar fasciitis, runner's heel, policemen's heel, calcaneodynia, and heel pain syndrome. It is one of the commonest problems experienced by athletes. The differential diagnosis of plantar heel pain is often difficult and has to address various different anatomic sites. The spectrum ranges from systemic conditions such as Reiter's syndrome, ankylosing spondylitis, or rheumatoid arthritis to medial plantar nerve entrapment or plantar fibromatosis. Most commonly, however, it is the running athlete who presents with complaints about plantar heel pain. A higher intensity of training sessions, weight gain, and return of overweight athletes to previous training schedules can be reasons. Furthermore, there are certain risk factors, such as high-impact aerobics or prolonged daily walking on hard surfaces (ie, construction workers, orthopedic residents). To understand the underlying pathology it is necessary to understand the anatomy and function of the plantar fascia.

The plantar fascia is a strong collagenous structure that originates on the anteromedial aspect of the calcaneus and inserts at the base of each proximal phalanx. The fascia is divided such that the flexor tendons can perforate the fascia to reach the toes. This results in 10 individual insertions of the plantar fascia. Overlying the plantar fascia is the plantar fad pad, which is approximately 2–3 cm thick.

The biomechanical function of the plantar fascia is a continuation of the Achilles tendon around the calcaneus resulting in the "windlass" mechanism. This mechanism enables the foot to stabilize itself in midstance due to a tightening of the longitudinal foot arch.

The tibial nerve splits into its final branches at the level of the medial malleolus. In particular, the first branch of the lateral plantar nerve, the posterior branch or "Baxter's nerve," can be a source of pain if it becomes trapped between the abductor hallucis and the quadratus planti muscle.

Clinical Findings

A. Symptoms

Patients report that they have sharp stabbing pain with the first steps in the morning. The pain eases during the day and toward the evening the entire heel is sore.

B. Signs

Physical examination has to address the underlying pathology and starts with an evaluation of the gastrocsoleus and TA complex. Almost all patients with plantar fasciitis have a tight heel chord and lack dorsiflexion up to, or past, neutral. Furthermore, the forefoot needs to be evaluated. A pronated or plantar flexed first ray can lead to plantar fasciitis in itself. Typically patients have palpable pain directly anteromedially on the plantar surface of the tuber calcanei. If a nerve entrapment is suspected there should be a positive Tinel's sign over the medial aspect of the heel just beneath the medial malleolus. Furthermore, a careful palpation of the plantar fascia should be performed to rule out single or multiple plantar fibromata.

C. Imaging Studies

Radiographs do not usually show the pathology. There may be a "bone spur" along the anterior aspect of the calcaneus, however, this bone spur actually arises within the aponeurosis of the flexor digitorum brevis and is not involved in the development of plantar fasciitis. An MRI scan can be helpful in detecting abnormalities of the plantar fascia. It will show increased fluid uptake in the T2-weighted images along the anteromedial border of the plantar fascia (Figure 4–9). It may also show a plantar fibroma or a neuroma of Baxter's nerve. An MRI scan may also indicate occult stress fractures that could be the cause of plantar foot pain such as an anterior process of the calcaneus fracture.

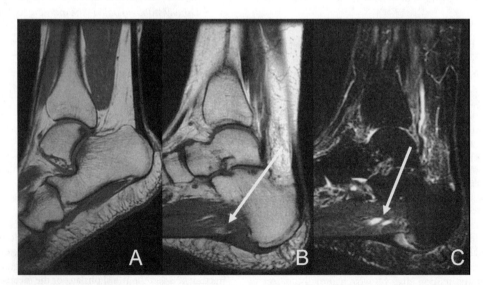

Figure 4–9. These MRI images show a sagittal view of a T1-weighted image of a normal foot on the left (**A**). The T1-weighted image in the middle (**B**) shows a calcification inside the plantar fascia (***arrow***). The T2-weighted image on the right (**C**) shows that these calcifications are inside a zone of edema in the plantar fascia signifying plantar fasciitis.

Treatment

The treatment for plantar fasciitis is focused on addressing the underlying disorder. Patients need to be counseled so that they understand that this condition is self-limiting and that successful treatment can take up to a year. The chronic tightness of the plantar fascia leads to a contracture of the fascia during sleep. The first steps in the morning stretch this contracted fascia and cause microtears that subsequently scar during the next rest period until the plantar fascia has eventually elongated to a point at which no more microtears occur. To break this cycle the first line treatment is stretching of the plantar fascia and the TA. A short heel chord leads to overuse of the windlass mechanism and consequently results in overtightening of the plantar fascia. Patients therefore should be instructed to stretch the TA multiple times during the day. In addition, they can be provided with night splints that prevent the contraction of the plantar fascia and keep the foot in neutral dorsiflexion during sleep. Furthermore, heel cups help to cushion the hard impact on the heel. There is some debate about the usefulness of full arch supports. It has been shown that they work as well as simple heel cups as long as they are utilized in conjunction with stretching exercises. In severe cases of plantar fasciitis it may be helpful to treat the patient with a cast or cast-boot for a few weeks to rest the plantar fascia before a rigorous stretching program is started.

We discourage steroid injections into the plantar fascia. Although the literature provides conflicting data on the success of steroid injections, there is clear evidence that use of steroid injections is associated with a high risk of a tear of the plantar fascia, which results in a catastrophic flat foot deformity that is essentially not correctible.

If the source of pain is entrapment of Baxter's nerve an electromyogram (EMG) should be obtained. If the EMG and nerve conduction studies suggest a nerve entrapment the first line of treatment is orthotics that correct any present foot deformity (overpronation, pes planus, pes planovalgus etc).

SURGICAL TREATMENT

Surgical release of the plantar fascia is reserved for very rare severe cases of plantar fasciitis in which there is intractable pain for 1 or more years. Various techniques have been used to release the plantar fascia. It is important that this is done under direct visualization. The medial aspect of the plantar fascia needs to be partially excised. A complete release will result in a deficiency of the plantar fascia and an uncorrectable flatfoot deformity. If a release of a plantar fascia is performed it is prudent to include a release of Baxter's nerve. This is important for two reasons. First, the nerve needs to be visualized so as not to cut it and second, there may be an element of both pathologies that can easily be addressed through one approach.

Return to Play

Athletes who are pain free can return to their previous exercise program. Running athletes are advised to maintain the stretching program in their warm-up routine.

Linz JC et al: Foot and ankle injuries. In: *Sports Injuries: Mechanism, Prevention, Treatment.* Fu FHg, Stone DA (editors). Lippincott Williams & Wilkins, 2001.

Williams SK, Brage M: Heel pain-plantar fasciitis and Achilles enthesopathy. Clin Sports Med 2004;23(1):123.

TURF TOE

ESSENTIALS OF DIAGNOSIS

- *Mechanism of injury [hyperplantar/hyperdorsiflexion of the first metatarsophalangeal (MTP) joint].*
- *Tenderness with ROM of the first MTP joint.*
- *Swelling.*
- *Pain with weight bearing.*

Pathogenesis

Sprains of the first MTP joint have been described as "turf toe" injuries since it was noted that athletic competition on artificial turf resulted in an increased incidence of soft tissue injuries to the great toe. Injuries to the first MTP joint occur in football and soccer but can happen during any athletic activity that forces the first MTP joint into hyperplantar or hyperdorsiflexion. Injuries to the first MTP joint are by no means benign and carry a significant short- and long-term morbidity. Despite the usual perception that this is a "trivial" injury, overall estimates of loss of playing time rank MTP joint injuries first, at the same level as ankle sprains even though they occur far less frequently.

The mechanism of injury is a hyperdorsiflexion injury that usually happens when the foot is planted and the first MTP joint is maximally dorsiflexed. The dorsal edge of the proximal phalanx is cocked against the articular surface of the metatarsal head. The capsuloligamentous structures are maximally stretched in this position. Forcing the first MTP joint into greater hyperdorsiflexion will lead to a structural failure of either the volar capsule or the collateral ligament or a fracture of either the dorsal phalanx or the metatarsal head. Classically this situation occurs when an offensive lineman plants his foot for maximal traction and another player falls onto his heel forcing his forefoot into greater hyperdorsiflexion. It also occurs when the foot, in maximal plantar flexion with the first toe pointed, is struck from behind, driving the first MTP joint into greater hyperplantar flexion.

To prevent these injuries the first MTP joint can be taped to limit dorsiflexion and plantar flexion. The variability in ROM of the first MTP joint is great. Normal ROM can range from 3–43 degrees of dorsiflexion to 40–100 degrees of plantar flexion. Individuals with a naturally limited ROM are at increased risk for "turf toe" injuries and should be taped. There is some evidence that the use of an orthotic (eg, Morton extension) or a 0.51-mm spring steel insert may help prevent these types of injuries.

Clinical Findings

Injuries to the first MTP joint vary widely. The spectrum of injury ranges from a simple sprain to complete avulsions of the dorsal or volar plate with or without associated fractures of the metacarpal head or base of the phalanx. In addition, the sesamoid bones can be involved in the injury if the flexor tendons are part of the injury.

A. SYMPTOMS

The trainer or physician on the sideline must keep a close eye on players who come off the field with a limp. Turf toe injuries are often treated as a minor injury by players. This leads to prolonged recovery and problems later on. Patients complain of first MTP joint pain and difficulty pushing off the injured foot.

B. SIGNS

A physical examination of the first MTP joint should include a study of active and passive ROM. The results of the examination have to be compared to the results from the opposite side and it needs to be noted if either active or passive ROM is painful. The normal examination should be painless. Pain at the extremes of ROM may indicate whether the injury is volar or dorsal. Strengths of the flexor hallucis longus as well as the extensor hallicus longus need to be tested to rule out an avulsion injury. Stability of then first MTP joint in valgus and varus stress also needs to be evaluated to rule out collateral ligament damage.

C. CLASSIFICATION

A classification system has been designed that is helpful in assessing the severity of the damage.

Grade 1 sprains represent stretch injuries:

- Localized pain.
- Minimal swelling, little ecchymosis.

- ROM mildly limited with minimal pain.
- Minimal pain with weight bearing.

Grade 2 sprains represent a partial tear of the capsuloligamentous complex:

- More intense tenderness and diffuse pain.
- Moderate swelling with ecchymosis.
- Moderately decreased ROM.
- Mild to moderate pain with weight bearing.
- Athlete limps clearly.

Grade 3 sprains are complete disruptions of the capsuloligamentous complex with or without bony avulsions and osteochondral fractures:

- Very intense and diffuse tenderness around the entire MTP joint.
- Severe swelling and ecchymosis.
- Very limited ROM and very painful.
- Inability to ambulate normally.

Once the clinical diagnosis of a turf toe injury is made further diagnostic tools may be needed to clearly delineate the severity of the injury. We believe that any turf toe injury that is significant enough to cause pain with ROM should be evaluated with radiographs. Further diagnostic tools should be used if it is suspected that the severity of the injury is greater.

D. IMAGING STUDIES

Radiographs reveal avulsion fractures, osteochondral incongruencies in the metatarsal head or base of the phalanx, migration of the sesamoids, widening of the bipartite sesamoids, or subchondral bone resorption that can be seen with chondral injuries. If a collateral ligament or a purely ligamentous volar/dorsal plate injury is suspected, stress radiographs should be performed in valgus or maximal plantar/dorsiflexion of the MTP joint. If a stress fracture of a sesamoid is suspected, a bone scan can be obtained. An MRI can be used for diagnosis of ligament avulsions, particularly of the volar plate (Figure 4–10).

Treatment

Treatment of turf toe injuries is primarily nonsurgical. The initial treatment protocol adheres to the RICE principle followed by cryotherapy during the first 48 hours after the injury. The most important factor for rehabilitation following these injuries is rest until painless ROM is obtained. For simple grade 1 sprains without any structural damage the athlete can usually return to light stretching and functional rehabilitation within the painless ROM. Taping and toe spacers can be used to counter the initial injury mechanism.

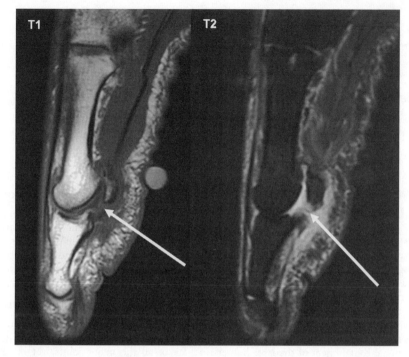

Figure 4–10. These T1- and T2-weighted MRI images of a turf toe injury show the disruption of the plantar plate at the first matatarsophalangeal joint (***arrows***).

For more severe grade 2 sprains athletes may miss between 5 and 14 days of training and game time. The treatment follows the same rules as for grade 1.

For grade 3 sprains the treatment depends on the anatomy of the injury. The initial treatment is the same as for grade 1 and 2 sprains. Athletes often require crutches for a few days to immobilize the toe.

In grade 3 injuries, surgical treatment may be necessary. Although capsular avulsions and collateral ligament injuries usually heal with nonoperative treatment, fractures, osteochondral avulsions, and nonreducible dislocations need to be addressed surgically. Late sequelae such as osteochondral nonunions, sesamoid nonunions, loose bodies, or late acquired deformities such as hallux varus or rigidus almost always require surgical intervention if conservative measures have failed.

Return to Play

For simple grade 1 sprains, once the athlete is pain free return to play is possible. For grade 2 sprains, it is imperative that the athlete is pain free before return to play. After a grade 3 injury, an athlete may need between 4 and 8 weeks to return to play. These injuries can be career ending, so it is not desirable to push a return to play until the athlete is completely pain free throughout all required drills.

Katcherian DA: Pathology of the first ray. In: *Orthopaedic Knowledge Update (OKU)2.* Mizel M et al (editors). American Academy of Orthopaedic Surgeons, 1998.

Mullen JE, O'Malley MJ: Sprains: residual instability of subtalar, Lisfranc joints, and turf toe. Clin Sports Med 2004;23(1):97.

Watson TS et al: Periarticular injuries to the hallux metatarsophalangeal joint in athletes. Foot Ankle Clin 2000;5(3):687.

Shoulder Injuries

5

Leslie S. Beasley Vidal, MD, Armando F. Vidal, MD, & Patrick J. McMahon, MD

■ SHOULDER INJURIES

The shoulder is the third most commonly injured joint during athletic activities, after the knee and the ankle. Sports-related injuries of the shoulder may result from a direct traumatic event or repetitive overuse. Any activity that requires arm motion, particularly overhead arm motion such as throwing, may stress the soft tissues surrounding the glenohumeral joint to the point of injury. The shoulder is the most mobile joint in the body partly as a result of minimal containment of the large humeral head by the shallow and smaller glenoid fossa. The trade-off for this mobility is less structural restraint to undesirable and potentially damaging movements. Thus, a fine balance must be struck to maintain full range of shoulder motion and normal glenohumeral joint stability.

Kim DH et al: Shoulder injuries in golf. Am J Sports Med 2004;32(5):1324.

THE SHOULDER

Anatomy

A. THE BONY ARTICULATION OF THE GLENOHUMERAL JOINT

The glenohumeral joint is a modified ball-and-socket joint. The glenoid fossa is a shallow inverted, comma-shaped, articular surface one-fourth the size of the humeral head. The articular surface of the humeral head is retroverted approximately 30° relative to the transverse axis of the elbow. Because the scapula is oriented anterolaterally about 30° on the thorax, relative to the coronal plane of the body, the face of the glenoid fossa matches the humeral head retroversion. The scapula rotates to direct the glenoid superiorly, inferiorly, medially, or laterally to accommodate changing humeral head positions. As a result, the humeral head is centered in the glenoid throughout most shoulder motions. When this centered position is disturbed, instability may result.

B. THE CLAVICLE AND ITS ARTICULATIONS

The clavicle articulates medially with the sternum at the sternoclavicular joint and laterally with the acromion of the scapula at the acromioclavicular joint. The clavicle rotates on its long axis and acts as a strut to stabilize the glenohumeral joint, serving as the only bone connecting the appendicular upper extremity to the axial skeleton.

C. THE GLENOHUMERAL JOINT CAPSULE, LIGAMENTS, AND LABRUM

The capsule of the glenohumeral joint may be the most lax of all the major joints, yet in certain positions it makes an important contribution to stability. The capsuloligamentous structures and the glenoid labrum share a common insertion. The anterior capsule is composed of the coracohumeral and superior glenohumeral ligaments, the middle glenohumeral ligament, and the inferior glenohumeral ligament (Figure 5–1). There is a variable relationship between the anterior capsuloligamentous structures and the labrum, such that certain anatomic variations may be associated with joint instability more often than others. For example, an antero-superior sublabral hole is variably present within the glenohumeral joint, connecting with the subscapularis bursa that lies between the subscapularis tendon and the capsule.

The glenoid labrum acts not only as an attachment site for the capsuloligamentous structures but also as an extension of the articular cavity. Its presence deepens the glenoid socket by nearly 50% and removal of the labrum decreases joint stability to shear stress. In this way, the triangular cross section of the labrum acts as a chock-block to help prevent subluxation.

D. THE SHOULDER MUSCULATURE

The muscles around the shoulder may be divided into three functional groups: glenohumeral, thoracohumeral, and those that cross both the shoulder and the elbow.

1. Glenohumeral muscles—Four muscles compose the rotator cuff: the supraspinatus, subscapularis, infraspinatus, and teres minor. The supraspinatus originates on the

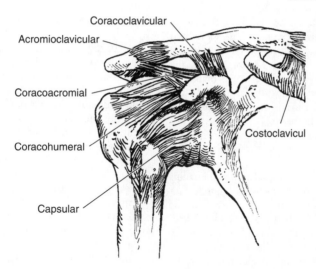

Figure 5–1. Ligaments about the shoulder girdle. (Reprinted with permission from McMahon PJ, Skinner HB: Sports medicine. In: Skinner HB (editor): *Current Diagnosis & Treatment in Orthopedics,* 3rd ed. McGraw-Hill, 2003.)

posterosuperior scapula, superior to the scapular spine. It passes under the acromion, through the supraspinatus fossa, and inserts on the greater tuberosity with an extended attachment of fibrocartilage. The supraspinatus is active during the entire arc of scapular plane abduction; paralysis of the suprascapular nerve results in an approximately 50% loss of abduction torque. The infraspinatus and the teres minor muscles originate on the posterior scapula, inferior to the scapular spine, and insert on the posterior aspect of the greater tuberosity. Despite their origin below the scapular spine, their tendinous insertions are not separate from the supraspinatus tendon. These muscles function together to externally rotate and extend the humerus. Both account for approximately 80% of external rotation strength in the adducted position. The infraspinatus is more active with the arm at the side, whereas the teres minor activates mainly with the shoulder in 90° of elevation. The subscapularis muscle arises from the anterior scapula and is the only muscle to insert on the lesser tuberosity. The subscapularis is the only anterior component of the rotator cuff and functions to internally rotate and flex the humerus. The tendinous insertion of the subscapularis is continuous with the anterior capsule so that both provide anterior glenohumeral stability.

The deltoid is the largest of the glenohumeral muscles. It covers the proximal humerus on a path from its tripennate origin at the clavicle, acromion, and scapular spine to its insertion midway on the humerus at the deltoid tubercle. Abduction of the joint results from activity of the anterior and middle portions. The anterior portion is also a forward flexor. The posterior portion extends the humerus. The deltoid is active throughout

the entire arc of glenohumeral abduction; paralysis of the axillary nerve results in a 50% loss of abduction torque. The deltoid muscle can fully abduct the glenohumeral joint with the supraspinatus muscle inactive.

The teres major muscle originates from the inferior angle of the scapula and inserts on the medial lip of the bicipital groove of the humerus, posterior to the insertion of the latissimus dorsi. The axillary nerve and the posterior humeral circumflex artery pass superior to it through the quadrilateral space also bordered by the teres minor, the triceps, and the humerus. It contracts with the latissimus dorsi muscle and the two muscles function as a unit in humeral extension, internal rotation, and adduction.

2. Thoracohumeral muscles—The pectoralis major and the latissimus dorsi muscles are powerful movers of the shoulder and, hence, contribute to the joint force, which, in turn, usually stabilizes the glenohumeral joint. The pectoralis major muscle arises as a broad sheet of two distinct heads with the lowermost fibers of the sternal head inserting most proximally on the humerus.

Muscles that originate on the thorax contribute to glenohumeral stability, but may have roles in instability as well. When the shoulder is placed in horizontal abduction, similar to the apprehension position, the lowermost fibers of the sternal head of the pectoralis major muscle are stretched to an extreme. Because anterior instability also occurs from forcible horizontal abduction of the shoulder, the humeral head may be pulled out of the glenoid by passive tension in the pectoralis major and latissimus dorsi muscles.

3. Biceps brachii muscle—Both heads of the biceps brachii muscle originate on the scapula. The short head originates from the coracoid, and with the coracobrachialis muscle forms the conjoined tendon. The long head of the biceps originates just superior to the articular margin of the glenoid from the posterosuperior labrum and the supraglenoid tubercle, and is inside the synovial sheath of the glenohumeral joint. It traverses the glenohumeral joint, passing over the anterior aspect of the humeral head to the bicipital groove, where it exits the joint under the transverse humeral ligament.

Its origin on the scapula and insertion of the radius provides the long head of the biceps brachii muscle with the potential to function at both the shoulder and the elbow. Its function at the elbow, as well established, includes both flexion and supination. The role of the active biceps, long considered a depressor of the humeral head, has recently been questioned as electromyographic studies have shown that there is little or no activity of the biceps when elbow motion is controlled. This does not preclude a passive role or an active role associated with elbow motion, as tension in the tendon may then contribute to glenohumeral joint stability.

E. THE NEUROVASCULAR SUPPLY

The axillary artery traverses the axilla, extending from the outer border of the first rib to the lower border of the teres minor muscle, forming the brachial artery. The axillary artery lies deep to the pectoralis muscle, but is crossed in its mid-region by the pectoralis minor tendon, just before the tendon inserts on the coracoid process. The axillary vein travels with the axillary artery, and branches of the axillary artery supply most of the shoulder girdle. The brachial plexus consists of the ventral rami of the fifth through eighth cervical nerves and the first thoracic nerve. This network of nerve fibers begins with the joining of the ventral rami proximally in the neck and continues anteriorly and distally, crossing into the axillary region obliquely underneath the clavicle at about the junction area of the distal one-third and proximal two-thirds. Clavicular fractures in this area may potentially injure the brachial plexus. The plexus then lies inferior to the coracoid process, where its cords form the peripheral nerves that continue down the arm. Muscles of the shoulder girdle are supplied by the nerves arising at all levels of the brachial plexus.

Eberly VC et al: Variation in the glenoid origin of the anteroinferior glenohumeral capsulolabrum. Clin Orthop 2002;400:26.

Enad JG: Bifurcate origin of the long head of the biceps tendon. Arthroscopy 2004;20(10):1081.

Price MR et al: Determining the relationship of the axillary nerve to the shoulder joint capsule from an arthroscopic perspective. J Bone Joint Surg Am 2004;86-A(10):2135.

History & Physical Examination

A. GENERAL APPROACH

The history of shoulder complaints must include age, arm dominance, location, intensity, duration, temporal occurrence, aggravating and alleviating factors, radiation of discomfort, level of physical activity, occupation, and the mechanism of injury. Previous responses to treatment will help to characterize their efficacy and establish a pattern of disease or injury progression. The physical examination begins with the patient undressing so that both shoulders are fully exposed. Patients should be examined first in the standing position. The surface anatomy should be checked for asymmetry, atrophy, or external lesions. It is particularly important to examine the supraspinatus and infraspinatus fossae for atrophy. The area of pain should be pointed out by the patient prior to the physician manipulating the shoulder to avoid hurting the patient unnecessarily. A thorough neurovascular examination of the upper extremity should be performed.

B. SHOULDER RANGE OF MOTION

1. Types of movement—Many terms may be used to describe movements of the shoulder joint (Figure 5–2 and Table 5–1). Flexion occurs when the arm begins at the side and elevates in the sagittal plane of the body anteriorly. Extension occurs when the arm starts at the side and elevates in the sagittal plane of the body posteriorly. Adduction occurs when the arm moves toward the midline of the body, with abduction occurring as the arm moves away from the midline of the body. Internal rotation occurs when the arm rotates medially, inward toward the body, and external rotation occurs as the arm rotates laterally or outward from the body. Horizontal adduction occurs as the arm starts at 90° of abduction and adducts forward and medially toward the center of the body, and horizontal abduction occurs as the arm starts at 90° of abduction and moves outward, away from the body. Elevation is the angle made between the thorax and arm, regardless of whether it is in the abduction plane, flexion plane, or in between.

2. Evaluation of movement—Range of motion of the injured shoulder should be compared with range of motion of the opposite shoulder, along with the strength during abduction and rotation. This should be done both passively and actively. The shoulder should be inspected for any changes in synchrony, such as scapular winging, elevation of the scapula, muscle fasciculations indicating abnormal function, and any other irregular or asymmetric movements of the scapula. Information may be gained on loss of flexibility and instability resulting from muscle imbalance, fibrosis, and tendon, capsular, or ligament

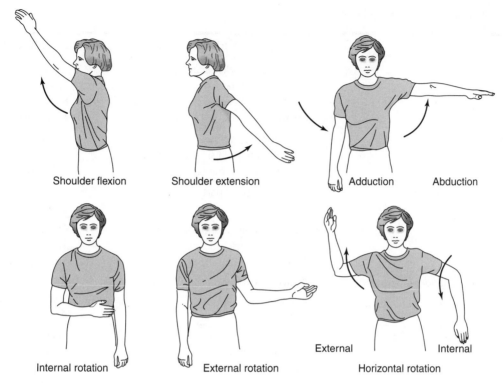

Figure 5–2. Description of shoulder motion. (Reprinted with permission from McMahon PJ, Skinner HB: Sports medicine. In: Skinner HB (editor): *Current Diagnosis & Treatment in Orthopedics,* 3rd ed. McGraw-Hill, 2003.)

contractures. Loss of flexibility usually occurs in the capsular tissues of the glenohumeral joint. Sudden pain or clicking may indicate an intraarticular problem. Loss of motion in either internal or external rotation is suggestive of a chronic anterior or posterior dislocation, respectively.

3. Provocative tests—Specific tests are then performed that aid in making the correct diagnosis. The specific tests for instability, impingement syndrome, bicipital tendinitis, and superior capsulolabral/biceps anchor lesions are discussed below.

Imaging & Other Studies

Many varieties of radiologic views and projections are available to examine shoulder injuries. An initial radiographic evaluation of the shoulder should consist of an anteroposterior view of the glenohumeral joint in both internal and external rotation, and an axillary lateral view. Additional plain radiographic views depend on the underlying pathologic factors. Magnetic resonance imaging (MRI) may be indicated in evaluating rotator cuff disorders recalcitrant to conservative treatment. An

MR arthrogram may be useful in detecting labral pathology. Traditional arthrography is rarely indicated because it is invasive and has little or no advantage to MRI. Ultrasonography is also useful in the diagnosis of rotator cuff injury, but it is operator dependent. Electromyographic examination can be useful in identifying shoulder pain of cervical origin.

Arthroscopic Evaluation

A. INDICATIONS

Indications for arthroscopic examination of the shoulder include the following:

1. impingement syndrome including subacromial bursitis, rotator cuff tendinitis, and rotator cuff tears;

2. acromioclavicular joint osteoarthritis;

3. loose bodies;

4. chronic synovitis;

5. glenohumeral instability;

6. superior capsulolabral/biceps anchor lesions; and

7. adhesive capsulitis (frozen shoulder).

Table 5–1. Motion at the shoulder joint.

Movement	Muscles[1]	Nerve Supply[2]
Flexion	Pectoralis major, clavicular part	Pectoral nerves
	Deltoid, clavicular part	Axillary
	Biceps, short head	Musculotaneous
	Coracobrachialis	Musculocutaneous
Extension	Deltoid, posterior part	Axillary
	Latissimus dorsi (if shoulder flexed)	Thoracodorsal
	Teres major (if shoulder flexed)	Subscapular
Abduction	Deltoid, acromial part	Axillary
	Supraspinatus	Suprascapular
Adduction	Pectoralis major, sternocostal part	Pectoral
	Latissimus dorsi	Thoracodorsal
	Teres major	Subscapular
External rotation of the humerus	Pectoralis major	Axillary
	Infraspinatus	Suprascapular
	Teres minor	Axillary
Internal rotation of the humerus	Pectoralis major	Pectoral
	Latissimus dorsi	Thoracodorsal
	Deltoid, clavicular part	Axillary
	Teres major	Subscapular
	Subscapularis	Subscapular
Stabilization[3]	Subscapularis	Subscapular
	Supraspinatus	Suprascapular
	Infraspinatus	Suprascapular
	Teres minor	Axillary
	Triceps, long head	Radial
	Biceps, long head	Musculocutaneous

[1] The actions of the muscles listed presuppose a fixed scapula. If the arm is flexed, muscles passing from the shoulder girdle to the arm will move the girdle on the trunk. If the shoulder joint is fixed, muscles passing from the trunk to the humerus will move the girdle on the trunk at the sternoclavicular joint.

[2] At the shoulder joint no movement is controlled by one nerve alone. However, some movements have their major muscle (or muscles) innervated by a single nerve and so are severely affected by damage to that nerve, eg, the axillary nerve in abduction, extension, and external rotation. Thus, destruction of the axillary nerve leads to the shoulder being held in a position of adduction, internal rotation, and flexion.

[3] All the muscles of stabilization are attached close to the shoulder joint, have a poor mechanical advantage over it, and are more effective in holding the joint that in moving it.

B. TECHNIQUE

With the patient either in the lateral decubitus or the beach chair position, the arthroscope is inserted into a posterior portal, medial and inferior to the posterolateral corner of the acromion. With visualization of the glenohumeral joint, an anterior portal immediately lateral to the coracoid allows entrance of additional instruments. Distal clavicle excision, removal of loose bodies, and capsular release of adhesive capsulitis can be performed. An additional anterior portal inferior to the first may aid in instability repair with an arthroscopic technique. The arthroscope is then removed from the joint and placed into the subacromial bursa. Portals lateral to the acromion allow subacromial decompression and rotator cuff repair to be carried out with arthroscopic techniques.

C. STEPS IN EVALUATION

Examination of shoulder range of motion and stability with the patient under anesthesia is helpful in the diagnosis and treatment of shoulder injuries. This should be performed in the operating room prior to arthroscopy. The steps in arthroscopic examination should then include the following:

1. glenohumeral articular surfaces;
2. rotator cuff from inside the joint;
3. labrum including the biceps anchor;
4. anterior capsuloligamentous structures;
5. rotator cuff from the subacromial bursal space;
6. coracoacromial ligament;
7. acromion; and
8. acromioclavicular joint.

Applegate GR et al: Chronic labral tears: value of magnetic resonance arthrography in evaluating the glenoid labrum and labral-bicipital complex. Arthroscopy 2004;20(9):959.

Kaplan LD et al: Internal impingement: findings on magnetic resonance imaging and arthroscopic evaluation. Arthroscopy 2004;20(7):701.

Lee DH et al: The double-density sign: a radiographic finding suggestive of an os acromiale. J Bone Joint Surg Am 2004; 86-A(12):2666.

Lindauer KR et al: MR imaging appearance of 180-360 degrees labral tears of the shoulder. Skeletal Radiol 2005;34(2):74.

Magee T et al: Shoulder MR arthrography: which patient group benefits most? Am J Roentgenol 2004;183(4):969.

Middleton WD et al: Sonography of the rotator cuff: analysis of interobserver variability. Am J Roentgenol 2004;183(5):1465.

Porcellini G et al: Arthroscopic treatment of calcifying tendinitis of the shoulder: clinical and ultrasonographic follow-up findings at two to five years. J Shoulder Elbow Surg 2004;13(5):503.

■ SHOULDER TENDON & MUSCLE INJURY

ROTATOR CUFF TENDON INJURIES

Injury to the rotator cuff, a common cause of shoulder pain and disability, has a high prevalence during athletic activities. Injury to the rotator cuff may result in pain, weakness, and decreased range of motion. Symptoms are often worsened by activity, especially when the hand is positioned overhead. Night pain is also common, and many patients complain of awakening after rolling onto

the affected shoulder. Although shoulder weakness and decreased range of motion usually result from a rotator cuff tendon tear, pain alone from subacromial bursitis or rotator cuff tendinitis may also be the cause. Each of these entities most often results from impingement syndrome.

IMPINGEMENT SYNDROME

Any prolonged repetitive activity involving overhead motion such as tennis, pitching, golf, or swimming may cause compromise of the space between the humeral head and the coracoacromial arch, which includes the acromion, the coracoacromial ligament, and the coracoid process. Impingement causes microtrauma to the rotator cuff, resulting in local inflammation, edema, cuff softening, pain, and poor function. These problems may even cause greater impingement, producing a continuous vicious cycle (Figure 5–3). This cycle may be precipitated by acute injury to the rotator cuff tendon itself. Blood supply to this tendon is precarious, thus decreasing its capacity for healing.

1. Subacromial Bursitis

ESSENTIALS OF DIAGNOSIS

- *History of repetitive overhead activity.*
- *Mild pain with overhead shoulder motion.*
- *No gross atrophy or profound weakness.*
- *Pain is relieved with a subacromial lidocaine injection.*

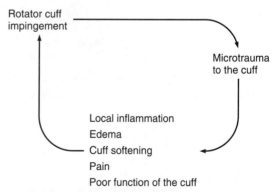

Figure 5–3. The cycle of injury and reinjury resulting from rotator cuff impingement. (Reprinted with permission from McMahon PJ, Skinner HB: Sports medicine. In: Skinner HB (editor): *Current Diagnosis & Treatment in Orthopedics,* 3rd ed. McGraw-Hill, 2003.)

Prevention

Limiting repetitive overhead activities and maintenance of good rotator cuff strength are keys to prevention. Additionally, overall conditioning and stretching and strengthening with careful attention paid to technique can be helpful in minimizing many injuries resulting from overuse.

Clinical Findings

Bursitis of the shoulder refers to an inflammation of the subacromial bursa. It has the mildest signs and symptoms of shoulder impingement. Pain is present with activity involving overhead motion and there is usually no pain or only mild pain with the arm at the side.

Active range of shoulder motion may be limited by pain. No atrophy of the shoulder muscles is present and manual muscle testing demonstrates mild weakness. Passively, when the internally rotated shoulder is moved into forward flexion, the patient will experience discomfort. This is called the Neer impingement sign (Figure 5–4). This pain then resolves and there is a dramatic increase in strength and range of motion with the Neer impingement test (10 mL of lidocaine is injected into the subacromial space).

Radiographic views of the subacromial space such as the supraspinatus outlet view may show a spur on the undersurface of the acromion, causing narrowing of the subacromial space. In recent years, advances in imaging methods such as ultrasonography and MRI have aided in the diagnosis of subacromial bursitis, rotator cuff tendinitis, and rotator cuff tendon tear (Figure 5–5).

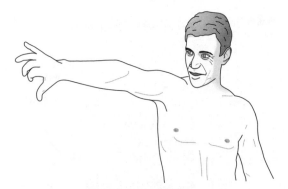

Figure 5–4. Evaluating for impingement of the supraspinatus with the Neer impingement sign. (Reprinted with permission from McMahon PJ, Skinner HB: Sports medicine. In: Skinner HB (editor): *Current Diagnosis & Treatment in Orthopedics,* 3rd ed. McGraw-Hill, 2003.)

Treatment

Treatment for impingement syndrome starts with conservative measures such as activity modification, physical therapy, and oral nonsteroidal antiinflammatory drugs (NSAIDs). Modalities such as heat and cold, iontophoresis or phonophoresis, and microelectric nerve stimulation may also be helpful. Only with normal function of the rotator cuff tendons will glenohumeral mechanics be improved and the impingement syndrome cease. If this treatment fails, a subacromial injection of corticosteroids may be helpful.

Surgical intervention is indicated only after failure of a prolonged conservative treatment program (a minimum of 3 months). If the subacromial space is narrow, shaving the undersurface of the acromion may result in relief of symptoms. This procedure can be done arthroscopically to decrease postoperative discomfort and minimize the complication of deltoid muscle rupture from the acromion.

Prognosis

Most patients respond well to nonoperative management, and those who require surgical decompression are usually able to return to pain-free activities as well.

2. Rotator Cuff Tendinitis

ESSENTIALS OF DIAGNOSIS

- *History of repetitive overhead activity.*
- *Similar to subacromial bursitis.*
- *Moderate pain with overhead shoulder motion.*
- *No gross atrophy or profound weakness.*
- *Pain is relieved by a subacromial lidocaine injection.*

Prevention

As with subacromial bursitis, limiting repetitive overhead activities and maintenance of good rotator cuff strength are keys to prevention. Additionally, overall conditioning and stretching and strengthening with careful attention paid to technique can be helpful in minimizing many overuse injuries.

Clinical Findings

Of the four rotator cuff muscles, the supraspinatus tendon is most often initially involved. Rotator cuff

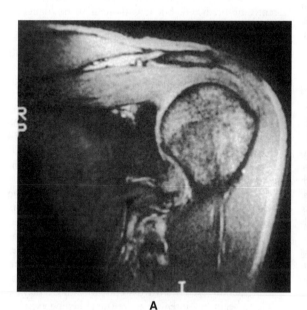

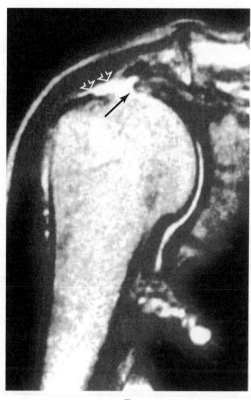

A   B

Figure 5–5. MRI demonstrating (**A**) normal shoulder anatomy and (**B**) cystic changes at the greater tuberosity with rotator cuff tear. (Reprinted with permission from McMahon PJ, Skinner HB: Sports medicine. In: Skinner HB (editor): *Current Diagnosis & Treatment in Orthopedics,* 3rd ed. McGraw-Hill, 2003.)

tendinitis also results from impingement syndrome and is characterized by pain with activity involving overhead motion. The patient may occasionally be awakened by pain at night. Active shoulder range of motion is limited by pain. Typically, no atrophy of the shoulder muscles is present and manual muscle testing demonstrates mild weakness. The Neer impingement sign is positive and the pain resolves with a subacromial injection of lidocaine.

Treatment & Prognosis

Radiographic evaluation and treatment are similar to management of subacromial bursitis. An exception is the young athlete with glenohumeral instability and secondary tendinitis. In this case, the instability should be treated first and the rotator cuff tendinitis will then resolve.

3. Rotator Cuff Tendon Tear

ESSENTIALS OF DIAGNOSIS

- *Pain with activity involving overhead motion.*
- *Night pain.*
- *Progressive loss of strength.*
- *Progressive atrophy of rotator cuff muscles.*

Prevention

Maintenance of overall body conditioning with regular stretching and strengthening of the rotator cuff and scapular stabilizing muscles can help prevent rotator cuff injuries.

Clinical Findings

A rotator cuff tendon tear is characterized by pain with activity involving overhead motion. However, the patient is often awakened at night with pain as well. The athlete with a chronic rotator cuff tear may experience a gradual loss of strength. Pain may be persistent, occurring even when the arm is at the side. Active range of shoulder motion is limited, and if the tear is severe, there will be atrophy of the shoulder muscles. Manual muscle testing demonstrates weakness. The Neer impingement sign is positive and the pain resolves with a subacromial injection of lidocaine. Radiographic evaluation is similar to that for subacromial bursitis and rotator cuff tendinitis.

Treatment

Radiographic evaluation and treatment are similar to subacromial bursitis management. Unlike acute tears, chronic rotator cuff tears often present insidiously, with slow progression from subacromial bursitis to rotator cuff tendinitis and eventual tendon tear. Differentiating severe rotator cuff tendinitis from partial or small full-thickness chronic rotator cuff tears may be difficult.

There are two important considerations in treating an individual with a rotator cuff tear—the current symptoms and the risk of the tear progressing. Although the lesion location and size are helpful in describing a rotator cuff tear, symptoms do not correlate with these factors alone. Some individuals are able to cope with the symptoms of a rotator cuff tear and some may be completely asymptomatic. The severity of symptoms is influenced by a number of other factors including pain tolerance, the acute or chronic nature of the injury, the age and activity level of the individual, humeral head superior migration, shoulder muscle strength, muscle atrophy, fatty changes in the muscle, arthritis, and workman's compensation status.

Rest, rehabilitation, and taking NSAIDs, sometimes for as long as 4–9 months, may relieve symptoms. Range-of-motion and strengthening exercises are recommended, unless they cause significant discomfort. Stengthening the other shoulder muscles may increase the individual's ability to cope with the rotator cuff tear. Avoidance of activities that exacerbate the symptoms, such as activities involving overhead motion, is also recommended. Symptoms of pain, weakness, or decreased range of motion that persist after a nonoperative treatment program has been tried indicate the need for surgical intervention.

Because rotator cuff tears may progress in size over time, immediate repair may be warranted in some at-risk individuals. Both epidemiologic and imaging studies of the general population indicate a high incidence of partial-thickness rotator cuff tears at younger ages and full-thickness rotator cuff tears at older ages. The increasing prevalence of rotator cuff injuries in older individuals may be the best evidence that rotator cuff tears progress in severity. Specifically, about 25% of individuals over 60 years of age have a tear and in those over 80 years of age, there is a full-thickness rotator cuff tear in about 50% of individuals. The risk of a rotator cuff tear progressing to a more severe tear cannot currently be predicted, but it is thought to be higher in young, active individuals, partly because they have many more years to sustain an injury.

The thin degenerated tissue of a chronic rotator cuff tear makes surgical repair more difficult than repair of an acute tear. The repair can be accomplished with either an arthroscopic or an open technique. Surgical decompression of the subacromial space to remove spurs should also be considered. Some severe tears may be impossible to repair. This includes tears that are large to massive in size or that involve two or more rotator cuff tendons. Debridement of the rotator cuff and the subacromial spurs may diminish pain in such instances.

Rehabilitation after a repair lasts from 3 months to a year with gradual exercise progression needed to restore normal, or near normal, function and strength. This varies with the size of the tear that was repaired and the type of surgery performed. Typically, immediately after the procedure, passive motion and isometric strengthening exercises start, along with elbow-, hand-, and grip-strengthening exercises. At 6 weeks, the athlete may be able to begin low-intensity active strengthening exercises against gravity. The goals are to bring the athlete to normal strength with a functional, pain-free range of motion.

Prognosis

The prognosis following a rotator cuff tear depends on many factors as described above. There are few specific criteria governing return to sports following rotator cuff injuries. Determining factors must be individualized to the athlete, considering the nature and treatment of the rotator cuff injury as well as the desired sport. Patients must be pain free and have attained full range of motion with near full strength prior to returning to their sport to minimize reinjury.

4. Partial Thickness Rotator Cuff Tear

A partial articular sided tendon avulsion is much more common than a bursal side tear of the rotator cuff. As with other rotator cuff injuries, symptoms may resolve with appropriate physical therapy and analgesics. Yet, some individuals with a partial thickness tear have persistent or recurrent symptoms. If a conservative program of exercises and gradual return to activity do not lead to steady improvement, then further diagnostic evaluation with ultrasonography, MRI, or arthroscopy may be helpful. Whereas repair of the partial-thickness rotator cuff tear may be best in some, debridement of the abnormal cuff may diminish or relieve symptoms in others. Some clinicians use involvement of greater than 50% of the tendon thickness as an indication for repair. Repair necessitates a rehabilitation program similar to that described above for full-thickness rotator cuff tears. Following debridement, immediate resumption of range-of-motion and muscle-strengthening exercises begins. Typically, it requires 6–12 months for an athlete whose sport involves throwing to return to athletics following arthroscopic debridement of a partial-thickness rotator cuff tear.

Klepps S et al: Prospective evaluation of the effect of rotator cuff integrity on the outcome of open rotator cuff repairs. Am J Sports Med 2004;32(7):1716.

Lam F, Mok D: Open repair of massive rotator cuff tears in patients aged sixty-five years or over: is it worthwhile? J Shoulder Elbow Surg 2004;13(5):517.

Millstein ES, Snyder SJ: Arthroscopic evaluation and management of rotator cuff tears. Orthop Clin North Am 2003;34(4):507.

O'Holleran JD et al: Determinants of patient satisfaction with outcome after rotator cuff surgery. J Bone Joint Surg Am 2005;87-A(1):121.

Rebuzzi E et al: Arthroscopic rotator cuff repair in patients older than 60 years. Arthroscopy 2005;21(1):48.

Romeo AA et al: Shoulder scoring scales for the evaluation of rotator cuff repair. Clin Orthop 2004;1(427):107.

Sperling JW et al: Rotator cuff repair in patients fifty years of age and younger. J Bone Joint Surg Am 2004;86-A(10):2212.

BICEPS TENDON INJURIES

1. Bicipital Tendinitis

ESSENTIALS OF DIAGNOSIS

- *Pain localized to the anterior proximal humerus and shoulder joint.*
- *Pain with resisted forward flexion and supination.*
- *Pain may be relieved by a steroid injection into the sheath of the biceps tendon.*

Prevention

Similar to the prevention of rotator cuff injuries, general conditioning and stretching and strengthening before activities can help minimize injury to the biceps tendon.

Clinical Findings

The long head of the biceps muscle is an intraarticular structure deep in the rotator cuff tendon as it passes under the acromion to its insertion at the top of the glenoid. The same mechanism that initiates symptoms of impingement syndrome in rotator cuff injuries may inflame the tendon of the biceps in its subacromial position, causing bicipital tendinitis.

Tendinitis may also result from subluxation of the tendon out of its groove in the proximal humerus, which occurs with rupture of the transverse ligament. The symptoms of bicipital tendinitis, whether the result of impingement or tendon subluxation, are essentially the same. Pain is localized to the proximal humerus and shoulder joint, with resisted supination of the forearm aggravating the pain. Pain may also occur on manual testing of the elbow flexors and on palpation of the tendon itself. The Yergason test is used to determine instability of the long head of the biceps in its groove.

Treatment

If the tendinitis is associated with shoulder impingement, then therapy aimed at treating the impingement syndrome will relieve the bicipital tendinitis. If subluxation of the tendon within its groove is the cause of the irritation, conservative therapy includes NSAIDs and restriction of activities, followed by a slow resumption of activities after a period of rest. Strengthening of the muscles that assist the biceps in elbow flexion and forearm supination is also beneficial. Steroid injections into the sheath of the biceps tendon are helpful, but they may be hazardous if placed into the substance of the tendon because they will promote tendon degeneration. Persistent symptoms may warrant tenodesis of the biceps tendon directly into the humerus.

Prognosis

Recovery from biceps tenodesis is difficult, and it is doubtful if a competitive athlete could return to peak performance after treatment.

2. Biceps Tendon Rupture

ESSENTIALS OF DIAGNOSIS

- *"Popeye" appearance of the upper arm from the retraction of the biceps muscle mass.*
- *May or may not be painful and ecchymotic depending on the chronicity of the injury.*

Prevention

Similar to the prevention of rotator cuff injuries, general conditioning and stretching and strengthening before activities can help minimize injury to the biceps tendon.

Clinical Findings

The long head of the biceps tendon may rupture proximally, either from the supraglenoid tubercle of the scapula at the entrance of the bicipital groove proximally, or at the exit of the tunnel at the musculotendinous junction. The muscle mass moves distally, producing a bulging appearance to the arm. Rupture of the long head of the biceps is predictive of a rotator cuff tear. Rupture of the biceps distally at its insertion involves both heads and the muscle mass moves proximally. The mechanism is usually a forceful flexion of the arm and is more common in older athletes, or following direct trauma. Microtears probably serve to render the tendon vulnerable to an acute tearing event. The degree of ecchymosis is dependent on the location of the tear, with avascular areas having less and the musculotendinous junction producing quite a noticeable amount of ecchymosis. Diagnosis is usually easily accomplished, as the deformity is obvious.

Treatment

Surgical treatment of proximal ruptures, if indicated, is usually reserved for younger patients. Open surgical repair leaves a long scar and usually does not completely restore the underlying anatomy. The coiled-up distal end of the tendon is usually found beneath the attachment of the pectoralis major. A correlation exists between proximal biceps tendon rupture and rotator cuff tears in middle-aged and older athletes. Rupture of the distal biceps tendon often warrants surgical repair, due to loss of forearm flexion and supination strength. In this case, the tendon is usually found about 5–6 cm above the elbow joint, and care must be taken to avoid damage to the lateral antebrachial cutaneous nerve.

Prognosis

Athletes are permitted to return to full contact play once they have achieved maximal functional strength and range of elbow motion, which typically occurs 4–6 months following a distal biceps repair.

Cope MR et al: Biceps rupture in body builders: three case reports of rupture of the long head of the biceps at the tendon-labrum junction. J Shoulder Elbow Surg 2004;13(5):580.

Vidal AF et al: Biceps tendon and triceps tendon injuries. Clin Sports Med 2004;23(4):707.

PECTORALIS MAJOR RUPTURE

ESSENTIALS OF DIAGNOSIS

- Sudden pain.
- Ecchymosis and swelling along the pectoralis major muscle.

Prevention

Similar to the prevention of rotator cuff injuries, general conditioning and stretching and strengthening before activities can help minimize injury to the pectoralis major.

Clinical Findings

Rupture of the pectoralis major tendon is an uncommon injury, usually occurring during bench press exercises in weight lifting and caused by sudden unexpected muscle contraction during pulling or lifting. The athlete usually experiences sudden pain and develops local ecchymosis and swelling. As the swelling subsides, a sulcus and deformity may be visible, and the patient notices weakness of the arm in adduction and internal rotation.

Treatment

The rupture may be partial or complete, and nonoperative treatment usually results in satisfactory function for the activities of daily life. Surgery may be considered if the athlete wishes to return to heavy weight lifting.

Prognosis

Athletes are permitted to return to contact sports once they have achieved full strength and range of motion, which typically occurs 6 months following a pectoralis major repair.

Aarimaa V et al: Rupture of the pectoralis major muscle. Am J Sports Med 2004;32(5):1256.

GLENOHUMERAL JOINT INSTABILITY

To make the correct diagnosis the glenohumeral joint must be tested for anterior, posterior, and inferior instability. Different classifications of glenohumeral joint instability have been proposed, based on etiology, the direction of the instability, or on various combinations. TUBS is an acronym describing instability caused by a *t*raumatic event, which is *u*nidirectional, is associated with a *B*ankart lesion, and often requires *s*urgical treatment. AMBRI refers to *a*traumatic, *m*ultidirectional instability that may be *b*ilateral and is best treated by *r*ehabilitation. In this classification, the etiology of multidirectional instability is thought to be enlargement of the capsule from either a genetic or microtraumatic origin.

The positive sulcus sign has been used as the diagnostic hallmark for multidirectional instability, but we now know that the sulcus sign is sometimes found in shoulders of asymptomatic individuals with increased laxity. Laxity or joint play is a trait of body constitution that differs from one individual to another. Individuals

Table 5–2. Classification of glenohumeral instability based on the direction of instability and the
presence or absence of hyperlaxity.

| Laxity | Direction | |
	UDI (Unidirectional Instability)	*MDI (Multidirectional Instability)*
Normal	Very common	Very rare
	60%	3%
Increased	Common	Rare
	30%	7%

Adapted, with permission, from Gerber C: Observations of
the classification of instability. In: *Complex and Revision
Problems in Shoulder Surgery.* Warner JJ et al (editors).
Lippincott-Raven, 1997, pp. 9–18.

may be loose or tight jointed. A shoulder is hyperlax if
the examiner can easily subluxate the humeral head out
of the glenoid in the anterior, posterior, and inferior
directions without eliciting symptoms. Unfortunately,
this makes classification of instability based on etiology,
or direction alone, extremely difficult. Instead, classification is best based on the direction of instability that
elicits symptoms and the presence or absence of hyperlaxity (Table 5–2).

Gerber C, Nyffeler RW: Classification of glenohumeral instability.
Clin Orthop 2002;400:65.

1. Glenohumeral Joint Instability Evaluation

Anterior Instability

The apprehension test is performed to assess anterior
instability. The test applies an anterior-directed force to
the humeral head from the back with the arm in abduction and external rotation (Figure 5–6). A positive test
results from the patient's apprehension that the joint
will dislocate. This maneuver mimics the position of
subluxation, or dislocation, and causes reflex guarding.
Conversely, the relocation test is positive if relief is
obtained by applying a posterior-directed force to the
humeral head (Figure 5–7).

Posterior Instability

No single test has high sensitivity and specificity for
posterior instability. The posterior apprehension test is
performed by applying a posterior-directed force to the
forward flexed and internally rotated shoulder. To perform the circumduction test the patient is instructed to

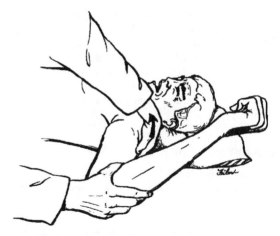

Figure 5–6. The apprehension test for anterior insta-
bility. (Reprinted with permission from McMahon PJ,
Skinner HB: Sports medicine. In: Skinner HB (editor):
Current Diagnosis & Treatment in Orthopedics, 3rd ed.
McGraw-Hill, 2003.)

actively move the shoulder in a large circle starting
from a flexed, internally rotated and cross-body position, then to forward flexion, then to an abducted and
externally rotated position, and lastly to the arm at
the side. The examiner stands behind the patient and
palpates the posterior shoulder. If positive, the joint

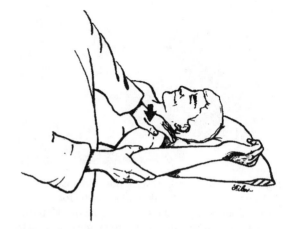

Figure 5–7. The relocation test is positive if relief is
obtained by applying a posterior directed force to the
humeral head. (Reprinted with permission from
McMahon PJ, Skinner HB: Sports medicine. In: Skinner HB
(editor): *Current Diagnosis & Treatment in Orthopedics,* 3rd
ed. McGraw-Hill, 2003.)

subluxes in the flexed, internally rotated and cross-body position, and reduces as the shoulder is moved. For the Jahnke test, a posteriorly directed force is applied to the forward flexed shoulder. The shoulder is then moved into the coronal plane as an anterior directed force is applied to the humeral head. A clunk occurs as the humeral head reduces from the subluxed position (Figure 5–8).

Inferior Instability

The sulcus sign is used to evaluate laxity and inferior instability. The test is performed with the athlete in a sitting position with the arm at the side. A distraction force is applied longitudinally along the humerus. If positive, discomfort or apprehension of instability is experienced as the skin just distal to the lateral acromion hollows out (Figure 5–9).

2. Glenohumeral Dislocation

When the shoulder is forced beyond the limit of its normal range of motion, the articular surface of the humeral head may be displaced from the glenoid to varying degrees. The majority of glenohumeral dislocations, or subluxations, are in the anteroinferior direction.

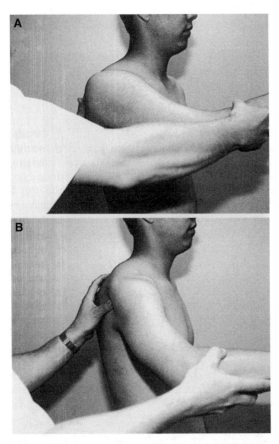

Figure 5–8. The Jahnke test for posterior instability. **A:** A posterior directed force applied to the forward flexed shoulder. **B:** The shoulder is then moved into the coronal plane as an anterior directed force is applied to the humeral head. A clunk occurs as the humeral head reduces from the subluxed position. [Reprinted with permission from Hawkins RJ, Boker DJ: Clinical evaluation of shoulder problems. In: Rockwood CA et al (editors) *The Shoulder.* WB Saunders, 1998.]

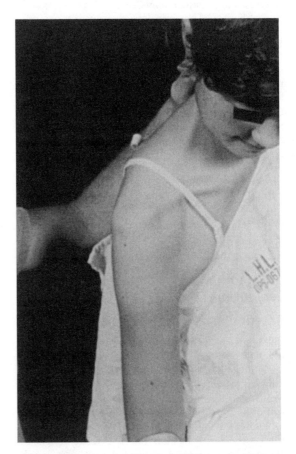

Figure 5–9. The sulcus sign for inferior instability. With the elbow grasped, inferior traction is applied. Dimpling of the skin below the acromion may be seen. Palpation reveals widening of the subacromial space between the acromion and the humeral head. [Reprinted with permission from Hawkins RJ, Boker DJ: Clinical evaluation of shoulder problems. In: Rockwood CA et al (editors): *The Shoulder.* WB Saunders, 1998.]

3. Anterior Dislocation

ESSENTIALS OF DIAGNOSIS

- The arm is typically held supported at the side.
- A visible dimple may be seen under the acromion due to the absence of the humeral head.
- The humeral head may be palpable under the coracoid or in the axilla.
- Range of motion will be extremely painful and limited.
- Appropriate radiographs will confirm the direction of dislocation and possible associated injuries.

ANATOMICAL LESIONS

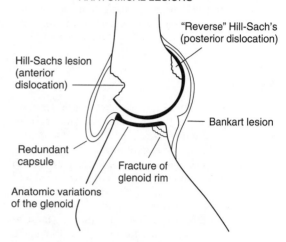

Figure 5–10. Anatomic lesions associated with shoulder instability. (Reprinted with permission from McMahon PJ, Skinner HB: Sports medicine. In: Skinner HB (editor): *Current Diagnosis & Treatment in Orthopedics*, 3rd ed. McGraw-Hill, 2003.)

Prevention

Shoulder dislocations are typically the result of an acute traumatic injury. Therefore, although avoiding injury to the shoulder is the best form of prevention, minimizing the risk of dislocation following a blow can be achieved with regular stretching and strengthening of the rotator cuff musculature.

Clinical Findings

Anterior glenohumeral dislocation occurs from either an external rotation, or abduction force on the humerus, a direct posterior blow to the proximal humerus, or a posterolateral blow on the shoulder strong enough to displace the humeral head. The anterior capsule is either stretched or torn within its attachment to the anterior glenoid. The head may be displaced into a subcoracoid, subglenoid, subclavicular, or intrathoracic position. Two major lesions are typically seen in patients with recurrent anterior dislocations (Figure 5–10). First is the Bankart lesion, an anterior capsular injury associated with a tear of the glenoid labrum off the anterior glenoid rim. The Bankart lesion may occur with fractures of the glenoid rim. Such fractures are often minimally displaced, and treatment is usually dictated by the joint instability. The second major lesion associated with recurrent anterior dislocations is the Hill–Sachs lesion, a compression fracture of the posterolateral articular surface of the humeral head. It is created by the sharp edge of the anterior glenoid as the humeral head dislocates over it. When large, both the Bankart and the Hill-Sachs lesions predispose to recurrent dislocations when the arm is placed in abduction and external rotation. If the glenoid rim fracture involves more than 20% of the glenoid diameter, then the joint becomes prone to instability and treatment with open reduction and internal fixation is best. If the fracture is old, or the glenoid rim is worn to a similar level, then corticocancellous bone grafting of the glenoid rim is indicated.

Other injuries associated with anterior dislocation may occur. These include avulsion of the greater tuberosity from the humerus, caused by traction from the rotator cuff, and injury to the axillary nerve, which may be stretched or torn. Permanent loss of axillary nerve function results in denervation of the deltoid muscle and loss of sensation over the proximal lateral aspect of the arm. Axillary nerve palsy may also occur during reduction of the dislocation, and therefore should be tested both before and after reduction. The deltoid extension lag sign, described in the section on Axillary Nerve Injury, may be the best way to assess function of this nerve. Lastly, the dead arm syndrome may occur after anterior joint instability. For example, a pitcher may report a sudden inability to throw, with the arm going numb and becoming extremely weak after ball release. The symptoms are transient, resolving within a few seconds to minutes.

Athletes who sustain a shoulder dislocation will try to hold the injured extremity at their side, gripping the forearm with the opposite hand. Most athletes know their shoulder is dislocated, and will immediately seek help. On physical examination of an anterior dislocation, the examiner will note a space underneath the acromion where the humeral head should lie and a palpable anterior mass representing the humeral head in the anterior axilla.

Treatment

Acute and recurrent anterior glenohumeral dislocations must be distinguished, as an acute dislocation sustains severe trauma with the increased probability of associated injuries. The recurrent dislocation may occur with minimal trauma, and reduction may be accomplished with much less effort. Anterior dislocations may be reduced by one of several techniques. Longitudinal traction may be exerted on the affected arm with external rotation, followed by internal rotation of the arm. Care must be taken to avoid direct pressure on the neurovascular structures. Another method is to have the patient lie face down on the table and tie or tape a bucket to the injured arm and slowly fill it with water. This allows the musculature around the shoulder to relax from the force of the weight, and effect a spontaneous reduction.

Following reduction of an initial dislocation, the shoulder should be immobilized in internal rotation for 2–6 weeks. Healing will generally take at least 6 weeks. Before returning to athletics, the patient should have normal range of motion without pain and normal strength in the shoulder. Emphasis must be placed on strengthening the rotator cuff muscles to compensate for the laxity of the ligamentous support. When weight training is begun, military press, fly exercises, a narrow grip while bench pressing, and deep shoulder dips must be excluded until considerable time has elapsed and healing is complete.

Recurrent dislocations should be treated with minimal immobilization until the pain subsides, followed by range-of-motion and muscle-strengthening exercises. Many restraining devices are available to help prevent recurrent dislocations during sporting activities, focusing on keeping the arm from going into abduction and external rotation. These orthotics may be effective, but because they limit the athlete's range of shoulder motion, their use is limited for certain competitive activities.

If an athlete has sustained multiple dislocations and is unresponsive to conservative treatment, surgical reconstruction of the shoulder joint may be indicated. The orthopedic literature presents a wide variety of procedures to correct the instability, with most involving repair of the labral defect, and tightening of the anterior capsule and ligamentous structures through an anterior incision (Table 5–3).

For most surgical procedures, aggressive range-of-motion exercises do not start until at least 3 weeks postoperatively. The goal is to have full abduction and 90° of external rotation. By 12 weeks, patients have often progressed well into their initial programs and may begin a variety of weight training exercises, avoiding exercises that strain the anterior capsule.

Table 5–3. Surgical procedures for the treatment of shoulder instability.

Bankart procedure
Du Toit procedure
Viek procedure
Eyre–Brook procedure
Moseley procedure
Muscle and capsule placation
Putti–Platt procedure
Symeonides procedure
Muscle and tendon sling procedures
Magnuson–Stack procedure
Bristow–Helfet–Latarjet procedure modifications
Boytchev procedure
Nicola procedure
Gallie–LeMesurier procedure
Boyd transfer of long head of biceps (for posterior dislocation)
Bone block
Eden–Hybbinette procedure
DeAnquin procedure (through a superior approach to the shoulder)
Osteotomies
Weber (humeral neck)
Saha (humeral shaft)

Prognosis

Young patients are at a high risk for redislocation after a primary traumatic anterior shoulder dislocation if treated conservatively with rehabilitation. Surgical stabilization should be considered in these cases. In general, despite surgical stabilization, patients have up to a 10% chance of redislocation if returning to play in contact sports.

4. Posterior Dislocation

ESSENTIALS OF DIAGNOSIS

- *Posterior dislocations are more difficult to diagnose than anterior dislocations.*
- *The arm is typically held in internal rotation, and is not able to be externally rotated.*
- *Appropriate radiographs will confirm the direction of dislocation and possible associated injuries.*

Prevention

Shoulder dislocations are typically the result of an acute traumatic injury. Therefore, while avoiding injury to the shoulder is the best form of prevention, the risk of dislocation following a blow can be minimized with regular stretching and strengthening of the rotator cuff musculature.

Clinical Findings

Posterior glenohumeral dislocations result from the posterior capsule being torn, stretched, or disrupted from the posterior glenoid. A reverse Hill–Sachs lesion (Figure 5–10) may appear on the anterior articular surface of the humerus. With a posterior dislocation, the subscapularis, or its insertion on the lesser tuberosity, may be injured. Posterior dislocations are often difficult to diagnose, as the patient may have a normal contour to the shoulder or the deltoid of a well-developed athlete may mask signs of a displaced humeral head. The patient holds the injured shoulder in internal rotation and the examiner cannot externally rotate it. Anteroposterior and axillary radiographs must be obtained to diagnose a posterior dislocation.

Treatment

Applying traction in the line of the adducted humerus, with an anterior directed force to the humeral head, reduces a posterior dislocation. Anesthesia often helps decrease the trauma of reduction. Following reduction, the shoulder is immobilized for 2–6 weeks in external rotation and a small amount of abduction. Surgical treatment should be considered if these measures fail to provide the desired results.

Prognosis

Patients with an acute posterior dislocation are often able to return to their sport following a course of rehabilitation emphasizing range-of-motion and rotator cuff strengthening.

MULTIDIRECTIONAL INSTABILITY

ESSENTIALS OF DIAGNOSIS

- *Symptomatic global instability of the shoulder.*
- *Nonspecific shoulder pain, fatigue, apprehension, or paresthesias may be present.*
- *Increased translation on the load and shift test in more than one direction.*
- *Positive sulcus sign.*
- *Must be evaluated for signs of hyperlaxity and distinguished from instability.*

Clinical Findings

Some patients will have instability in both the anterior and posterior directions, which is most often subluxation and not dislocation. This may result in a painful shoulder, especially if rotator cuff strength decreases. The pain is often primarily a result of rotator cuff inflammation, likely from attempts to stabilize the humeral head during activity. Patients may complain of vague symptoms including upper extremity fatigue, discomfort, pain, apprehension, and paresthesias. They may describe frank episodes of instability. Physical examination should include evaluation for signs of generalized hyperlaxity, which include hyperextension of the metacarpophalangeal joints, elbows, and knees and the ability to adduct the thumb to the ipsilateral wrist. Generalized hyperlaxity does not necessarily indicate symptomatic instability of the shoulder. The shoulder examination should include tests for anterior, posterior, and inferior instability as described above. MRI can be a useful adjunct to plain radiographs and may reveal an enlarged axillary pouch and labral or rotator cuff pathology.

Treatment & Prognosis

The mainstay of treatment for multidirectional instability involves a conservative program, which leads to successful results in the vast majority of cases. This includes patient education, modification of activity, and a strengthening program for the rotator cuff and scapular stabilizing muscles.

Brophy RH, Marx RG: Osteoarthritis following shoulder instability. Clin Sports Med 2005;24(1):47.

Good CR, Macgillivray JD: Traumatic shoulder dislocation in the adolescent athlete: advances in surgical treatment. Curr Opin Pediatr 2005;17(1):25.

Kim SH et al: Painful jerk test: a predictor of success in nonoperative treatment of posteroinferior instability of the shoulder. Am J Sports Med 2004;32(8):1849.

Kim SH et al: Loss of chondrolabral containment of the gleno-humeral joint in atraumatic posteroinferior multidirectional instability. J Bone Joint Surg Am 2005;87-A(1):92.

Kirkley A et al: Prospective randomized clinical trial comparing the effectiveness of immediate arthroscopic stabilization versus immobilization and rehabilitation in first traumatic anterior dislocations of the shoulder: long-term evaluation. Arthroscopy 2005;21(1):55.

Krishnan SG et al: A soft tissue attempt to stabilize the multiply operated glenohumeral joint with multidirectional instability. Clin Orthop 2004;(429):256.

Safran O et al: Posterior humeral avulsion of the glenohumeral ligament as a cause of posterior shoulder instability. A case report. J Bone Joint Surg Am 2004;86-A(12):2732.

GLENOID LABRUM INJURY

ESSENTIALS OF DIAGNOSIS

- *Pain or clicking as the arm is taken through a range of motion.*
- *Pain or apprehension when the arm is brought into the abducted externally rotated position, often relieved by a posteriorly directed froce on the humeral head.*
- *Discomfort with horizontal adduction of the shoulder.*
- *MRI (with or without intraarticular contrast) can aid in the diagnosis.*

Prevention

As labral injuries can result from repetitive activity or an acute traumatic event, it is important to maintain good strength and flexibility of the shoulder to minimize these injuries.

Clinical Findings

The glenoid labrum is a fibrocartilaginous rim around the glenoid fossa that deepens the socket and provides stability for the humeral head. It is also a connection for the surrounding capsuloligamentous structures. Glenoid labrum tears may occur from repetitive shoulder motion or acute trauma. In the athlete with repeated anterior subluxation of the shoulder, tears of the anteroinferior labrum may occur, leading to progressive instability.

Weight lifters may also develop glenoid labrum tears as a result of repetitive bench pressing and overhead pressing. Weakness in the posterior rotator cuff may aggravate this condition. Tears of the glenoid labrum may also occur from acute trauma such as falling on an outstretched arm, but are also seen in the leading shoulders of golfers and batters when they ground their clubs or bats.

Patients with glenoid labrum injuries may describe pain that interrupts the smooth functioning of the shoulder during specific activities. On examination, they may have discomfort on forced external rotation at 90° of abduction, with the pain typically not increasing as the arm goes into further abduction. Frequently, a labrum disruption may be felt as a "pop" or "click" on forced external rotation. The patient may also experience discomfort on forced horizontal adduction of the shoulder. Manual muscle testing may show associated weakness in the rotator cuff muscles. Diagnostic tests such as a computed tomography (CT) scan and MRI following injection of contrast dye into the shoulder joint may allow early detection of glenoid labrum lesions.

Treatment

Range-of-motion exercises and gradual return to activity are often successful in relieving symptoms. However, if nonoperative management fails, arthroscopic intervention may be indicated to debride a torn, symptomatic labrum. During arthroscopy, care must be taken not to debride the inferior labrum, as this may result in increased anterior shoulder instability escalating the probability of anterior shoulder dislocation. Immediately following surgery, range-of-motion exercises and strengthening training begin.

Prognosis

Usually within 2–3 weeks following arthroscopic debridement, the athlete may begin a throwing program. Baseball pitchers may be ready to throw 3 months postoperatively.

SLAP LESIONS

The use of shoulder arthroscopy in the diagnosis and treatment of shoulder disorders has led to increased awareness of superior labrum anterior posterior (SLAP) lesions. SLAP lesions involve the origin of the long head of the biceps brachii (biceps anchor) and the superior capsulolabral structures. A type I lesion involves degeneration or fraying of the labrum without instability. Type II lesions are most common, accounting for over 50% of patients with a SLAP lesion, and involve detachment of the superior labrum from the glenoid. A type III lesion involves a bucket-handle tear of the superior labrum with firm attachment of the remainder of the labrum. In type IV lesions attachment to the labrum remains, but there is an associated bucket-handle tear of the labrum that extends into the biceps tendon (Figure 5–11).

Types V–VII SLAP lesions were later added to this initial four-part classification. A type V lesion is an anterior–inferior Bankart lesion that continues superiorly to include separation of the biceps tendon. A type VI lesion includes a biceps separation with an unstable flap tear of the labrum. Finally, a type VII lesion involves a superior labrum–biceps tendon separation that extends anteriorly beneath the middle glenohumeral ligament.

ESSENTIALS OF DIAGNOSIS

- *Nonspecific shoulder pain usually associated with activities involving overhead motion.*
- *Pain with resisted forward flexion with the arm in the internally rotated and slightly adducted position, relieved by externally rotating the arm.*
- *MR arthrography can aid in the diagnosis.*

Prevention

As labral injuries can result from repetitive activity or an acute traumatic event, it is important to maintain good strength and flexibility of the shoulder to minimize these injuries.

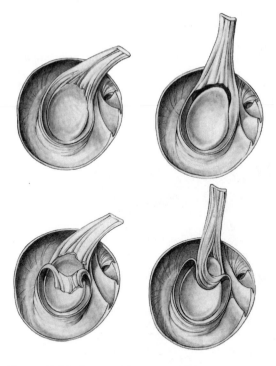

Figure 5–11. The initial four types of the SLAP lesions include fraying of the superior capsulolabrum (type 1), detachment of the superior capsulolabrum and the biceps anchor (type 2), bucket-handle tearing of the superior capsulolabrum (type 3), and detachment of the superior capsulolabrum and tearing into the biceps anchor (type 4). (Reprinted with permission from McMahon PJ, Skinner HB: Sports medicine. In: Skinner HB (editor): *Current Diagnosis & Treatment in Orthopedics,* 3rd ed. McGraw-Hill, 2003.)

Clinical Findings

Patients present with nonspecific shoulder pain associated with activity. A complicating factor in making the diagnosis is that the majority of SLAP lesions are associated with other shoulder pathology such as rotator cuff tears, acromioclavicular joint pathology, and instability. Less than 28% of SLAP lesions are isolated.

No single test is both sensitive and specific for the diagnosis of SLAP lesions. MR arthrography can be helpful. However, diagnostic arthroscopy remains the best means to definitively diagnose SLAP lesions. The active compression test may prove to be the most useful single provocative maneuver. The internally rotated shoulder is forward flexed to 90° and is then brought across the body in horizontal abduction about 10°. The test is positive if the patient has pain with resisted forward flexion that is relieved by external rotation of the shoulder.

Treatment

Treatment of SLAP lesions can be simplified by noting whether the lesion would contribute to detachment of either the biceps anchor or the anterosuperior capulolabrum. Lesions producing meaningful detachment of the anterior capsuloligamentous structures generally require repair of these structures back to the bony glenoid rim. Lesions producing significant defects extending into the biceps tendon may require biceps tenotomy, with or without tenodesis.

Holtby R, Razmjou H: Accuracy of the Speed's and Yergason's tests in detecting biceps pathology and SLAP lesions: comparison with arthroscopic findings. Arthroscopy 2004; 20(3):231.

Musgrave DS, Rodosky MW: SLAP lesions: current concepts. Am J Sports Med 2001;30(1):29.

Parentis MA et al: Disorders of the superior labrum: review and treatment guidelines. Clin Orthop 2002;400:77.

SHOULDER STIFFNESS

ESSENTIALS OF DIAGNOSIS

- *Very painful and/or limited range of motion of the shoulder.*
- *May be idiopathic or posttraumatic.*
- *Loss of active and passive range of motion, most notably internal rotation.*
- *Arthrography can aid in the diagnosis.*

Prevention

Most patients have some sort of antecedent trauma to their shoulder, be it minimal or severe. Initiating gentle range of motion and strengthening exercises immediately after the traumatic event is essential to minimizing the likelihood of developing shoulder stiffness.

Clinical Findings

Often called adhesive capsulitis or frozen shoulder, shoulder stiffness is a painful condition characterized by significant restriction in both active and passive range of motion. The shoulder is characterized as being stiff when the articular surfaces are normal and the joint is stable, yet there is a restriction in range of motion. Stiffness may also result from pathologic connections between the articular surfaces, soft tissue contracture, bursal adhesions, or a shortened muscle–tendon unit. Often of uncertain etiology, the restrictions of shoulder motion are global. That is, none of the shoulder planes of motion is spared.

Shoulder stiffness may be separated into idiopathic and posttraumatic etiologies. Idiopathic shoulder stiffness is most common in older individuals, especially women between 40 and 60 years of age. Other factors that predispose to idiopathic shoulder stiffness include cervical, cardiac, pulmonary, neoplastic, neurologic, and personality disorders. Patients with diabetes mellitus are also at a high risk of developing shoulder stiffness, with 10–35%

of diabetics having restriction of shoulder motion. Diabetics who have been insulin dependent for many years have the greatest incidence and bilateral involvement. The pathophysiology of idiopathic shoulder stiffness remains uncertain, but the pathoanatomy is commonly limited to contracture of the glenohumeral capsule (Figure 5–12). Most prominently involved is the rotator interval, which includes the coracohumeral ligament.

Although all patients can recall some traumatic event that preceded their shoulder stiffness, those with distinct trauma such as a prior fracture, rotator cuff tear, or surgical procedure have a posttraumatic etiology. Stiffness after shoulder surgery is typical and usually resolves with time and appropriate rehabilitation. But the shoulder should not be neglected after any surgery about the shoulder girdle. This includes axillary or cervical lymph node dissections, especially when combined with radiation therapy, cardiac catheterization in the axilla, and coronary artery bypass grafting with sternotomy and thoracotomy. All surgeons should be aware that these procedures may result in restricted shoulder motion.

The clinical presentation of idiopathic shoulder stiffness is classically described as having three phases. The first phase is the painful, freezing phase. The pain is typically achy in nature and sudden jolts or attempts at rapid motion exacerbate the chronic discomfort. The pain may begin at night and shoulder motion becomes progressively limited. Patients often hold their arm at their side and in internal rotation with the forearm across

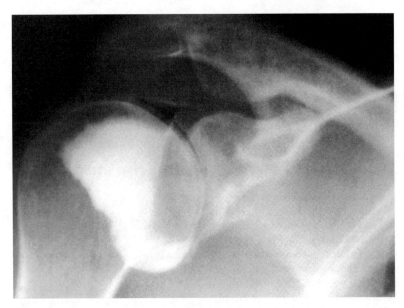

Figure 5–12. Arthrogram of the shoulder demonstrating the classic findings of adhesive capsulitis. Note the small irregular joint capsule with addition of contrast material. (Reprinted with permission from McMahon PJ, Skinner HB: Sports medicine. In: Skinner HB (editor): *Current Diagnosis & Treatment in Orthopedics,* 3rd ed. McGraw-Hill, 2003.)

the belly. They may also be treated for nonspecific shoulder pain with a sling in this position. This inflammatory phase often lasts between 2 and 9 months.

The second phase of progressive stiffness lasts between 3 and 12 months. Stiffness progresses to a point at which shoulder motion is restricted in all planes. Essentially, the shoulder has undergone fibrous arthrodesis. Fortunately, pain progressively decreases from the initial, inflammatory phase. With time, patients are able to use the shoulder with little or no pain, within the restricted range of motion, but attempts to exceed this range are accompanied by pain. The patient's symptoms then plateau. Unfortunately, this phase may be persistent with symptoms lasting for extended periods. In the resolution, or thawing phase, the shoulder slowly and progressively becomes more supple. It can be as short as a month, but typically lasts 1–3 years.

On clinical examination, there is loss of both active and passive range of shoulder motion. Often the first motion to be affected is internal rotation, demonstrated by an inability to bring the arm up the back to the same level as the normal shoulder. Radiographic confirmation of adhesive capsulitis may be done by arthography, which will demonstrate marked reduction in the capacity of the joint. Often the affected shoulder will not take more than 2–3 mL of dye, although normal capacity is 12 mL.

Treatment

Treatment varies, but conservative modalities and progressive range-of-motion exercises seem effective. Range-of-motion exercises for external rotation and abduction will help minimize the length of restriction in motion and dysfunction. Manipulation under anesthesia, long the mainstay of intervention, is being replaced by selective arthroscopic capsular release. Short-term results indicate a quicker return of motion.

Prognosis

Whether treated with rehabilitation alone, or with capsular release, a return of about 80% shoulder range of motion is usual.

Nicholson GP: Arthroscopic capsular release for stiff shoulders: effect of etiology on outcomes. Arthroscopy 2003;19(1):40.

Omari A, Bunker TD: Open surgical release for frozen shoulder: surgical findings and results of the release. J Shoulder Elbow Surg 2001;10(4):353.

Wolf JM, Green A: Influence of comorbidity on self-assessment instrument scores of patients with idiopathic adhesive capsulitis. J Bone Joint Surg Am 2002;84-A(7):1167.

FRACTURES ABOUT THE SHOULDER

1. Clavicular Fracture

The clavicle is one of the most commonly fractured bones in the body, with direct trauma being the usual cause in athletic events (Figure 5–13). Football, wrestling, and ice hockey are the sports most commonly involved in clavicular fractures, which is not surprising as all three are associated with high-speed contact between players.

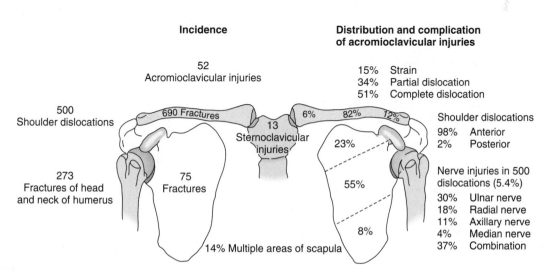

Figure 5–13. Analysis of 1603 shoulder girdle injuries showing the frequency and location of fractures and dislocations. (Reprinted with permission from McMahon PJ, Skinner HB: Sports medicine. In: Skinner HB (editor): *Current Diagnosis & Treatment in Orthopedics,* 3rd ed. McGraw-Hill, 2003.)

ESSENTIALS OF DIAGNOSIS

- *History of injury to the shoulder.*
- *Swelling and ecchymosis overlying the injured clavicle.*
- *Pain and crepitation upon palpation of the fracture site.*
- *Pain and limited range of motion of the arm, specifically in forward flexion and abduction.*
- *Appropriate radiographs will define the location and severity of the fracture.*

Clinical Findings

Despite the proximity of vital structures, clavicular fractures that occur during athletic activities are rarely associated with neurovascular damage, and accompanying soft tissue disorders are uncommon. The patient will usually give a history of falling in the area of the shoulder or receiving a blow to the clavicle, experiencing immediate pain and an inability to raise the arm. Radiography will usually confirm the clinical impression, and must show the entire clavicle, including the shoulder girdle, upper third of the humerus, and sternal end of the clavicle.

Of clavicular fractures, midclavicular fractures account for 80%, distal fractures for 15%, and proximal fractures for 5%. Most fractures of the shaft of the clavicle heal well. However, some neurovascular complications, such as a tear of the subclavian artery or a brachial plexus injury, are serious, although rare. Therefore, when evaluating and treating clavicular fractures, an initial neurovascular examination is very important. Pulses in the distal part of the upper extremity, strength, and sensation must be carefully evaluated.

Because the clavicle is the only bone structure that fixes the shoulder girdle to the thorax, a fracture through the clavicle causes the shoulder to sag forward and downward. The pull of the sternocleidomastoid muscle may displace the proximal fragment superiorly. These forces tend to hinder the initial reduction and maintenance of reduction. In addition, distal fractures, which are more common in older age groups, may involve tears in the coracoclavicular ligament, which allows the proximal clavicle to ride up superiorly, mimicking an acromioclavicular dislocation. Delayed union is much more common in this type of fracture than in other clavicular fractures.

Treatment

Mid and proximal clavicular fractures are usually treated with a short period of rest, with a sling on the affected side to support the extremity. Immobilization is usually discontinued at 3–4 weeks, and once the clavicular fracture has healed, range-of-motion and strengthening exercises should begin.

Prognosis

Onset of exercises prior to healing may result in nonunion. Athletes should not be allowed to return to play until shoulder strength and range of motion return to preinjury levels. Generally, no special braces or pads are required when the athlete returns to play.

Grassi FS et al: Management of midclavicular fractures: comparison between nonoperative treatment and open intramedullary fixation in 80 patients. J Trauma 2001;50(6):1096.

Robinson CM, Cairns DA: Primary nonoperative treatment of displaced lateral fractures of the clavicle. J Bone Joint Surg Am 2004;86-A(4):778.

Robinson CM et al: Estimating the risk of nonunion following nonoperative treatment of a clavicular fracture. J Bone Joint Surg Am 2004;86-A(7):1359.

2. Proximal Humerus Fracture

Fractures of the proximal humerus, which represent approximately 4–5% of all fractures, are a relatively uncommon sports injury. They most often present in young adolescents with open growth plates or in elderly osteoporotic patients. When they do occur in the athlete, they are typically the result of a high-energy impact injury or are secondary to an underlying pathologic bone condition.

ESSENTIALS OF DIAGNOSIS

- *History of trauma to the shoulder.*
- *Swelling and ecchymosis overlying the shoulder that may extend down to the elbow.*
- *Tenderness and crepitation over the fracture site.*
- *Pain with attempted range of motion of the shoulder.*
- *Appropriate radiographs will define the location and severity of the fracture.*

Clinical Findings

The proximal humerus consists of four major bony components: the humeral head, the greater tuberosity, the lesser tuberosity, and the humeral shaft. Fractures, which can occur between any or all of these regions, are traditionally defined by the location and displacement of the fracture fragments (Figure 5–14). The patient

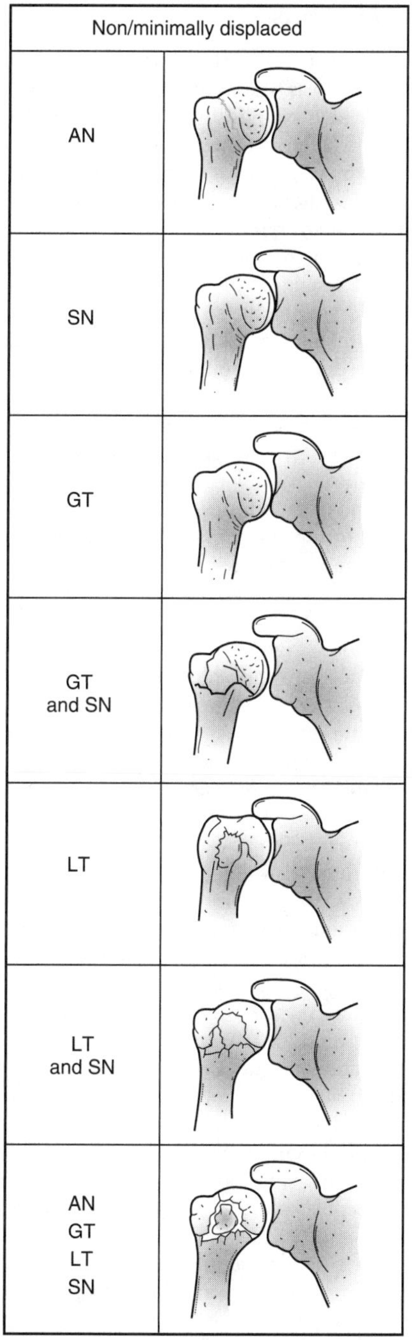

Non/minimally displaced	
AN	
SN	
GT	
GT and SN	
LT	
LT and SN	
AN GT LT SN	

Figure 5–14. Four part classification for fractures of the proximal humerus. AN, anatomic neck; SN, surgical neck; GT, greater tuberosity; LT, lesser tuberosity. [Reprinted with permission from Norris TR, Green A: Proximal humerus fractures and fracture-dislocations. In: Browner BD et al (editors): *Skeletal Trauma: Fractures, Dislocation and Ligamentous Injuries.* Elsevier, 1998.]

with a proximal humerus fracture will usually be able to report the mechanism of injury and will complain of pain, swelling, and an inability to use the shoulder. A physical examination will often reveal loss of the normal contour of the shoulder, tenderness about the shoulder, ecchymosis that may extend down to the elbow, and crepitus on attempted range of motion. A thorough neurovascular examination is essential, as brachial plexus and axillary nerve injuries have been reported in association with proximal humerus fractures. Because the axillary nerve is the nerve most commonly injured in these cases, sensation to light touch and pin-prick over the lateral aspect of the upper arm and deltoid muscle function must be tested. An accurate radiographic evaluation is necessary to confirm the type and severity of the fracture and is essential in determining the treatment plan. Anteroposterior and lateral views in the plane of the scapula as well as an axillary view to rule out an associated glenohumeral dislocation are necessary.

Treatment

Most proximal humerus fractures are minimally displaced and can be treated nonoperatively with sling immobilization and early passive range of motion. However, about 20% need to be treated operatively. Many factors contribute to this decision-making process including fracture type and degree of displacement, bone quality, activity level, and associated injuries. Surgical options range from closed reduction and percutaneous pinning to open reduction with internal fixation to humeral head replacement.

Prognosis

For minimally displaced fractures, the prognosis is generally good. Loss of motion is the most common complication. It can take 12–18 months to attain the maximal result, so range-of-motion exercises should be continued for an extended period of time.

Guttmann D et al: Injuries of the proximal humerus in adults. In: *Orthopaedic Sports Medicine: Principles and Practice.* DeLee JC et al (editors). Saunders, 2003, pp. 1096–1118.

Iannotti JP et al: Nonprosthetic management of proximal humeral fractures. J Bone Joint Surg Am 2003;85:1578.

3. Proximal Humeral Epiphyseal Fracture

In young athletes, epiphyseal fractures of the proximal humerus may occur. The separate growth centers of the articular surface, greater tuberosity, and lesser tuberosity coalesce at approximately age 7 years, with the remaining growth plates closing at 20–22 years of age. Therefore, fracture separations may occur at any age until the growth plates have closed. Fortunately, fractures in this area usually do not arrest growth.

ESSENTIALS OF DIAGNOSIS

- *Proximal humerus pain.*
- *Widening of the proximal humeral physis on radiographs.*

Clinical Findings

Injury can occur to the shoulder in the growing musculoskeletal system of young athletes engaged in sports that involve overhead throwing. Proximal humerus pain associated with widening of the proximal humerus epiphysis, especially while throwing, has been termed "little league shoulder." Although widening of the proximal humerus epiphysis can be an adaptive change to throwing, when painful it may represent a fracture resulting from overuse.

Treatment

Cessation of throwing is the first step in treatment. Once pain has resolved, range of motion and strengthening exercises can be initiated. Ultimately, throwing can be resumed as long as the patient is pain free.

Dobbs MB et al: Severely displaced proximal humeral epiphyseal fractures. J Pediatr Orthop 2003;23(2):208.

Karatosun V et al: Treatment of displaced, proximal, humeral, epiphyseal fractures with a two-prong splint. J Orthop Trauma 2003;17(8):578.

ACROMIOCLAVICULAR JOINT INJURY

ESSENTIALS OF DIAGNOSIS

- *Pain and swelling over the acromioclavicular joint.*
- *May have visible elevation or displacement of the clavicle relative to the acromion (asymmetric to the contralateral shoulder).*
- *Pain with forward elevation of the arm.*
- *Appropriate radiographs can be confirmatory.*

Prevention

Avoiding activities that may result in a downward blow to the tip of the shoulder is the best way to prevent these injuries.

Clinical Findings

Acromioclavicular dislocations or subluxations, commonly referred to as separations, vary in severity depending on the extent of injury to the stabilizing ligaments and capsule. The typical mechanism of injury is a direct downward blow to the tip of the shoulder. Clinically, pain at the top of the shoulder over the acromioclavicular joint is the predominant symptom, with varying decreases in motion depending on the severity of the injury. The athlete who has sustained this type of injury will typically leave the field holding the arm close to the side.

When checking for instability of the acromioclavicular joint, the examiner should manipulate the midshaft of the clavicle, rather than the acromioclavicular joint to rule out pain from contusion to the acromioclavicular area. For milder acromioclavicular injuries, the patient should put the hand of the affected arm on the opposite shoulder, and the examiner may then gently apply downward pressure at the patient's affected elbow, noting if this maneuver causes pain at the acromioclavicular joint.

Acromioclavicular joint injuries were initially divided into grades I–III (Figure 5–15). Grade I injuries are typically produced by a mild blow causing a partial tear of the acromioclavicular ligament. When the acromioclavicular ligament is completely torn, but the coracoclavicular ligament remains intact, a grade II injury that involves subluxation or partial displacement results. When the force of injury is severe enough to tear the coracoclavicular and acromioclavicular ligaments in addition to the capsule, a grade III injury occurs.

Three additional injuries were later added to the classification. In grade IV injuries, the clavicle is displaced posterior and buttonholed through the fascia of the trapezius muscle. Grade V injuries demonstrate severe inferior displacement of the glenohumeral joint, with the clavicle often 300% superior to the acromion. Lastly, in grade VI injuries the distal end of the clavicle is locked inferior to the coracoid.

Acromioclavicular joint displacement is often obvious on physical examination, but it is best classified by radiography. An anteroposterior radiograph that is aimed 10° cephalad allows visualization of the acromioclavicular joint. A radiograph of the entire upper thorax allows the vertical distance between the coracoid and the clavicle on both the involved and uninvolved sides to be compared. Anteroposterior radiographs with weights applied to the upper extremities are usually unnecessary. An axillary lateral radiograph is also essential for proper classification.

Treatment

Management of acromioclavicular joint injuries depends on their severity. Grade I and grade II injuries may be treated with a sling until discomfort dissipates,

A

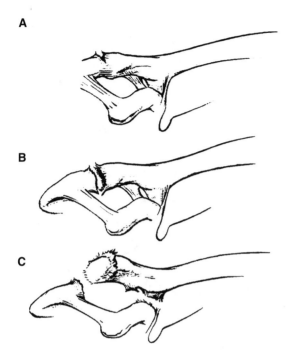

B

C

Figure 5–15. Grades of acromioclavicular (AC) joint separations. **A:** Type I, partial tear of the AC ligament. **B:** Type II, complete tear of the AC ligament; the coracoclavicular (CC) ligaments remain intact. **C:** Type III, disruption of the AC and CC ligaments. (Reprinted with permission from McMahon PJ, Skinner HB: Sports medicine. In: Skinner HB (editor): *Current Diagnosis & Treatment in Orthopedics,* 3rd ed. McGraw-Hill, 2003.)

usually within 2–4 weeks. Next a rehabilitation program starts and normal range of motion and strength to the upper extremity begins to be restored. The treatment of grade III injuries or complete dislocations in athletes is controversial. Although most believe that grade III injuries are best managed nonoperatively, others advocate operative treatment. Grade IV–VI injuries are best treated with open reduction and internal fixation along with reconstruction of the coracoclavicular ligament.

Nonsurgical treatment may either involve a sling for comfort or an acromioclavicular sling to try to achieve reduction. The device must be fit to apply pressure to the distal clavicle sufficient to afford reduction, but not great enough to compromise the skin. Ice and other modalities are used for an acute acromioclavicular injury to reduce soreness and swelling. Pain is the limiting factor in beginning range-of-motion and isometric muscle-strengthening exercises. It should be used as a guide for gradual initiation and escalation of these physical therapy regimes. Isotonic exercises may then follow because

isometric exercises are more effective earlier when range of motion is limited.

Before resuming athletic activities, the patient must have full range of pain-free motion and no tenderness upon direct palpation of the acromioclavicular joint or pain when manual traction is applied.

Prognosis

Athletes who do not need to elevate their arms, such as soccer or football players, tend to return to sports earlier than players engaged in sports that require overhead arm activity, such as tennis, baseball, and swimming.

Dumonski M et al: Evaluation and management of acromioclavicular joint injuries. Am J Orthop 2004;33(10):526.

Su EP et al: Using suture anchors for coracoclavicular fixation in treatment of complete acromioclavicular separation. Am J Orthop 2004;33(5):256.

CORACOID FRACTURE

Fractures of the coracoid process are rare; they are usually seen in professional riflemen and skeet shooters, though they have also been reported in baseball and tennis players. They are identified on radiographs, and conservative treatment, including cessation of activity, usually results in uncomplicated healing after 6–8 weeks.

STERNOCLAVICULAR JOINT INJURY

In the skeletally mature adult athlete, injury to the sternoclavicular joint usually involves the surrounding soft tissue and capsule tearing, leading to subluxation or dislocation. The mechanism of injury is either a blow to the point of the shoulder, which predisposes the athlete to anterior dislocation, or a direct blow to the clavicle or chest with the shoulder in extension, which predisposes the athlete to posterior dislocation. The injury may range from a symptomatic sprain to a complete sternoclavicular dislocation with disruption of the capsule and its restraining ligaments.

1. Anterior Dislocation

ESSENTIALS OF DIAGNOSIS

- *History of trauma to the upper chest wall.*
- *Painful prominence overlying the proximal end of the clavicle.*
- *Appropriate radiographs or CT scan can be diagnostic.*

Clinical Findings

The most common type of sternoclavicular dislocation is anterior dislocation. This is recognized clinically by an anterior prominence of the proximal clavicle on the involved side. Radiographic documentation of an anterior sternoclavicular dislocation is difficult because the rib, sternum, and clavicle overlap at the joint, but may be confirmed by oblique views. A CT scan is very sensitive and should be done if the radiograph appears normal but a dislocation is suspected.

Treatment

Although dislocation of the anterior sternoclavicular joint may cause considerable distress initially, the symptoms usually subside rapidly, with no loss of shoulder function. A variety of surgical and nonsurgical approaches have been advocated, but surgery for anterior dislocations often results in significant complications. Closed treatment modalities vary from using a sling to attempted closed reduction, which may be successful initially but is difficult to maintain.

2. Posterior Dislocation

ESSENTIALS OF DIAGNOSIS

- *History of trauma to the upper chest wall.*
- *Pain in the region of the proximal end of the clavicle.*
- *Patient may present with hoarseness, dysphagia, or severe respiratory distress.*
- *Appropriate radiographs or CT scan can be diagnostic.*

Clinical Findings

Posterior sternoclavicular dislocation is much less common, but is associated with more complications because of the potential for injury to the esophagus, great vessels, and trachea. Presenting symptoms range from mild to moderate pain in the sternoclavicular region to hoarseness, dysphagia, severe respiratory distress, and subcutaneous emphysema from tracheal injury.

Treatment

In most instances, closed reduction of posterior dislocations, if performed early, is successful and stable. To effect reduction, a pillow is placed under the upper back

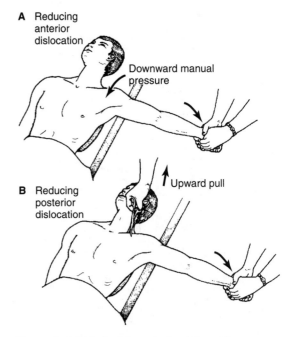

Figure 5–16. Method for reducing (**A**) anterior sternoclavicular and (**B**) posterior sternoclavicular dislocation. (Reprinted with permission from McMahon PJ, Skinner HB: Sports medicine. In: Skinner HB (editor): *Current Diagnosis & Treatment in Orthopedics,* 3rd ed. McGraw-Hill, 2003.)

of the supine patient and gentle traction is applied with the shoulder held in 90° of abduction and at maximum extension (Figure 5–16). Rarely, closed reduction under general anesthesia or open reduction is required.

After reduction, the patient is put in an immobilization splint and is instructed to use ice and oral NSAIDs. Once the joint has healed sufficiently, usually within 2–3 weeks, range-of-motion exercises may begin. Elevation of the arm should not be attempted until 3 weeks after injury.

Medial Clavicular Epiphyseal Fracture

In athletes younger than 25 years of age, sternoclavicular injuries may not result in true dislocations, but rather in fractures through the growth plate of the proximal clavicle. These clavicular epiphyseal fractures may appear clinically as dislocations, particularly if some displacement is present, and may be treated conservatively. Typically, these are not associated with growth deformities, and reduction of the fracture is not needed unless there is severe displacement. Symptomatic treatment for pain will usually suffice. Sometimes an adolescent presents with an enlarging mass at the sternoclavicular joint, accompanied by parents with worries of cancer. A careful history reveals trauma several weeks earlier and the mass represents the callus of a healing clavicular epiphyseal fracture that can be demonstrated radiographically.

Battaglia TC et al: Interposition arthroplasty with bone-tendon allograft: a technique for treatment of the unstable sternoclavicular joint. J Orthop Trauma 2005;19(2):124.

SHOULDER NEUROVASCULAR INJURY

1. Brachial Plexus Injury

ESSENTIALS OF DIAGNOSIS

- *Often preceded by a fall onto the shoulder.*
- *Paresthesias and/or motor loss in the affected extremity that can be transient or permanent.*
- *Electromyography can help localize the lesion and aid in prognosis.*

Clinical Findings, Treatment, & Prognosis

Brachial plexus injuries are typically caused by a fall on the shoulder as seen in acromioclavicular joint injuries. Most brachial plexus injuries do not involve motor loss and exhibit paresthesias, which resolve in a period of minutes to weeks, although some cases may persist for months or years. Early in the course of the injury, a transient slowing of conduction across the plexus or a mild prolongation of nerve latency may be seen. The "burner" or "stinger" is one of the most common brachial plexus injuries encountered in athletes. The key to diagnosis is a short duration of upper extremity paresthesias and shoulder weakness, with pain-free range of motion of the cervical spine. Players may return to competition after shoulder strength and full, pain-free range of motion have returned.

Rarely, a severe injury will occur (eg, from motorcycle racing). Chronic injuries result in instability of the shoulder that may be treated with trapezius transfer. Arthrodesis is an alternative, initially or after failed muscle transfer.

Safran MR: Nerve injury about the shoulder in athletes. Part 2: Long thoracic nerve, spinal accessory nerve, burners/stingers, thoracic outlet syndrome. Am J Sports Med 2004;32:1063.

2. Long Thoracic Nerve Injury

ESSENTIALS OF DIAGNOSIS

- *Palsy of the serratus anterior results in medial winging of the scapula.*

Clinical Findings, Treatment, & Prognosis

Traction incidents may cause a long thoracic nerve palsy, with subsequent serratus anterior paralysis and winging of the scapula. Traction and blunt trauma may also cause injury to the spinal accessory nerve, another cause of winging of the scapula. These can be differentiated on physical examination by the position of the scapula. With serratus anterior palsy, the inferior portion of the scapula tends to go medially, whereas the opposite occurs with spinal accessory nerve palsy. Treatment is usually conservative, with return of function in weeks if the nerve has not been divided.

Aquino SL et al: Nerves of the thorax: atlas of normal and pathologic findings. Radiographics 2001;21(5):1275.

Safran MR: Nerve injury about the shoulder in athletes. Part 2: Long thoracic nerve, spinal accessory nerve, burners/stingers, thoracic outlet syndrome. Am J Sports Med 2004; 32:1063.

3. Suprascapular Nerve Injury

ESSENTIALS OF DIAGNOSIS

- *Poorly localized pain and weakness in the posterolateral shoulder.*
- *Weakness and atrophy of the supraspinatus ± infraspinatus muscles.*
- *MRI may reveal the presence of a cyst in the suprascapular or spinoglenoid notch.*
- *Electromyography/nerve conduction velocity (EMG/NCV) can aid in the diagnosis.*

Clinical Findings, Treatment, & Prognosis

Entrapment of the suprascapular nerve is often associated with activities such as weight lifting, baseball pitching, volleyball, and backpacking. Traction and repetitive shoulder use are the mechanisms of injury. Compression of the nerve may occur from entrapment at the anterior suprascapular notch of the scapula or at the level of the spinoglenoid notch. The latter occurs in volleyball players and baseball players and is likely caused by rapid overhead acceleration of the arm. Compression is associated with poorly localized pain and weakness in the posterolateral aspect of the shoulder girdle. This may be followed by atrophy of the supraspinatus or infraspinatus muscles. Eventually, there is weakness of forward flexion and external rotation of the shoulder. The diagnosis is confirmed by electromyography and nerve conduction studies.

Conservative therapy consists of rest, NSAIDs, and physical therapy designed to increase muscular tone and strength. If this is unsuccessful, then surgical exploration is indicated, which may reveal hypertrophy of the transverse scapular ligament, anomalies of the suprascapular notch, and ganglion cysts. Results of surgery vary with the lesion discovered, but many patients return to full function postoperatively.

Safran MR: Nerve injury about the shoulder in athletes. Part 1: Suprascapular nerve and axillary nerve. Am J Sports Med 2004;32:803.

4. Musculocutaneous Nerve Injury

ESSENTIALS OF DIAGNOSIS

- *Weak or absent biceps muscle function with sensory loss in the lateral forearm.*
- *EMG/NCV may aid in the diagnosis and prognosis.*

Clinical Findings, Treatment, & Prognosis

This nerve is susceptible to direct frontal blows or surgical procedures. Injury is associated with numbness in the lateral forearm to the base of the thumb and weak to absent biceps muscle function. Most injuries seen in sports are transient and respond to conservative treatment in a matter of days to weeks.

Klepps SJ et al: Anatomic evaluation of the subcoracoid pectoralis muscle transfer in human cadavers. J Shoulder Elbow Surg 2001;10(5):453.

5. Axillary Nerve Injury

ESSENTIALS OF DIAGNOSIS

- *Present following a shoulder dislocation or proximal humerus fracture.*
- *Weakness or absence of deltoid muscle function.*
- *Positive deltoid extension lag sign.*
- *EMG/NCV can aid in diagnosis and prognosis.*

Clinical Findings, Treatment, & Prognosis

The usual mechanism of injury is trauma either by direct blow to the posterior aspect of the shoulder or following dislocation of the shoulder or fracture of the proximal humerus. Axillary nerve injury occurs in many sports such as football, wrestling, gymnastics, mountain climbing, rugby, and baseball. The degree of injury to the nerve varies because the initial presentation may be mild weakness during elevation and abduction of the arm with or without numbness of the lateral arm. The deltoid extension lag sign is indicative of axillary nerve injury. To perform this test the examiner elevates the arm into a position of near full extension, asks the patient to hold the arm in this position, and then releases the arm. If there is complete deltoid paralysis, the arm will drop. For partial nerve injuries, the magnitude of the angular drop, or lag, is an indicator of deltoid strength. Approximately 25% of all dislocated shoulder injuries are associated with axillary nerve traction injuries, which respond well to rest, physical therapy, and time. If recovery is not complete within 3–6 months, surgical intervention is recommended with exploration, utilizing neurolysis or grafting, or both, as necessary. Results of surgery are usually favorable, with sensory recovery occurring before motor recovery.

Steinmann SP, Moran EA: Axillary nerve injury: diagnosis and treatment. J Am Acad Orthop Surg 2001;9(5):328.

THORACIC OUTLET SYNDROME

ESSENTIALS OF DIAGNOSIS

- *Symptoms are often nonspecific and may be neurologic, venous, or arterial, and may include edema, pallor, or coolness as well as paresthesias.*
- *Doppler examination and EMG/NVC studies can assist in the diagnosis.*

Clinical Findings, Treatment, & Prognosis

The symptoms resulting from thoracic outlet compression may be neurologic, venous, or arterial in nature. Obstruction of the subclavian vein may lead to stiffness, edema, and even thrombosis of the limb. Arterial obstruction may be the result of direct compression and manifests with pallor, coolness, and forearm claudication. Doppler examination reveals changes in arterial and venous flow. Electromyography and nerve conduction studies are also helpful in diagnosis.

Nonoperative treatment is recommended for less severe forms of this syndrome, and once the pain subsides, an exercise program to strengthen the pectoral girdle muscles is beneficial. Special exercises to strengthen the upper and lower trapezius, along with the erector spinae and serratus anterior muscles, yield good results. Correcting poor posture and an ongoing maintenance program are mandatory once improvement is reached. Progression of symptoms or failure of nonoperative treatment is an indication for surgical exploration and correction of the pathologic factors encountered.

Connolly JF, Ganjianpour M: Thoracic outlet syndrome treated by double osteotomy of a clavicular malunion: a case report. J Bone Joint Surg Am 2002;84:437.

Wiesler ER et al: Humeral head fracture-dislocation into the thoracic outlet: case report and review of the literature. J Shoulder Elbow Surg 2004;13(5):576.

Elbow, Wrist, & Hand Injuries

6

Alexandre Rasouli, MD, & Ranjan Gupta, MD

■ ELBOW PAIN

ANATOMY

The elbow has articulations between three bones: the humerus, ulna, and radius. The humeroulnar articulation is a hinge joint between the trochlea of the medial humeral condyle and semilunar notch of the proximal ulna. The coronoid and olecranon processes of the ulna deepen the semilunar notch and increase contact at the humeroulnar joint. The humeroradial articulation is between the radial head and the capitellum of the lateral humeral condyle. The radius and ulna also articulate with each other to create the proximal radioulnar joint, between the radial head and the sigmoid notch of the ulna. These joints, together with their ligamentous and musculotendinous attachments, allow flexion and extension of the elbow, and pronation and supination of the forearm.

Musculotendinous Attachments

To achieve coordinated motion at each joint, muscle forces are usually balanced to provide precise, controlled motion. The brachialis muscle inserts on the coronoid process anteriorly whereas the triceps inserts broadly on the olecranon process posteriorly. The dorsal extensor mass originates from the lateral humeral epicondyle and includes the extensor carpi radialis longus, extensor carpi radialis brevis, extensor communis, and extensor carpi ulnaris. On the other side of the distal humerus, the pronator–flexor mass originates from the medial epicondyle and medial supracondylar ridge. It includes the pronator teres, flexor carpi radialis, palmaris longus, flexor digitorum superficialis, and flexor carpi ulnaris.

Ligamentous Attachments

Portions of each joint capsule, thickened to provide joint stability, are defined as ligaments. Complex ligamentous structures occur around every component of the elbow joint. A complex of four ligaments stabilizes the lateral elbow. They are all thickenings of the joint capsule and include, from deep to superficial, the lateral collateral ligament (LCL), the annular ligament, the accessory LCL, and the lateral ulnar collateral ligament (LUCL). The LCL attaches to the lateral epicondyle and expands distally to combine with the deep fibers of the annular ligament. The LCL confers varus stability to the elbow and tethers the annular ligament. The annular ligament attaches to the anterior and posterior aspects of the sigmoid notch, forming a ring around the radial head and neck, and provides stability during pronation–supination. The accessory LCL attaches distally to the tubercle of the ulnar supinator crest and merges with and tethers the annular ligament proximally. The LUCL attaches proximally to the lateral humeral epicondyle and distally to the supinator crest, deep to the fascia of the supinator muscle. It stabilizes the lateral elbow against rotary stresses and provides a posterior buttress for the radial head.

The medial side of the elbow is also stabilized by a complex of ligaments formed by capsular thickening. These structures include the anterior band, the posterior band, and the transverse ligament of Cooper. Of these, the anterior band is the most important in stabilizing against valgus stress. It attaches to the medial epicondyle of the humerus and the sublime tubercle of the coronoid process. It provides static and dynamic stability during the throwing arc of motion, from 20° to 120° of flexion. The posterior band stabilizes the medial elbow against internal rotary stress. Its attachments are the lateral humeral epicondyle and the olecranon process. Together with the humeroulnar articulation, the LCL and medial collateral ligament complexes are the three primary stabilizers of the elbow. Injury to any of these primary stabilizers places increased demand on the secondary elbow stabilizers, which include the radial head, the anterior and posterior elbow joint capsule, the extensor–supinator origin, the flexor–pronator origin, the anconeus, the triceps, and the brachialis.

Neural Structures

The elbow is the causeway for the three major nerves of the distal upper extremity: the radial (and posterior interosseous) nerve, which courses anterolaterally, the median nerve, which courses along the anterior midline, and the ulnar nerve, which lies posteromedially. The radial nerve, formed by the posterior cord of the brachial plexus (roots C6, C7, C8, and T1), innervates the triceps, supinator, and wrist and digital extensors. The ulnar nerve, arising from the medial cord of the brachial plexus (roots C8 and T1), innervates the flexor carpi ulnaris, ulna-two flexor digitorum profundi, ulnar-two lumbricals, dorsal and volar interossei, adductor pollicis, and the hypothenar muscles (oppenes digiti minimi, abductor digiti minimi, and flexor digiti minimi). The median nerve is formed by the lateral and medial cords of the brachial plexus (roots C6, C7, C8, and T1) and innervates the palmaris longus, pronator teres, flexor carpi radialis, flexor digitorum profundus of the index and middle fingers, flexor digitorum sublimis, flexor pollicis longus, pronator quadratus, first and second lumbricals, and the thenar muscles (opponens pollicis, abductor pollicis, and flexor pollicis).

Compression of these nerves along their dedicated anatomic paths is a common and often treatable cause of elbow pain. Potential sites of compression for the radial nerve include the fibrous arch of the lateral head of the triceps, the arcade of Frohse, the origin of the extensor carpi radialis brevis, and neighboring structures (see the section on Radial Tunnel Syndrome). The ulnar nerve can undergo compression at the supracondylar humeral process, the arcade of Struthers, the origin of the flexor carpi ulnaris, and in Guyon's canal at the wrist (see the section on Cubital Tunnel Syndrome). Medial nerve compression can occur at the supracondylar process, ligament of Struthers, flexor digitorum arch, lacertus fibrosis, pronator teres, and the carpal tunnel.

Jobe MT, Martinez SF: Peripheral nerve injuries. In: *Campbell's Operative Orthopaedics,* 10th ed. Canale ST (editor). Mosby, 2003.

Mehta JA, Bain GI: Posterolateral rotatory instability of the elbow. J Am Acad Orthop Surg 2004;12:405.

LATERAL ELBOW PAIN

1. Lateral Epicondylitis (Tennis Elbow)

ESSENTIALS OF DIAGNOSIS

- *A history of repetitive activity or overuse.*
- *Pain that localizes to the lateral epicondyle with radiation to the forearm.*

- *Tenderness localized to extensor carpi radialis brevis (ECRB) origin, maximal 2 mm anterior and distal to the center of the lateral epicondyle.*
- *Elbow range of motion is preserved.*
- *Radiographs are often unremarkable.*
- *Differential diagnosis includes cervical radiculopathy, radial tunnel syndrome, posterior interosseous nerve compression syndrome, elbow arthritis, osteochondral defect, and forearm tendonitis.*

Prevention

Recreational and occupational activities that involve repetitive motions predispose to lateral epicondylitis. Prevention involves attention to technique, equipment, and environmental factors. In the case of racket sports, there are several key activities that may help to prevent the development of lateral epicondylitis including (1) avoidance of poor stroke techniques (such as leading with a flexed elbow, striking the ball off center, using a single hand backstroke), (2) the use of proper grip size, (3) the appropriate racket weight, (4) looser string tension, (5) the limitation of play time to less than 2 hours, and (6) play on softer surfaces. With most work-related conditions, attention to the work station to ensure appropriate ergonomics is important in helping to prevent the development of this condition.

Clinical Findings

Most patients will complain of chronic pain in the elbow of the dominant arm, with insidious onset and localization to the lateral epicondyle. Palpation will elicit tenderness over the common extensor origin and more specifically over the origin of the ECRB. Wrist and middle finger extension against resistance with the elbow extended will replicate the primary complaint. Range of motion typically is not affected nor is sensation. Any distal motor weakness should be attributable only to pain. If there is muscle atrophy or true muscle weakness, alternative diagnoses should be explored. To address radiculopathic, arthritic, or neurologic sources that may also produce lateral elbow pain, a thorough examination of the entire upper extremity and neck should be performed. Plain radiographs of the elbow are obtained to rule out other etiologies, but will usually appear normal in the case of lateral epicondylitis. Some cases may exhibit inconsequential calcification of tissue around the lateral epicondyle. If classical signs are not present, cervical radiographs and/or electrodiagnostic tests may be performed to explore other causes of elbow pain as mentioned above.

Gross pathological specimens of debrided tissue have revealed partial or complete tears in the origin of an extensor tendon, most often that of the extensor carpi radialis brevis. The pathologic changes are consistent with a chronic degenerative inflammatory process: edema, fibrillation, granulation, and loss of parallel collagen fiber orientation.

Treatment

Nonoperative intervention is the mainstay of treatment. Most conservative modalities aim to relieve pain, reverse inflammation, and strengthen the extensor mass. The offending activity should be either suspended or modified significantly, but cessation of all activity is to be avoided. Oral antiinflammatory agents are instituted. Poor technique and equipment are identified and should be rectified. Counterforce bracing, which increases force distribution across the extensor mass, can be adopted with a lateral arm strap. A rehabilitation program to stretch and strengthen the forearm extensor muscles is started, initially with isometric and then with progressively concentric and eccentric resistive exercises. It is often quite helpful for the patient to abduct the shoulder to 90° and have the offending arm held in extension. With the nonaffected arm, flex the wrist of the offending arm. Three sets of 10 stretches of this gradual stretching exercise should be performed four times a day. If these exercises fail to ameliorate the problem, modalities such as ultrasonography and electrical stimulation may have some utility. If pain persists, a corticosteroid injection may be administered deep to the ECRB origin, into the subaponeurotic recess. Superficial injections or injections into the substance of the tendon should be avoided.

Although most compliant patients will respond completely to a nonoperative program, persistent cases will require surgery. Surgical indications include failure of a conservative trial that lasts at least 1 year with the elimination of other possible etiologies. All surgical techniques must address the inflamed tendon. Historically, four techniques have been used: release of the common extensor origin (Hohmann tension relieving technique), lengthening of the extensor carpi radialis, intraarticular synovial and annular ligament excision, and debridement of pathological tendinous tissue with reattachment to the lateral epicondyle. The fourth technique allows resolution of symptoms and avoids some of the strength deficits reported after the classical Hohmann technique. With this technique, the extensor origin is subperiosteally detached, its inflammatory portions are sharply debrided, and it is then reattached to decorticated lateral epicondyle by sutures through transosseous tunnels. After brief postoperative immobilization, progressive range of motion is begun; light resistance exercises and strengthening exercises are started at 4 and 6 weeks postoperatively, respectively.

Complications

Complications of surgical intervention include strength deficits, recalcitrant pain, and functional limitation in activities such as heavy lifting.

Prognosis

Outcome in both nonsurgical and surgical cases is excellent, with up to 90% of patients reporting near to complete resolution of symptoms and return to previous level of activity.

Return to Play

A patient capable of rapid repetitive motion exercises without pain may return to normal activity with progressive increase in duration and load. Return to play usually occurs by 16 weeks.

Miller MD: Sports medicine. In: *Review of Orthopaedics*, 3rd ed. Miller MD (editor). W.B. Saunders, 2000.

2. Radial Tunnel Syndrome

ESSENTIALS OF DIAGNOSIS

- *Compression of the posterior interosseous nerve with pain as the primary complaint; there is no motor or sensory dysfunction as with posterior interosseous nerve compression syndrome.*
- *Pain is localized to the lateral elbow, over the anterior radial neck.*
- *Provocative maneuvers include the resisted supination test and the long finger extension test.*
- *Electromyographic and nerve conduction velocities are usually negative.*
- *Differential diagnosis includes lateral epicondylitis and posterior interosseous nerve compression syndrome.*
- *Lateral epicondylitis may coexist with 5% of cases.*

Prevention

Radial tunnel syndrome affects individuals whose activities involve repetitive elbow extension, forearm pronation, and wrist flexion for prolonged durations. Prevention is aimed at ergonomic optimization in those settings.

Clinical Findings

Patients will complain only of pain, with tenderness to palpation most severe 2–3 cm distal to the radial head along the radial tunnel. The radial tunnel transmits the posterior interosseous nerve and runs from the distal aspect of the radiohumeral joint to the distal extent of the supinator muscle. The anatomic structures along the course of the tunnel can cause compression of the nerve: the fibrous margin of the ECRB, fibrous bands at the radiohumeral joint, branches of the radial recurrent artery, the arcade of Frohse, and the distal end of the supinator muscle.

The area of maximal lateral elbow tenderness is slightly distal to that observed in lateral epicondylitis. Diagnosis relies on two provocative tests. The resisted forearm supination test will reproduce the nature and location of the pain. The long finger extension test will also produce forearm pain and is elicited by resisted extension of the long finger with pressure over the P1 pulley while the forearm is supinated and the wrist extended. Although radial tunnel syndrome involves the same nerve and the same sites of compression as posterior interosseous nerve compression syndrome, there will be no reports or findings consistent with motor or sensory deficits. Consequently and in contrast to posterior interosseous nerve compression syndrome, electromyographic and nerve conduction velocity studies will be negative. In this respect, radial tunnel syndrome is unique in that its clinical manifestations have little to do with the distribution of the nerve involved.

Treatment

Nonoperative management is begun and includes rest, antiinflammatory medication, activity modification, stretching, and temporary splinting in neutral elbow position. If pain persists after 12 weeks of conservative therapy, a corticosteroid injection around the nerve at the site of maximal tenderness may be administered.

Surgical release of the compressed nerve has equivocal results and is reserved for confirmed refractory cases after at least 12 months of conservative management. Both a transverse and Thompson approach to the radial tunnel have been described. All potential sites of compression along the radial tunnel should be released. Brief postoperative immobilization is followed by increased range of motion and extensor stretching exercises.

Return to Play

Return to previous activity is permitted when provocative tests are no longer positive. For operative cases, gradual return to play may take between 6 and 12 weeks, but maximal recovery postoperatively may not occur for up to 18 months.

Lubahn JD, Cermak MB: Uncommon nerve compression syndromes of the upper extremity. J Am Acad Orthop Surg 1998;6:378.

MEDIAL ELBOW PAIN

1. Medial Epicondylitis (Golfer's Elbow)

 ESSENTIALS OF DIAGNOSIS

- *A history of advanced-level activity in which the elbow undergoes valgus stress, such as in golf or pitching or other throwing activities.*
- *Pain along the medial elbow, worsened by throwing and resisted forearm pronation.*
- *Tearing and degeneration of the flexor pronator group, usually of the pronator teres and flexor carpi ulnaris origins.*
- *The range of motion is usually preserved.*
- *Differential diagnosis includes medial collateral ligament instability or sprain, cubital tunnel syndrome, arthritis, and cervical radiculopathy.*

Prevention

Prevention relies on optimal pitch or stroke technique, adequate conditioning, and proper preactivity stretching and warm-up.

Clinical Findings

Medial epicondylitis is a less common cause of elbow pain in athletes than lateral epicondylitis. The primary complaint is gradual onset medial elbow pain usually without limitation in range of motion, strength, or sensation. Tenderness is maximal distal and lateral to medial epicondyle, over the origins of the two muscles that arise from the supracondylar ridge: pronator teres and flexor carpi ulnaris. Resisted forearm pronation or wrist flexion will reproduce the primary complaint. The physical examination must include an assessment of medial elbow stability, as collateral ligament sprains can mimic symptoms of epicondylitis. Ulnar nerve compression at the cubital tunnel can also replicate and may coexist with the clinical spectrum of medial epicondylitis. Radiographs may show medial collateral ligament calcification in some athletes, but are otherwise unremarkable. Magnetic resonance imaging (MRI) is useful in cases in which the diagnosis is less certain or is obfuscated by coexisting syndromes, and can be used in situations in which conservative management has failed. MRI will reveal increased signal intensity within the involved tendinous structures, consistent with an inflammatory degenerative process.

Treatment

As with lateral epicondylitis, treatment is initially nonoperative and employs the usual modalities of rest, ice, antiinflammatory medications, temporary counterforce bracing, and perhaps adjuncts such as electrical stimulation. Limited corticosteroid injections around the area of the involved tendons may provide relief if pain persists. Modification and enhancement of the throwing technique are then initiated, along with flexor and pronator group stretching. Isometric exercises are gradually added to the rehabilitation program and when strength has improved, additional more intensive resistance exercises are started. In cases in which supervised conservative management has been attempted for at least 6 months and has failed, surgical intervention is indicated. Current techniques not only address the inflamed myotendinous structures, but also aim to preserve flexor–pronator strength. In one technique, debridement and reapproximation of the flexor–pronator mass are performed. An oblique incision is made over the medial epicondyle. The flexor–pronator origin is incised (without violation of the medial collateral complex) and elevated, and inflamed tissue is sharply debrided. The origin is then securely reapproximated to the medial epicondyle to preserve the strength afforded by the muscle group. After brief postoperative immobilization, gentle range of motion is begun in the elbow and wrist. At 6 weeks, resisted wrist flexion and forearm pronation exercises are started, with a strengthening program to follow.

Complications

Complications occur infrequently but include weakening of the flexor–pronator mass despite the best efforts to preserve its origin and reattach the flexor–pronator mass to the distal humerus.

Prognosis

Both conservative and surgical approaches lead to excellent results in about 90% of patients.

Return to Play

Gradual return to activity is permitted in nonoperative cases if resistive exercises and occupational simulation can be performed without pain. In operative cases, return to play is usually permitted by the fourth postoperative month.

Chen FS et al: Medial elbow problems in the overhead-throwing athlete. J Am Acad Orthop Surg 2001;9:99.

2. Cubital Tunnel Syndrome

ESSENTIALS OF DIAGNOSIS

- *There is compression, traction, or irritation of the ulnar nerve as it passes through the structures of the medial elbow.*
- *The primary complaint is medial elbow pain exacerbated by throwing.*
- *Additional complaints involve paresthesias in the ring and little fingers.*
- *Provocative maneuvers reveal a positive Tinel sign over the cubital tunnel and a positive elbow flexion test.*
- *Associated with both medial epicondylitis and medial collateral ligament injury.*
- *Differential diagnosis includes medial epicondylitis, ulnar collateral ligament injury, and cervical radiculopathy.*

Prevention

Prevention relies on sound throwing techniques that minimize the valgus load on the elbow. Correction of known causes of nerve irritation including valgus instability of the elbow may also prevent the syndrome.

Clinical Findings

The cubital tunnel proper is formed by the medial epicondyle anteriorly, the elbow joint laterally, and the two heads of the flexor carpi ulnaris medially. There are structures proximal to, within, and distal to the tunnel that can cause compression, entrapment, traction, subluxation, or irritation of the ulnar nerve. Proximally, these structures include the arcade of Struthers (not to be confused with the *ligament* of Struthers, which is associated with median neuropathy) and the medial head of the triceps; within the groove they include the medial epicondyle, the epicondylar groove, the anconeus epitrochlearis, the two heads of the flexi carpi ulnaris, and their interconnecting ligament of Osborne; distally, offending structures include the deep flexor–pronator fascia. Regardless of cause or site, the final common pathway of cubital tunnel syndrome is the onset of nerve ischemia and fibrosis.

The syndrome will initially produce varying degrees of medial elbow pain with occasional radiation to the medial forearm. Paresthesias may occur in the ulnar two fingers. Athletes will often present before onset of weakness. Care must be taken to evaluate for ulnar collateral ligament injury, which may occur concomitantly with cubital tunnel syndrome. Mechanical complaints such as snapping may occur with nerve subluxation. The diagnosis is primarily clinical and relies on two provocative tests. Most patients will exhibit a positive Tinel's sign over the course of the pathology. The elbow flexion test is performed by placing the elbow in full flexion and the wrist in maximal extension. A test is positive if pain or paresthesias are elicited after 1 minute. Sensory changes can be detected with Semmes–Weinstein monofilament testing, and in more advanced cases, with two-point discrimination tests. Motor deficits often occur late and are thus infrequently observed in athletes. Changes include asymmetric hypothenar atrophy, decreased pinch and grip strength, abducted small finger or Wartenberg's sign, Froment's sign, and clawing of the ulnar two fingers. Motor deficits may not be present, even in late cases, if the intrinsic muscles of the hand receive innervation from the median nerve–the result of an anatomic variant known as the Martin–Gruber anastomosis.

A thorough examination of the neck and proximal upper extremity is performed to eliminate neuropathic etiologies with similar manifestations such as cervical radiculopathy, brachial plexopathy (of the medial cord), and thoracic outlet syndrome.

Plain radiographs including special views such as a cubital tunnel view may reveal derangements in osseous anatomy that cause compression. Similarly, MRI may identify soft tissue abnormalities with mass effect against the nerve. Electromyographic and nerve conduction velocity studies will be negative in more than 50% of patients with the syndrome. Slowing of conduction velocities to less than 50 m/s when the elbow is flexed is indicative of disease. Reduction in sensory nerve action potential also confirms early neuropathy.

Treatment

Treatment of ulnar neuropathy at the cubital tunnel is initially nonoperative: rest, ice, antiinflammatory medication, and padded splinting at 30–45° elbow flexion. Nighttime extension splinting is often quite helpful in reducing symptoms early in the disease process. Corticosteroid injections are not recommended due to the superficial position of the nerve. Conservative management will often fail in athletes due to high biomechanical demand and the potential of a subluxing ulnar nerve. Surgical indications include failed nonoperative management, ulnar nerve subluxation, and predisposing elbow pathology such as medial instability. Several techniques have been used: simple decompression, medial epicondylectomy, subcutaneous transposition, and submuscular transposition. With each technique, the ulnar nerve should be released at all possible sites of compression, from the ligament of Struthers proximally, through the cubital tunnel, past the two heads of the flexor carpi ulnaris.

Although each technique has potential complications and each has an approximately 85% success rate with primary surgery, the submuscular technique is the technique currently used for athletes. Simple decompression alone may lead to recurrence, as the medial epicondyle remains a potential offending structure. Medial epicondylectomy alone may destabilize the ulnar nerve and may disturb the medial ligamentous complex. As such, a subtotal medial epicondylectomy has been recommended in select patients. A subcutaneous transposition may leave the ulnar nerve vulnerable to direct trauma. The submuscular technique decompresses the nerve, relieves tension by transposition, and confers protection via placement between the flexor mass and pronator mass. It does require extensive dissection and may weaken the flexor–pronator musculature by altering the muscle mass origin. The flexor mass is incised to prepare the transposition bed and is reattached after anterior transposition of the released nerve. After brief postoperative immobilization, passive and then active range of motion is begun (by 4 weeks). Strengthening and throwing exercises are started by the eighth postoperative week.

Complications

Complications are uncommon but include injury to the medial antebrachial cutaneous nerve, injury to the medial collateral ligament complex, and perineural scarring. Coexisting medial elbow pathology may also limit the success of surgical intervention.

Prognosis

Conservative therapy has excellent results except in high-demand athletes. Results of surgical intervention vary inversely with the degree of preoperative nerve involvement. This can be a career-ending insult to a throwing athlete if the pathology had been present for a prolonged time prior to treatment.

Return to Play

Many patients with good to excellent results return to unrestricted play by 6 months postoperatively.

Chen FS et al: Medial elbow problems in the overhead-throwing athlete. J Am Acad Orthop Surg 2001;9:99.

Dinh PT, Gupta R: Subtotal medial epicondylectomy as a surgical option for treatment of cubital tunnel syndrome. Tech Hand Upper Extremity Surg 2005;9(1):52.

3. Ulnar Collateral Ligament Sprain & Valgus Instability

ESSENTIALS OF DIAGNOSIS

- *Tears and degenerative inflammation in the medial (ulnar) collateral ligament complex, usually involving the anterior band.*
- *Acute onset of medial elbow pain after throwing.*

- *The pain is greatest at the late cocking and acceleration phase of throwing.*
- *Tenderness is maximal posterior to flexor–pronator origin.*
- *Provocative maneuvers that place valgus stress on the elbow replicate symptoms.*
- *Varying degrees of valgus elbow instability are present.*
- *Ulnar neuropathy and posteriomedial elbow impingement may coexist.*
- *Medial epicondylitis and cubital tunnel syndrome are present.*

Prevention

Proper throwing technique and exercises that enhance flexibility help minimize the risk of ligament injury during play.

Clinical Findings

A patient with acute medial collateral injury will have sudden moderate to severe pain at the posteromedial elbow and will not be able to resume activity until treated. Patients may report feeling a "pop" at the time of injury and some patients may be unable to resume throwing. Activities of daily living are not affected, however, and most patients will report pain only during the act of throwing. Mechanical symptoms such as locking may also occur if loose bodies are present. In addition to palpation, physical examination relies on valgus stressing of the elbow to reproduce the primary complaint. Valgus stressing is performed with the elbow in 30° of flexion, which specifically stresses the anterior band. Increased medial space opening, lack of a firm endpoint, apprehension, and/or elicitation of pain all suggest medial collateral ligament failure. The crucial posterior aspect of the anterior band can be stressed using the "milking maneuver," in which valgus force is applied to the maximally flexed elbow (>90°) with the forearm in supination. Joint space opening, apprehension, or replication of medial side pain reveals ligament injury. Chronically affected athletes may exhibit limitation in elbow extension due to flexion contractures caused by the inflammatory process. Patients with chronic injury may exhibit signs and symptoms consistent with ulnar neuropathy from secondary cubital tunnel syndrome secondary to traction forces.

Stress radiographs are used to quantify the degree of joint space opening. The threshold above which medial collateral ligament incompetence is suspected is 3 mm of gapping. Standard plain films are obtained to rule out other pathology and to identify the presence of loose bodies secondary to injury. Calcification of ligament structures is expected in chronic cases. Furthermore, chronic medial instability will overload the lateral aspect of the elbow at the radiocapitellar joint. Plain films should be evaluated to determine if joint space narrowing and asymmetry are present. MRI can verify the diagnosis and may help to characterize the nature of the injury as avulsion or tear.

Treatment

In about 50% of injured athletes, nonoperative intervention is effective. Rest and antiinflammatory medication are used to address the pain. A rehabilitation program consisting of flexor–pronator mass strengthening is then started to enhance dynamic elbow stabilization. Throwing exercises are then started at 3 months, with gradual return to play when the symptoms do not recur. In cases in which the athlete does not respond to nonoperative therapy by 3 months or in acute cases of total ligament rupture or major avulsion, surgical intervention is indicated. Avulsion is treated by repair of the ligament back to its respective attachment. Ligament reconstruction, usually with the palmaris longus tendon, is employed in more chronic cases or with midsubstance tears. In ligament reconstruction, the elbow is approached through a medial incision centered at the epicondyle and the flexor–pronator origin is left intact. The flexor mass is longitudinally split and the ligament and capsule are then incised; transosseous tunnels in the coronoid and epicondyle are created. The harvested graft is then applied and appropriately tensioned in a figure-of-eight configuration. Ulnar nerve transposition is performed only if there is evidence of attendant ulnar nerve irritation or subluxation.

Complications

Complications include graft rupture or fatigue, ulnar nerve injury, medial antebrachial cutaneous nerve injury, and, rarely, donor site morbidity when grafts other than the palmaris longus are used. Postoperative immobilization is brief, with active range of motion started early. Strengthening exercises are started by 4–6 weeks postoperatively.

Prognosis

Some athletes treated nonoperatively will be able to return to play by 3 months. Those who eventually require surgery usually have good to excellent results.

Return to Play

Return to play is gradual. Valgus stressing of the elbow is to be avoided until 4 months, at which time gentle throwing exercises are begun. Throwing intensity is slowly increased with a return to the previous level of play not occurring until about 12–18 months postoperatively.

Cain EL Jr et al: Elbow injuries in throwing athletes: a current concepts review. Am J Sports Med 2003;31:621.

Chen FS et al: Medial elbow problems in the overhead-throwing athlete. J Am Acad Orthop Surg 2001;9:99.

POSTERIOR ELBOW PAIN

1. Posterior Impingement

ESSENTIALS OF DIAGNOSIS

- *Posterior elbow pain during terminal extension of the throwing arm.*
- *Impingement of the olecranon osteophytes against the olecranon fossa and trochlea.*
- *Examination reveals loss of elbow extension and tenderness along the posterior or posteromedial olecranon.*
- *Pain is elicited with forced rapid elbow extension in the presence of valgus load.*
- *Posterior and posteromedial olecranon osteophytes are sometimes visible on plain films.*
- *Associated with valgus extension overload and valgus instability.*
- *Differential diagnosis includes triceps tendonitis and posteromedial shear syndrome.*

Prevention

Development of a sound throwing technique and proper conditioning of the flexor–pronator mass will minimize excessive stress on the posteromedial elbow during throwing. Early identification of valgus elbow instability may prevent secondary impingement.

Clinical Findings

The acceleration and follow-through phases of throwing place enormous stress on the medial collateral ligament complex of the elbow. Overuse and lack of support from a properly conditioned flexor–pronator mass will lead to valgus extension overload: microtears in the medial collateral ligament complex allow transient valgus elbow subluxation during extension (late-phase throwing), whereby excessive force is transmitted to the posterior aspect of the elbow. The altered biomechanics create abnormal cyclic impaction of the olecranon against the olecranon fossa and trochlea, which produces hypertrophy and osteophyte formation on these structures. The resulting limitation in joint space leads to posterior impingement.

Patients will complain of posterior elbow pain during terminal extension. Catching and locking may be present if the osteophytes have become loose bodies. Physical examination will reveal tenderness to palpation along the posteromedial olecranon. Range of motion is limited at the extremes of extension, and rapid extension with valgus stress on the elbow will reproduce the primary complaint (the valgus extension overload test). An assessment of gross elbow valgus stability should also be performed as posterior impingement is associated with instability and will recur if the instability is not addressed. Plain radiographs, especially the true lateral elbow view, may demonstrate olecranon or olecranon fossa osteophytes, although such osteophytes are often not detected with radiography. Stress views and MRI are used to evaluate for medial collateral ligament failure. The latter can also reveal loose bodies when intraarticular contrast is used.

Treatment

Throwing is initially avoided. A treatment regime of rest, ice, antiinflammatory medication, and flexor–pronator mass strengthening is initiated. If the pain ceases, an interval-throwing plan is started. Athletes whose symptoms persist despite extended rehabilitation or whose pathology is secondary to established valgus laxity are candidates for surgery. Surgery usually involves arthroscopic excision of olecranon osteophytes, removal of loose bodies, and debridement of areas with chondromalacia. Lesions of the medial collateral complex can also be visualized for later open repair. Excision should be limited to the osteophyte itself, as removal of additional normal bone will lead to increased valgus angulation of the elbow. Elbow range of motion is started the day of surgery, and strengthening exercises of the wrist and forearm are started shortly thereafter. Shoulder strengthening and interval-throwing exercises are implemented by 10 weeks.

Complications

The most serious complication is damage to neurovascular structures during arthroscopic portal introduction and debridement. Inadequate surgeon experience or knowledge of anatomic relationships will place the radial, median, ulnar, medial antebrachial cutaneous, and anterior interosseous nerves all at risk.

Prognosis

Outcome as measured by return to previous level of activity is excellent for most operative and nonoperative cases. Some patients may require further surgical procedures if there is recurrence. The precise recurrence rate is not known, but is higher when primary causes such as instability are not corrected.

Return to Play

In operative cases, unrestricted play is usually allowed by 12 weeks postoperatively.

2. Posteromedial Shear

ESSENTIALS OF DIAGNOSIS

- *Posterior elbow pain during the acceleration phase of throwing.*
- *Caused by traction between the posteromedial olecranon and olecranon fossa.*
- *The clinical spectrum is similar to posterior impingement.*
- *Associated with valgus extension overload and valgus instability.*

As with posterior impingement syndrome, posteromedial shear is secondary to valgus extension overload. The excessive valgus torque through the posteromedial elbow causes shear stress between the posteromedial olecranon and the olecranon fossa, which results in pain during the acceleration phase of throwing. Prevention, clinical findings, treatment, and prognosis are similar to those for posterior impingement syndrome (see above). Traction spurs on the medial aspect of the olecranon notch are especially common.

Cain EL Jr, Andrews JR: Arthroscopic management of posterior elbow impingement in throwers. Tech Shoulder Elbow Surg 2001;2:118.

3. Triceps Tendonitis

ESSENTIALS OF DIAGNOSIS

- *Posterior elbow pain during resisted elbow extension.*
- *Common in throwing sports or hammering.*
- *Tenderness at triceps insertion.*
- *Range of motion is decreased.*
- *Olecranon spur is observed on lateral radiographs.*
- *Differential diagnosis includes olecranon bursitis, triceps tendon avulsion, and posterior impingement.*

Prevention

Proper conditioning and throwing technique and avoidance of overuse are the fundamentals of prevention.

Clinical Findings

Patients are principally male and are involved in high-intensity throwing or heavy manual labor. The precipitating injury is traction of the tendon at its olecranon insertion site during resisted elbow extension. The primary complaint is posterior elbow pain with extension against resistance. Maximal tenderness is directly over the triceps insertion. Both of these clinical hallmarks distinguish this overuse syndrome from other causes of posterior elbow pain. Plain radiographs should be obtained, and will often reveal olecranon osteophytes at the insertion site. These osteophytes serve to exacerbate injury and perpetuate symptoms.

Treatment

Treatment is almost always nonoperative and consists of rest, ice packs, antiinflammatory agents, and temporary bracing. Stretching and strengthening exercises are started when acute pain subsides. Corticosteroid injections will weaken the triceps tendon and are contraindicated. If pain persists despite 3–6 months of conservative management and other causes have been ruled out, excision of the spur and repair of the triceps tendon (so as to avoid the complication of tendon rupture) may be performed. A rehabilitative regime similar to that of nonoperative treatment is then instituted.

Return to Play

Return to unrestricted activity is permitted when the patient no longer has symptoms associated with provocative maneuvers and has regained full extension strength and range of motion.

Gabel GT: Acute and chronic tendinopathies at the elbow. Curr Opin Orthoped 2000;11:56.

■ ELBOW INSTABILITY

VALGUS INSTABILITY

The essential features, diagnosis, treatment, and prognosis of valgus elbow instability are described in the section on Medial Elbow Pain and the section on Ulnar Collateral Ligament Sprain & Valgus Instability.

POSTEROLATERAL ROTARY INSTABILITY

ESSENTIALS OF DIAGNOSIS

- *Instability of the elbow due to failure of the lateral ulnar collateral ligament (LUCL).*
- *Causes recurrent three-dimensional elbow sub-luxation or dislocation.*
- *History of antecedent traumatic dislocation.*
- *Symptoms include giving way, locking, and clunking of the elbow during normal daily activity.*
- *No tenderness to palpation.*
- *Range of motion is preserved.*
- *Positive posterolateral rotary instability test.*
- *Standard varus/valgus instability tests are negative.*
- *Differential diagnosis includes valgus instability of the elbow.*

Prevention

In the athletic setting, posterolateral rotary instability (PLRI) is usually a sequela of elbow trauma, and prevention is less important than early detection, which comes from a meticulous history and physical examination. PLRI can also be an iatrogenic injury and may result from surgical approaches that violate the LCL (Kocher approach) or release the LCL from its distal attachment (Boyd approach). The incidence of PLRI decreases when the LCL is repaired or reattached during these procedures.

Clinical Findings

PLRI may have many causes including previous elbow dislocation, elbow sprains, destabilizing fractures of the radial head, fractures of the coronoid, global ligament laxity, and cubitus varus elbow alignment. The final common pathway is laxity or complete disruption of the LUCL, which renders the elbow unstable against the combined vector of axial compression, external rotation (or ulnar supination), and valgus force. As a result, the ulna can undergo an abnormal external rotary moment about the humerus, which causes the radial head to sublux behind the capitellum.

PLRI not only eliminates athletic performance, it also significantly affects regular daily activities of living. Patients may report recurrent subluxations/dislocations of the elbow, painful clicking, and mechanical symptoms. Apprehension is reported when the forearm is in extension and supination. Clinical examination will reveal no areas of tenderness and standard tests for varus or valgus laxity are unremarkable. Diagnosis depends on a positive

posterolateral rotary instability test, described by O'Driscoll et al. The patient is supine while the arm is placed over the head. The examiner holds the forearm in full supination and extension, and applies a gradual flexion, varus, and axial moment to the elbow. At mid-flexion, the elbow will undergo external rotary subluxation, with subluxation of the radial head that can be palpated posteriorly. Continued flexion will cause the triceps to reduce the radial head, which produces a noticeable clunk. The series of events, or apprehension during the provocative maneuvers, constitutes a positive test. This test may be positive only when the patient is evaluated under anesthesia. The supination chair push-up test and posterolateral rotary drawer test are also useful clinical indicators.

Plain radiographs may reveal abnormal humeroulnar joint widening and stress views or fluoroscopy during the PLRI test may show rotary subluxation.

Treatment

Nonsurgical management is rarely appropriate, particularly for the high-level athlete. Surgical correction relies either on (1) proximal advancement of the lateral collateral ligament complex if the tissue is structurally intact, or (2) reconstruction of the lateral complex using a palmaris longus graft with transosseous suture fixation in chronic cases or when sufficient ligamentous tissue is not present. Other autogenous graft sources may also be used. The approach in either case, as described by Mehta and Bain, is a lateral Z arthrotomy centered over the annular ligament to prevent further injury to lateral structures. Postoperative management consists of brief splinting of the elbow at 90° of flexion and the forearm in mid-pronation. A gradual increase in extension is allowed in a locking hinged elbow brace.

Complications

Complications include elbow flexion contracture, but this is often less than 20°.

Prognosis

Successful repair or reconstruction of the lateral complex allows return to play by 6 months in most cases.

Mehta JA, Bain GI: Posterolateral rotatory instability of the elbow. J Am Acad Orthop Surg 2004;12:405.

O'Driscoll SW et al: Posterolateral rotatory instability of the elbow. J Bone Joint Surg Am 1991;73:440.

▓ WRIST PAIN

ANATOMY

The wrist includes the distal radioulnar joint, radiocarpal joint, triangular fibrocartilaginous complex, and eight carpal bones. The carpal bones include the capitate, trapezoid, trapezium, scaphoid, lunate, triquetrum, hamate, and pisiform.

The ulnar head articulates with the distal radius at its lesser sigmoid notch to form the distal radioulnar joint. The joint is principally stabilized by the dorsal and volar radioulnar joints. The radius also articulates with the scaphoid and lunate at its respective facets to form the radiocarpal joint. These articulations are in turn stabilized by a series of extrinsic (wrist-spanning) ligaments: the radial collateral, radioscaphoid, radiolunate, radiotriquetral, radioscaphocapitate, radiolunotriquetral, and radioscapholunate. The radiocarpal joint alone transmits up to 75% of the axial load across the wrist.

Analogous to the articulation between the radius and carpus, the ulna is also intimately associated with the proximal carpal row via the triangular fibrocartilagenous complex (TFCC). The TFCC is a network of ligamentous and cartilagenous structures that spans the wrist between the ulna, radius, and carpus; it allows the ulna to bear 25% of the axial wrist load. The TFCC is composed of the ulnar collateral ligament, the dorsal and volar radioulnar ligaments, the sheath of the extensor carpi ulnaris, the articular disc, the meniscal homologue, and the ulnolunate and ulnotriquetral ligaments.

The carpal bones are organized into proximal (scaphoid, lunate, triquetrum, pisiform) and distal (trapezium, trapezoid, capitate, hamate) rows. Proper wrist kinematics and stability rely heavily on the numerous intrinsic (interosseous) ligaments that interconnect every and all carpal bones. Dorsally, these include the intercarpal, trapeziotrapezoid, dorsal capitotrapezoid, and dorsal capitohamate ligaments. Volarly, they include the volar capitohamate, volar capitotrapezoid, deltoid (between the trapezium and capitate and triquetrum and capitate), lunotriquetral, and scapholunate ligaments.

Gupta R et al: Kinematic analysis of the distal radioulnar joint after a simulated progressive ulnar-sided wrist injury. J Hand Surg 2002;27A:854.

Wright PE II: Wrist disorders. In: *Campbell's Operative Orthopaedics,* 10th ed. Canale ST (editor). Mosby, 2003.

SCAPHOID FRACTURE

ESSENTIALS OF DIAGNOSIS

- *History reveals a fall on an outstretched hand with hyperextension of the wrist.*
- *Classic complaint is pain on the dorsal aspect of the wrist after a fall.*
- *Physical examination and high index of suspicion are keys to the diagnosis.*
- *Maximal tenderness over the anatomic snuffbox and scaphotrapezial joint.*

- *Plain radiographs are often negative in acute nondisplaced cases.*
- *Differential diagnosis: wrist "sprain," distal radius fracture, distal radioulnar joint disruption, carpal ligament rupture with carpal instability, and lunate fracture.*

Prevention

Although scaphoid fractures cannot be avoided, early clinical detection and prompt treatment will prevent complications of fracture nonunion and wrist instability.

Clinical Findings

Athletes will complain of radial wrist pain (classically dorsal, but also volar), with swelling, and wrist stiffness after a fall on the outstretched hand. Tenderness is elicited over the anatomic snuffbox between the tendons of the extensor pollicis longus and brevis, or over the tubercle at the scaphotrapezial joint. A thorough radiographic assessment is essential, but will fail to detect fractures 36% of the time. The series should consist of posteroanterior (PA), lateral, and clenched fist ulnar deviation views. Lateral views should be reviewed for intrascaphoid angulation and the presence of carpal instability patterns [such as dorsal intercalary instability (DISI)], which indicate an unstable fracture. Although bone scans have historically been used to evaluate for occult scaphoid fractures, MRI is now more routinely used for immediate radiographic diagnosis. MRI also plays a role in assessing the viability of fracture fragments in the case of nonunions, particularly if the fracture involves the watershed region at or proximal to the scaphoid waist. Computed tomography (CT) scans are useful for assessing fracture union during treatment or in cases in which nonunion is suspected.

Treatment

Only stable scaphoid fractures—nondisplaced, nonangulated fractures without associated carpal instability—may be treated nonoperatively. A short arm thumb spica cast is applied for 12–16 weeks. Healing time approaches 12 weeks, but union rates approach 90% with appropriate treatment. Recent research has demonstrated that even stable fractures may be treated operatively with percutaneous screw fixation with minimal additional morbidity. In cases of elite athletes, the fracture can be percutaneously fixed and placed in a playing cast. Patients may return to competition in about 2 weeks but continue to wear the cast until healing is clinically and radiographically evident.

Unstable fractures, which have ≥1.0 mm displacement, are comminuted, are fractured at the proximal pole, have an intrascaphoid angulation >45°, or exhibit carpal instability patterns should undergo reduction and internal fixation. Without operative intervention, the risk of nonunion/malunion and disability is high. Union is often assessed by CT scan. Nonunions must undergo open treatment and internal fixation, with or without vascularized bone grafting, depending on the viability of the proximal fragments. Proximal pole fracture and nonunions are approached dorsally, whereas waist fractures are usually addressed volarly.

Prognosis

Both nonoperative and operative outcomes are very good. Highly comminuted fractures, nonunions that undergo correction, and cases with carpal instability have more variable results.

Return to Play

Return to play after fixation of unstable fractures depends on postoperative fracture stability. Unprotected play is allowed when the patient is no longer symptomatic, has regained full range of motion, and has exhibited complete healing on radiographs or CT scan.

Bond CT et al: Percutaneous screw fixation or cast immobilization for nondisplaced scaphoid fractures. J Bone Joint Surg Am 2001;83-A(4):483.

Morgan WJ, Slowman LS: Acute hand and wrist injuries in athletes: evaluation and management. J Am Acad Orthop Surg 2001;9:389.

Trumble TE et al: Management of scaphoid nonunions. J Am Orthop Surg 2003;11:380.

WRIST SPRAINS

1. Scapholunate Ligament

Injury to the scapholunate ligament occurs in contact/collision or after a fall on a hand with wrist extension and ulnar deviation (intercarpal supination). Patients will exhibit swelling and pain along the dorsum of the wrist. Tenderness is maximal at the scapholunate interval dorsally. The Watson's sign is elicited by placing dorsal pressure over the distal scaphoid while shifting the wrist from ulnar to radial deviation; the maneuver will result in pain and an audible click. With established, complete ligament tears, plain PA radiographs will show that the scapholunate interval or gap is 2 mm or greater, and the lateral view will demonstrate the characteristic DISI pattern. The clenched-fist view can also further demonstrate the injury. MRI can diagnose complete ligament tears with ease, but partial tears are harder to

appreciate and clinical acumen is required. Treatment involves arthroscopic confirmation of the diagnosis and then open repair or reconstruction. In cases in which the tear is incomplete, percutaneous pinning for 4–6 weeks may be employed. In acute cases, open repair of the ligament is performed with or without augmentation using the dorsal intercarpal ligament. Chronic cases may not be amenable to repair after 9 months and remain an unsolved problem. Salvage procedures include bone–ligament–bone graft reconstruction or partial carpal fusion. Untreated patients will invariably develop carpal collapse and wrist arthritis. Carpectomy or arthrodesis may need to be performed in these cases. Results are variable and depend on the severity and chronicity of the injury.

2. Lunotriquetral Ligament

Tears in the lunotriquetral ligament result from a fall on an outstretched hand, with the wrist in extension and radial deviation (intercarpal pronation). The patient will report ulnar-sided wrist pain, weakness, and other mechanical complaints. Tenderness is maximal over the lunotriquetral interval. Pain is reproduced with the lunotriquetral shear test, in which the pisiform and triquetrum are pressed in a dorsal direction while the lunate is pressed in a volar direction. Diagnosis in most cases is clinical. Radiographs are often normal but may show the characteristic volar intercalary instability (VISI), which will occur if the dorsal radiotriquetral ligament is also torn. MRI exhibits poor resolution of this ligament. Treatment by immobilization is successful in most patients, with return to play in a matter of weeks if the ligament is not completely torn. Surgery is reserved for only the most resistant cases, as return to play is lengthy, from 2 to 6 months. Procedures include bone–ligament–bone reconstruction, arthroscopic debridement, carpal fusion, and ulnar shortening osteotomy.

3. Midcarpal Instability

Instability between a proximal and distal row (carpal instability nondissociative) occurs when the ligamentous attachment between the capitate and the proximal carpal row is injured. Athletes will report ulnar wrist pain. The catch-up clunk is a diagnostic maneuver in which the proximal row does not move into dorsiflexion until late into a sweep from radial to ulnar deviation. The sudden shift is manifested as a clunk. Abrogation of the clunk with dorsally directed pressure over the pisiform secures the diagnosis. Radiographs may show a volar intercalary instability pattern. Treatment is usually non-operative, and employs ulnar carpus support splinting and antiinflammatory medication. Surgical procedures are reserved for severe cases, and include thermal shrinkage, ligament reconstruction, or midcarpal arthrodesis. Results are unimpressive.

4. Distal Radioulnar Joint & the Triangular Fibrocartilagenous Complex

Injuries to the distal radioulnar joint (DRUJ) and its closely associated structure, the TFCC, are common in a wide range of sports. Tears may be either traumatic or degenerative. Hypersupination, traction, and axial loading with rotational stress are possible mechanisms. Tenderness over the TFCC is best assessed by palpating between the ulnar styloid and pisiform. Damage to the DRUJ is often revealed by painful and excessive volar–dorsal shuck between the radius and ulna at the wrist, a provocative maneuver known as the piano key sign. The TFCC grind is another provocative maneuver performed with the wrist in ulnar deviation and dorsiflexion, while the carpus is rotated on the wrist by the examiner as an axial load is applied on the hand. Physical examination as described above is often the most reliable diagnostic modality. Plain radiographs may reveal ulnar styloid fractures, widened radioulnar joint space, and distal ulnar subluxation. Comparison CT images of the DRUJ with the forearm in supination and pronation may reveal abnormal excursion and hence instability. High-quality MR images may show TFCC tears, but are often equivocal based on the quality of the imaging system. Wrist arthroscopy is used to confirm the diagnosis and is considered the gold standard. For individuals with central lesions, early arthroscopic debridement of the TFCC is advocated, followed by splinting and early range of motion. Return to play with restrictions occurs by 6 weeks. With peripheral sided tears, arthroscopic repair is performed followed by immobilization for 6 weeks. A DRUJ that remains unstable after arthroscopic repair may be augmented by pinning the DRUJ with the forearm in maximum supination. Return to play is allowed at 4 months. Results for both groups are excellent. With chronic or degenerative injuries, a shift in wrist biomechanics occurs, with increased load through the radiocarpal joint. Abnormal ulnar variance may be present and ulnar shortening procedures along with carpal arthroscopy may be indicated.

Gupta R et al: Wrist anthroscopy: indications and technique. J Am Acad Orthop Surg 2001;9(3):200.

Gupta R et al: Kinematic analysis of the distal radioulnar joint after a simulated progressive ulnar-sided wrist injury. J Hand Surg 2002;27A:854.

Rettig AC: Athletic injuries of the wrist and hand, part 1: traumatic injuries of the wrist. Am J Sports Med 2003;31:1038.

■ HAND PAIN

ULNAR COLLATERAL LIGAMENT INJURY OF THE THUMB

 ESSENTIALS OF DIAGNOSIS

- *A history of contact sport or fall during skiing.*
- *Swelling and pain at the base of the thumb.*
- *Tenderness over the ulnar collateral ligament at the thumb metacarpophalangeal (MCP) joint.*
- *Identification and correction of Stener lesions.*

Clinical Findings

In addition to obtaining a history and performing a physical examination, careful palpation of the MCP base should be performed to identify the Stener lesion. This lesion occurs when there is complete detachment of the ulnar collateral ligament from the phalangeal base and displacement over the adductor pollicis. This interposition will prevent proper healing unless surgically corrected. Radiographic stress views will reveal MCP joint instability and the degree of ligament injury. A complete rupture is indicated by opening of 30° or more on multiple views.

Treatment

Nondisplaced avulsion fractures are treated with a thumb spica cast for 4 weeks, and the thumb is then protected in a custom-molded splint after return to play is allowed. In patients with complete ruptures and Stener lesions, surgical correction is required acutely. This is done by a tension band technique, interfragmentary screw, or the use of mini-Mitek suture anchors. Immobilization lasts for 4 weeks, after which a custom-molded splint is applied.

Prognosis

Outcomes for both nonoperative and successful operative cases are excellent, provided the patient is compliant with protection splinting and taping.

Return to Play

Return to play is permitted with a protection splint and rigid taping of the thumb MCP.

FINGER INJURIES

Mallet Finger & Jersey Finger

Mallet finger is a flexion deformity of the distal interphalangeal (DIP) joint that is the result of a disruption in the extensor mechanism. The unopposed force of the flexor digitorum profundus moves the terminal phalanx into flexion. Injury is usually the result of forcible flexion of the joint during active extension, usually when catching a ball, hence the injury is commonly called "baseball" or "drop finger." Two forms of mallet finger exist, one involving only the tendon and the other involving an avulsed fracture fragment. Three-view radiographs are recommended as bony mallets are difficult to diagnose by physical examination alone. Severe injuries may involve volar subluxation of the distal phalanx. Treatment includes extension splinting for 8 weeks with 80% achieving good to excellent results. If the injury is associated with a fracture or subluxation, reduction of the distal fragment should be performed. Mallet finger can be treated for up to 4 months after the initial injury. After that time, provided the joint is supple and without arthritis, reconstruction of the tendon may be a treatment option. In other cases, DIP fusion is recommended. Swan neck deformities may develop over time if there is laxity of the volar plate. Follow-up examinations should be performed every 2 weeks, and the finger retested. An additional 2–4 weeks of splinting may be required.

A Jersey finger is the result of the avulsion of the flexor digitorum profundus when a flexed DIP joint is forced into extension. Injuries can occur when a player grabs another jersey during a game, or when lifting a latch on a car door. The ring finger is most commonly affected. Patients are unable to flex the DIP joint and have swelling and prominence of the digit. Three-view radiographs are recommended to identify bony avulsions. Early diagnosis is important as the treatment for Jersey fingers is almost always operative. Delays can result in fibrosis and scarring of the tendon sheath. Pure tendinous injuries allow the flexor digitorum profundus to retract to the palm, whereas injuries with bone fragments tend to limit retraction to the level of the middle phalanx.

The Jersey finger is classified into four types: Type I, the tendon retracts to the palm with rupture of the vincula; Type II, the tendon retracts to the proximal interphalangeal joint and is held by the vinculum; Type III, a large bony fragment catches on a pulley at the middle phalanx; and Type IV, a bony avulsion with the tendon avulsed to the fragment.

Treatment varies by type. Type I injuries should be repaired in 7–10 days from the onset of injury as the tendon is dysvascular. Repair of Type II injuries can be done within 6 weeks. In Type III injuries, open reduction with internal fixation (ORIF) is performed. Type III injuries involve repair of the articular fragment with secondary repair of the distal phalanx. Type IV injuries involve dynamic rehabilitation of the tendon with passive flexion, dorsal block splint, and active extension exercises.

Spine

7

Frank Fumich, MD, Adam C. Crowl, MD & James D. Kang, MD

■ CERVICAL SPINE INJURIES IN ATHLETES

ANATOMY

The anatomy of the cervical spine must be understood to appreciate its susceptibility to injury in athletics. Mobility of the head is afforded at the cost of stability. The cervical spine is made up of seven vertebrae relying on bone and ligamentous and muscular attachments to confer stability to axial loads, rotational movements, and bending movements.

The architecture of the cervical spine protects the spinal cord circumferentially by the vertebral body and the paired lamina that make up the protective roof of the spinal canal. Each vertebral body articulates with the adjacent vertebra with an interposed intervertebral disk. The uncovertebral joints of Luschka form the anteromedial boundary of the neuroforamen, which is bordered posteriorly by the facet joint. Through this neuroforamen the nerve root exits (Figure 7–1). Anterior to the spine and covering the vertebral bodies and intervertebral disks the anterior longitudinal ligament (ALL) spans the length of the entire vertebral column. The posterior longitudinal ligament spans the posterior aspect of the vertebral bodies in a similar fashion. These osseous and ligamentous structures make up the anterior spinal column, provide axial support to load imparted to the head, provide protection to the neural structures, and allow mobility in rotation and bending movements. The posterior cervical spine is made up of the lamina, facet articulations, lateral masses, and spinous processes that give the posterior spinal column the ability to share axial loads and provide sites of attachment for muscles that control head and neck movement. Each vertebra has a paired set of facets that articulates superiorly and inferiorly with the adjacent vertebra.

Approximately one-half of the flexion and extension arc occurs through the atlantooccipital articulation and approximately one-half of neck rotation occurs between the atlas and axis. Each segment below the axis allows coupled rotation and lateral bending due to the unique shape of the uncovertebral articulation and facet joints, which further increases the functional range of cervical motion.

Static and dynamic restraints are of great importance due to the lack of intrinsic stability in the neck. The osseous anatomy of the cervical spine is connected by several ligaments that provide restraint to the extremes of neck motion. The primary static stabilizers of the cervical spine include the anterior longitudinal ligament, intervertebral disk, posterior longitudinal ligament, ligamentum flavum, facet capsules, and interspinous and supraspinous ligaments. These ligamentous structures function only as a checkrein at the end point of neck movements. The dynamic stabilization, which is the muscular support of the neck, includes the sternocleidomastoid, trapezius, and strap muscles and paraspinal musculature. The protective function of the neck musculature functions throughout the range of motion. Both the static and dynamic stabilizers of the neck are vulnerable to injury during sporting events that involve high-energy impact of the head or neck.

DIFFERENTIAL DIAGNOSIS

Most injuries to the cervical spine are minor. The most commonly diagnosed injuries are soft-tissue trauma including ligament sprains, muscle strains, and contusions of soft tissue. The magnitude and direction of force applied to the neck determine the type and severity of injury. Cervical strains are injuries to the musculotendinous portions of the neck and cervical sprains are injuries to the ligaments of the neck. Cervical strains are the most common neck injury of athletes. Differentiating these two injuries may be very difficult in the clinical setting. The most common mechanism of injury involves high-velocity contact sports. Two other common mechanisms include sudden deceleration of the body involving a whiplash of the head and overuse syndromes. Sporting accidents are second only to motor vehicle accidents as the leading cause of emergency department visits involving neck injuries.

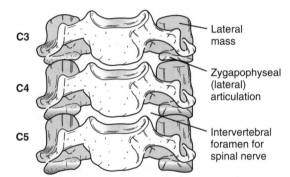

C3 — Lateral mass

C4 — Zygapophyseal (lateral) articulation

C5 — Intervertebral foramen for spinal nerve

Figure 7–1. Anterior view of cervical spine skeletal structure displaying uncovertebral joints and facet articulations.

CERVICAL STRAIN

ESSENTIALS OF DIAGNOSIS

- *Symptoms (history) and knowledge of mechanism of injury.*
- *Physical examination for tenderness and range of motion.*
- *Plain radiographs with flexion and extension views.*
- *Further imaging such as magnetic resonance imaging (MRI) with neurologic injury.*

Prevention

The prevention of neck injury such as a strain or sprain is best done through muscular conditioning and development. This includes isometric exercises to strengthen the paraspinal musculature. Other measures include proper education of the athlete concerning techniques of play and avoidance of spearing and facemask holding, for example.

Clinical Findings

A. SYMPTOMS

Muscle strains in the neck occur as a result of a blow to the head or neck during muscle contraction producing eccentric muscle loading. The complaint of pain following the described mechanism suggests injury to the musculotendinous junction of the involved muscle. These complaints may be preceded by amnesia to the event depending on the severity of impact or deceleration.

B. SIGNS

Painful limited cervical range of motion and tenderness over the involved neck muscles are the cardinal signs of cervical strain injury.

C. IMAGING STUDIES

Radiographic imaging of the cervical spine is necessary to rule out fractures and dislocations that make the cervical spine unstable. At a minimum, two orthogonal views with visualization from the occiput to the C7 to T1 junction are necessary. Instability may be suspected with findings of interspinous widening, vertebral subluxation, compression fracture, or loss of cervical lordosis. Other studies looking at the stability afforded by the ligaments of the spine have identified horizontal displacement of 3.5 mm or angular displacement of 11° or more as signs of instability (Figures 7–2 and 7–3).

In the acute setting lateral flexion and extension views may be of less benefit in patients experiencing

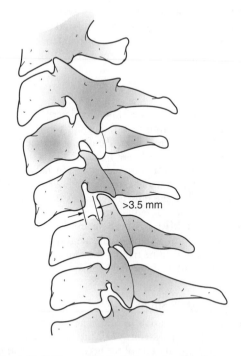

>3.5 mm

Figure 7–2. The method of measuring translatory displacement. A distance of 3.5 mm or greater is considered to be clinically unstable. (Reproduced, with permission, from White AA et al: Biomechanical analysis of clinical stability in the cervical space, Clin Orthop Relat Res 1975;120(109):85.)

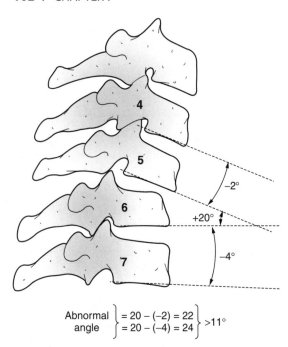

$$\left.\begin{array}{l} \text{Abnormal} \\ \text{angle} \end{array}\right\} \begin{array}{l} = 20 - (-2) = 22 \\ = 20 - (-4) = 24 \end{array}\Bigg\} >11°$$

Figure 7–3. A difference of 11° or greater than that of either adjacent interspace is considered clinically unstable. (From White AA 3rd et al: Spinal stability: evaluation and treatment. Instr Course Lect 1981;30:457.)

significant pain. Subacute instability describes patients who present with normal radiographs initially but demonstrate instability later. Paraspinal muscle spasm can mask instability acutely because it prevents adequate excursion on flexion and extension radiographs. Therefore the flexion and extension radiographs should be repeated when the muscle spasm has improved after a period of cervical immobilization with a collar.

The use of MRI has been reserved for situations involving cervical instability and neurologic compromise. For cervical spine trauma the rate of detection of cervical ligamentous injury and spinal cord injury with MRI is 100%.

D. Special Examinations

A thorough examination to find areas of cervical spine tenderness and the assessment of the fullest amount of pain-free range of motion of the neck are the foundation of an examination for a cervical muscular strain injury. As in all spinal injuries, assessment of mental status and neurologic examination of the extremities are of paramount importance in making decisions concerning the athlete's care and possible return to play. Otherwise, no other special examinations or tests are necessary to diagnose a muscle strain injury.

Treatment

A. Rehabilitation

Treatment is generally conservative requiring initial immobilization with a cervical collar. The collar is worn until muscle spasm is relieved. This usually takes 7–10 days, at which time follow-up flexion and extension radiographs may be obtained to rule out instability. During the period of immobilization antiinflammatory medications may be of benefit. With the resolution of spasm and determination from follow-up radiographs that serious injury has been ruled out a physical therapy program is instituted. The collar is weaned as gentle range of motion exercises and isometric strengthening are done. Prolonged immobilization results in muscular atrophy and deconditioning of healthy muscle fibers. Physical therapy prevents muscular deconditioning and postinjury stiffness. Advancement of activities is allowed with clinical improvement.

B. Surgery

Surgery is necessary only after severe injury that has resulted in instability. Ligamentous disruption may have been initially masked through muscular spasm. Surgical options in most cases involve arthrodesis of the destabilized segment, but this is quite rare.

Return to Play

Late complications of cervical strains include continued pain or discomfort. The prognosis is good and most athletes, upon resolution of symptoms and regaining of full and pain-free neck range of motion, return to play within weeks of the injury. For return to play in football the use of cervical orthoses has been shown to limit hyperextension of the cervical spine yet allow enough extension to prevent axial loading injuries.

Holmes JF et al: Variability in CT and magnetic resonance imaging in patients with cervical spine injuries. J Trauma 2002;53:524.

Jarvinen TA et al: Muscle strain injuries. Curr Opin Rheumatol 2000;12:155.

Kelley LA: In neck to neck competition are women more fragile? Clin Orthop 2000;(372):123.

Versteegen GJ et al: Neck sprain not arising from car accidents: a retrospective study covering 25 years. Eur Spine J 1998;7:201.

COMMON FRACTURES

Cervical fractures are much less common than fractures of the thoracolumbar spine. Anatomic differences in the shape of the vertebra and the increased range of motion of the neck account for this difference. The three most common minor fractures of the cervical spine due to athletic participation are compression fractures, spinous-process fractures, and isolated lamina fractures. Hyperflexion is believed to be the cause of cervical spine compression fractures. The amount of posterior ligamentous injury is directly proportional to the amount of force imparted to the neck at the time of fracture. Posterior ligamentous disruption present in combination with a fracture significantly increases the amount of instability of the neck and requires a careful work-up to determine its presence.

Spinous process fractures may occur in isolation, but as with compression fractures a thorough work-up must be completed to rule out ligamentous injury. The upper and lower cervical spinal segments are the most commonly involved levels of spinous process fracture. The most common mechanism of injury for spinous process fracture is contraction of the trapezius and rhomboid muscles causing an avulsion of the spinous process. Extreme hyperflexion and hyperextension as seen in the high-energy trauma of a collision may also produce a spinous process fracture by avulsion of the spinous process when pulled by the supraspinous and interspinous ligaments. Much less commonly a direct blow may cause a spinous process fracture.

An isolated lamina fracture is rare and is usually associated with a more complex mechanism of injury such as a burst fracture or a fracture dislocation of the cervical spine. Axial loads with or without rotation produce vertical lamina fractures and are usually associated with fracture of the vertebral body. Transverse fractures of the lamina are due to avulsion as the ligamentum flavum pulls during extreme hyperflexion. These transverse lamina fractures may be associated with instability.

ESSENTIALS OF DIAGNOSIS

- Symptoms (history) and knowledge of the mechanism of injury.
- Physical examination for tenderness and range of motion.
- Plain radiographs with flexion and extension views.
- Further imaging such as MRI with neurologic injury.

Clinical Findings

A. SYMPTOMS

The primary complaint associated with fracture of the cervical spine is pain. The onset of pain from fracture in the cervical spine correlates with time of injury and the magnitude of load imparted to the neck.

B. SIGNS

Resistance to movement of the neck is seen. Neurologic injury may be present depending on the nature of the

fracture, the presence of a facet fracture and/or associated dislocation, and the presence of disk or bone fragments impinging on the spinal cord or nerve roots.

C. IMAGING STUDIES

As with any trauma to the cervical spine a complete radiographic evaluation of the athlete injured during play is mandatory. Imaging of the cervical spine begins with anteroposterior and lateral views of the cervical spine, which allow visualization of the atlantooccipital articulation and the C7–T1 junction. If the cervicothoracic junction cannot be visualized with plain radiographs a computed tomography (CT) scan of this area may be done. Common cervical fractures associated with sporting accidents include compression, spinous process, and isolated lamina fractures.

D. SPECIAL TESTS/SPECIAL EXAMINATIONS

There are no special tests other than a standard history and physical examination assessing the mechanism of injury, energy imparted to the head or neck at the time of injury, and a thorough skeletal and neurologic examination to diagnose a cervical spine fracture.

Complications

The possible complications of a cervical fracture sustained during athletic participation depend on the nature of the fracture, the presence of neurologic compromise, the overall stability of the neck after injury, and the presence of other injuries sustained at the same time. Most fractures that occur in the neck from sports participation are minor in comparison to the entire scope of cervical fractures and heal uneventfully, especially in a young and motivated patient population. When fractures or ligamentous disruption have occurred that have gone unrecognized the athlete is at risk for future neurologic injury or posttraumatic deformity.

Treatment

A. REHABILITATION

Isolated compression fractures are usually treated with a semirigid collar for 8–10 weeks. Spinous-process fractures are benign and usually heal without any significant problem. Immobilization in a cervical collar for 4–6 weeks relieves pain. For both types of fractures flexion and extension radiographs should be taken at the end of the immobilization period to rule out a more serious ligamentous disruption.

Lamina fracture treatment is dictated by the stability of the cervical spine. When lamina fractures occur in isolation without any other ligamentous injury or fracture the neck may be immobilized in a cervical collar for 8–10 weeks. This is followed by lateral flexion and extension radiographs to rule out instability.

B. SURGERY

Surgery is necessary to stabilize the cervical spine when bony or ligamentous injury has occurred that cannot be treated with immobilization alone or to perform decompression when either bone or soft tissue such as disk material causes neurologic deficits. These are rare instances in athletes but surgery is necessary when the stability of the cervical spine has been compromised.

C. SPECIAL PROCEDURES

The procedures used to confer stability to the neck after a destabilizing injury in almost all circumstances involve performing an arthrodesis of the destabilized segments. Anterior and posterior approaches are available to accomplish this goal. The direction taken is influenced by the site of destabilization and the presence of neurologic compromise that may require decompression.

Return to Play

The athlete may be allowed to return to play after healing of the fracture and determining by lateral flexion and extension radiographs that instability is not present. In addition, a full rehabilitation course aimed at achieving full neck strength and range of motion will reduce discomfort and the possibility of recurrence when returning to full contact sports.

Laporte C et al: Severe hyperflexion sprains of the lower cervical spine in adults. Clin Orthop 1999;363:126.

Makan P: Neurologic compromise after an isolated laminar fracture of the spine. Spine 1999;24:1144.

NECK PAIN & PARESTHESIAS

A "burner" or "stinger" is a transient neurologic event characterized by pain or paresthesias in one upper extremity following an impact to the neck or shoulder.

ESSENTIALS OF DIAGNOSIS

- *Symptoms (history) and knowledge of the mechanism of injury.*
- *Physical examination for tenderness and range of motion.*
- *Plain radiographs with flexion and extension views.*
- *Further imaging such as MRI with neurologic injury.*

Prevention

An athlete who has sustained a previous stinger is at risk for sustaining a second occurrence. Protective equipment to restrain excessive movements in side bending and extension of the neck for play in football is recommended. The use of a strap that connects the helmet to the shoulder pads to limit cervical extension is not recommended.

Proper tackling technique and not dropping the shoulder also help to prevent injury by limiting the amount of neck extension. Maintaining eye contact with the opposing player results in a more upright position during tackling and thereby decreases the risk of sustaining a stinger.

Clinical Findings

A. SYMPTOMS

Athletes experience sensations of tingling, burning, or numbness in a circumferential distribution with an inability to move the involved extremity. The athlete is often seen either holding the affected arm with the other arm or trying to shake off the feeling of pain and numbness. The symptoms may localize to the neck or radiate to the hand on the affected side. A stinger differs from a radiculopathy, which involves symptoms in a single dermatomal pattern.

The injurious event usually involves the downward displacement of the shoulder with concomitant lateral neck flexion toward the contralateral shoulder applying stretch to the brachial plexus. Head rotation may also play a part in the etiology of stingers. Head rotation to the affected side narrows the neuroforamen causing compression of the exiting nerve root. Direct blunt trauma to Erb's point may also result in a stinger.

B. SIGNS

A patient who has sustained a stinger requires a thorough examination of the cervical spine with a complete neurologic assessment. The integrity of the neck's ligamentous and bony anatomy is determined by palpation for areas of tenderness and testing the active range of motion of the neck. Palpation is done to find tenderness, localized swelling, and deformity. Range of motion testing includes active rotation, lateral bending, forward flexion, and extension. The neurologic examination includes strength testing of all muscle groups, sensory examination over all dermatomes, deep tendon reflex and testing, and performing an upper motor neuron assessment with either the Hoffmann reflex test or the radial reflex test. The shoulder examination includes assessment of the clavicle, acromioclavicular joint, supraclavicular region, and glenohumeral joint. Percussion of Erb's point may elicit radiation of pain into the upper extremity when injury to the brachial plexus has occurred.

The player typically presents with an inability to move the involved upper extremity following a high-energy collision with another player. The on-field evaluation of the injured player shows arm weakness and a burning pain present in the involved extremity. Shoulder abductor, external rotation, and arm flexion are reliable indicators that the player has sustained a stinger. Weakness in the upper trunk of the brachial plexus including the deltoid, biceps, supraspinatus, and infraspinatus muscles is commonly seen. In most cases these symptoms resolve within minutes. Motor weakness may develop hours to days after the injury, therefore repeat examinations are necessary. When nerve-root injuries have occurred the athlete may maintain a slightly flexed posture of the neck to alleviate pressure from the affected nerve roots.

C. IMAGING STUDIES

The lateral cervical spine radiograph is most useful to determine if cervical stenosis is present. Encroachment of the facet articulations on the spinolaminar line is a positive indicator. The Torg ratio is determined by measuring the space available for the spinal cord from the posterior aspect of the vertebral body to the spinolaminar line and then dividing this distance by the anteroposterior width of the vertebral body at the same level (Figure 7–4). In most people this ratio is one. College athletes with a Torg ratio less than 0.8 have a three-fold increased risk of sustaining a stinger with cervical spine extension–compression injuries. In a group of high school athletes in which Torg ratios and foramen/vertebral body ratios were used to assess foraminal stenosis, athletes with cervical spinal canal or foraminal stenosis were demonstrated to be at an increased risk of sustaining a stinger.

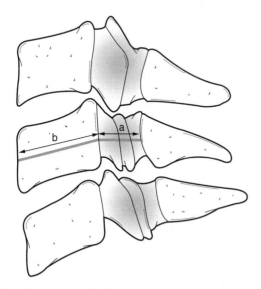

Figure 7–4. The Torg ratio is determined from the distance from the mid-point of the posterior aspect of the vertebral body to the nearest point on the corresponding spinolaminar line (**a**) divided by the anteroposterior width (**b**) of the vertebral body. (From Torg JS et al: Neuropraxia of the cervical spinal cord with transient quadriplegia. J Bone Joint Surg Am 1986;68A:1354.)

D. SPECIAL TESTS

Electrodiagnostic testing is rarely necessary as stingers are usually temporary. The abnormal spontaneous activity seen on electromyographic (EMG) testing is not evident for at least 2 weeks following injury and maximizes at 3–5 weeks. EMG testing is most useful for the evaluation of persistent weakness at 2–3 weeks. Evidence of nerve injury shows fibrillation potentials in the involved muscles. When nerve root injury is suspected an MRI is the study of choice. The MRI will show shifting of the cord away from an avulsed cervical nerve root when present.

Studies of electrodiagnostic testing for stinger syndrome have found that even though the patient's strength improved over time up to 80% of athletes continued to have abnormal EMG studies at 5 years postinjury. It therefore can be concluded that only in rare instances is EMG testing necessary following stingers and the most reliable criteria for return to play remain the physical examination and appropriate imaging studies.

E. SPECIAL EXAMINATIONS

The Spurling's maneuver may be used to assess foraminal narrowing and has been shown to reproduce arm symptoms in 70% of those who have experienced stingers. By laterally bending the neck with concomitant application of axial load a compressive load is produced on the neural foramen. When arm pain is reproduced the test is considered positive as this indicates that nerve root irritation has occurred.

Stingers involving the upper extremity are always unilateral and have not been reported to occur in the lower extremity. When bilateral symptoms and or deficits occur the possibility of a spinal cord injury must be ruled out. This clinical situation requires an assessment of motion and areas of tenderness. Reluctance to move the neck and severe tenderness are signs of a potentially serious injury. This requires immobilization of the patient and transport on a backboard to a nearby trauma center for a full work-up and radiologic testing.

Treatment

Isolated stingers are considered to be benign injuries. By definition stingers are transient injuries and usually do not require formal treatment other than observation and supportive care. The athlete should not be allowed to return to play until the symptoms completely resolve. For severe injuries, a sling should be worn while clinicians await the resolution of symptoms. Modalities in a physical therapy center and medications can be used as necessary to control pain. Rehabilitation should then ensue to strengthen all of the upper extremity muscles including those not involved in the injury.

Rehabilitation of the cervical spine after a stinger involves conditioning of the neck and shoulder musculature. Attaining full neck range of motion essentially clears the patient of nerve root irritation as an irritable nerve root will limit the ability to move the neck due to pain. The strengthening program should include isometrics with progression to isotonic exercises with inclusion of the shoulder and trapezius musculature.

Prognosis

A player should not be allowed to return to play when the risk of play outweighs the benefits for the player. The relative risk of a player sustaining a second stinger increases when compared to the risk of a player sustaining an initial stinger. Players should be excluded from further participation in contact sports when they remain symptomatic after a stinger or have persistently abnormal diagnostic studies.

Long-term muscle weakness with persistent paresthesias may result from severe or repeated stingers. Repeated stingers in athletes may result from a combination of cervical stenosis and degenerative disk disease.

Return to Play

Vaccaro and co-workers' return to play criteria for cervical spine injury in the athlete provide one of the most complete guidelines for managing players who have sustained a stinger. For a first time stinger an athlete may return to play only if neck range of motion is full and painless and the upper extremity strength is full. An athlete who has sustained three or fewer episodes of stingers in the past each of which has lasted fewer than 24 hours may also return to play on the day of injury. An athlete whose symptoms do not resolve on the sideline may not be allowed to return to play until either the symptoms resolve or further imaging studies are performed to determine the cause of the stinger.

The relative contraindications to return to play include a prolonged symptomatic burner lasting for more than 24 hours or more than three stingers that have occurred in the past. Absolute containdications to return to play include (1) more than two episodes of transient quadriparesis, (2) a clinical history, examination findings, or an imaging study that confirm cervical myelopathy, and (3) any continued neck discomfort, decreased range of motion, or any neurologic deficit sustained from any prior cervical spine injury.

Aldrige JW et al: Nerve entrapment in athletes. Clinics Sports Med 2001;20:95.

Bergeld JA et al: Brachial plexus injury in sports: a five year follow-up. Orthop Trans 1998;12:743.

Feinberg JH: Burners and stingers. Phys Med Rehab Clin North Am 2000;11:771.

Proctor MR, Cantu RC: Head and neck injuries in young athletes. Clinics Sports Med 2000;4:693.

Slipman CW et al: Symptom provocation of fluoroscopically guided cervical root stimulation: are dynamic maps identical to dermatomal maps? Spine 1998;23(20):2235.

Vaccaro AR et al: Cervical spine injuries in athletes: current return-to-play criteria. Orthopedics 2001;24:699.

Weinstein S: Assessment and rehabilitation of the athlete with a "stinger": a model for the management of noncatastrophic athletic cervical spine injury. Clinics Sports Med 1998; 17:127.

SPINAL CORD NEUROPRAXIA & TRANSIENT TETRAPLEGIA

ESSENTIALS OF DIAGNOSIS

- *Symptoms (history) and knowledge of the mechanism of injury.*
- *Physical examination for tenderness and range of motion.*
- *Plain radiographs with flexion and extension views.*
- *Further imaging such as MRI with neurologic injury.*

Temporary paralysis after a sports-related collision followed by the resolution of symptoms and a normal physical examination has been named spinal cord neuropraxia (SCN) or transient tetraplegia. Cervical spine radiographs of athletes show congenital spinal stenosis, believed to be the most significant contributing factor to the development of this entity. Hyperextension of the neck is believed to cause an infolding of the ligamentum flavum leading to a 30% reduction in the anteroposterior diameter of the spinal canal. As the neck extends the spine shortens, resulting in the infolding of the dura mater, thickening of the spinal cord, buckling of the ligamentum flavum, and narrowing of the subarachnoid space, known as the "pincher mechanism." Any one or a combination of these events effectively increases the pressure on the cervical spinal cord and decreases its blood flow contributing to an SCN episode. Congenital narrowing of the spinal canal increases the risk of injury as a lower functional reserve is available for the spinal cord to adapt during significant blows to the head or neck.

Episodes of SCN are described in terms of neurologic deficit, duration of symptoms, and anatomic distribution. The terms paresthesias, paresis, and plegia describe a continuum of neurologic deficits that ranges from sensory involvement alone, to sensory involvement with motor weakness, to episodes of complete paralysis. There are three grades of SCN injury. Grade I injury involves symptoms lasting fewer than 15 minutes. Grade II injuries last from 15 minutes to 24 hours. Grade III injuries persist longer than 24 hours. When all four extremities are involved the term "quad" is used to describe the pattern. The term "upper" indicates that both arms are affected and "lower" that both legs are affected. Involvement of one leg and arm on the same side constitutes a "hemi" pattern.

Prevention

The prevention of SCN begins with the education of athletes participating in contact sports emphasizing proper technique to avoid injury. The spearing of other helmeted players has been prohibited since 1976 when the National Federation of State High School Associations and the National Collegiate Athletic Association banned this style of play in football. These rules were implemented because cinematographic and epidemiologic data revealed that the majority of cervical spine injuries were caused by axial loading. As players have learned how to play without making contact with the crown of the helmet the incidence of catastrophic and permanent quadriplegia has significantly decreased.

Clinical Findings

A. Symptoms

Symptoms include sensory changes of burning pain, numbness, tingling, and loss of sensation with motor changes ranging from weakness to complete paralysis. These episodes are transient and complete recovery usually occurs in 10–15 minutes, although some patients may not recover until 36–48 hours after injury. Neck pain is usually not present at the time of injury except for burning paresthesias.

B. Signs

The basic principles of advanced trauma life support (ATLS) and immobilization of the spine may make the difference between an uneventful recovery and permanent deficit or injury when initiating the work-up and treatment of the athlete. Patients who are transiently paralyzed may require respiratory support if a high cervical cord injury has occurred. Respiratory support requires removal of the helmet and shoulder pads, which must be done while maintaining full immobilization of the spine. In the event of airway obstruction or need for immediate intubation the facemask may be removed with a screwdriver or clippers either on the field or in the hospital setting when control of the airway is imperative. The principals of ATLS are always maintained. A thorough neurologic examination of both the upper and lower motor neurons is the foundation of the assessment of an athlete who has sustained an SCN. This involves full assessment of both upper and lower extremity strength, sensation, and lower and upper motor neuron reflexes.

C. Imaging Studies

A complete set of cervical spine radiographs is the first priority in the radiographic work-up of a patient who has sustained a spinal cord neuropraxia. The lateral radiograph allows the dimension of the sagittal canal to be determined. A 15-mm anteroposterior cervical canal diameter is considered normal but a canal of less than 13 mm is considered stenotic. Differences may occur due to the radiographic technique, thereby making measurements of the canal diameter inconsistent. The Torg ratio, described in the section on burners and stingers, has also been used to diagnose developmental stenosis. In the collegiate and professional football leagues it has been found that the Torg ratio has a low positive predictive value due to the relatively larger vertebral bodies in this group of athletes.

An MRI of the cervical spine is mandatory following an episode of SCN. The space available for the spinal cord may be more accurately assessed with an MRI scan. Results of MRI have led to the concept of functional stenosis, as assessment of focal cord deformation and blockage of cerebrospinal fluid flow are made possible. Athletes who have experienced an episode of transient SCN and who also show functional stenosis on MRI should perhaps not be allowed to return to play. Signal changes in the spinal cord shown on MRI that suggest actual injury indicate that the athlete should be prohibited from returning to high-risk athletic participation.

D. Special Tests

There are no special tests necessary to diagnose an SCN such as EMG. Plain radiographs and MRI, in addition to the physical examination, are the only tests routinely necessary. Only in very rare instances, such as when patient size, severe claustrophobia, or metallic implants prohibit obtaining an MRI, is it necessary to obtain a CT myelogram of the cervical spine to evaluate the spinal canal.

E. Special Examinations

No special examinations other than a thorough musculoskeletal, spinal, and neurologic examination are required to diagnose an SCN.

Complications

The most serious complication of an SCN, aside from its recurrence, is the possibility of a devastating and permanent neurologic injury resulting in quadriplegia. The patient is predisposed to such injury with any significant blow to the head that results in a fracture at the area of stenosis. This may occur as a result of a fall, motor vehicle accident, or even return to play, depending on the energy imparted to the head and neck at the time of collision.

Treatment

A. Rehabilitation

Rehabilitation after an episode of SCN is initiated by ensuring that all neurologic symptoms and deficits have resolved. A physical therapy program that focuses on attaining a full and pain-free range of motion of the neck and extremities ensures that ligamentous and bony injury will not predispose the athlete to further injury. Muscular conditioning to regain a preinjury level of strength in the extremities and neck ensures that all neurologic deficits have been eliminated and also assists in prevention of injury.

Throughout the rehabilitation process the athlete should be counseled on the risk of recurrent injury. Only after receiving an explanation of the injury process and the possible predisposition to recurrence based on radiographs and MRI studies and after being fully informed of their risk and the serious consequences of neurologic injury can athletes and their families make an informed decision about return to play.

B. SURGERY

Surgery is reserved for destabilizing injuries. There has been no long-term study investigating the efficacy of spinal cord decompression such as a canal expansive laminoplasty in preventing a recurrent episode of SCN.

C. SPECIAL PROCEDURES

No special surgical procedures have been widely accepted for the purpose of returning an athlete to play. In circumstances of severe cervical spine canal stenosis and the development of myelopathy, surgery is necessary. In a younger patient population normal cervical lordosis should be maintained and in the absence of severe neck pain a canal expansive laminoplasty may be an option. Cervical laminoplasty has proven useful in expanding the space available for the spinal cord, obviating the need for a much more aggressive anterior procedure that may require a multilevel corpectomy or a posterior laminectomy with fusion. Unfortunately, it decreases range of motion of the neck due to the arthrodesis required at each level performed.

Prognosis

An estimate of the incidence of SCN in a group of collegiate football players in 1984 was 0.06%. Interestingly, five of the seven players who returned to play sustained a second episode of SCN. In another study, 35 of 62 athletes who returned to play after sustaining an SCN experienced second episodes of SCN.

Return to Play

Just as important as the initial management of the injured athlete, a thorough physical examination must be completed and pertinent radiographic studies must be reviewed before allowing the athlete who has sustained an SCN to return to play. Only after all studies remain normal, the athlete is completely asymptomatic, and the physical examination is unremarkable for injury may the athlete return to play. Controversy exists when the physical examination is normal but the radiographs or MRI scan show evidence of cervical stenosis. This situation requires careful counseling of players and their families about the possible consequences of a second injury before returning to play.

Cantu RC: The cervical spine stenosis controversy. Clinics Sports Med 1998;17:121.

Muhle C et al: Dynamic changes of the spinal canal in patients with cervical spondylosis at flexion and extension using magnetic resonance imaging. Invest Radiol 1998;33(8):444.

Torg JS et al: Cervical cord neuropraxia: classification, pathomechanics, morbidity, and measurement guidelines. J Neurosurg 1997;87(6):843.

Wilberger JE: Athletic spinal cord and spine injuries. Clinics Sports Med 1998;17:111.

■ LUMBAR SPINE INJURIES IN ATHLETES

LUMBAR SPRAIN

ESSENTIALS OF DIAGNOSIS

- Low back pain.
- Absence of neurologic symptoms.
- Range of motion and paraspinal muscle spasm are common.
- Imaging studies are negative except for degenerative changes.
- Persistent, chronic, or recurrent symptoms should prompt further work-up.

Pathogenesis

Low back pain has been reported to affect approximately 85–90% of the population at least once during their lifetime. The incidence in the athletic population has been reported to be 1–30% and is one of the most common reasons for missed playing time in professional sports. Unfortunately, the specific etiology of the athlete's back pain often remains elusive. Muscle strain is the most common etiology of low back pain in adolescent, collegiate, and adult athletes. It is also the most common diagnosis in both acute and chronic low back pain.

Prevention

Strategies for prevention of lumbar strains and sprains have focused on increasing flexibility of the lumbar spine. It is thought that improved lumbar flexibility improves responses to high-energy demands and prevents episodes of low back pain in athletes. Although a definitive relationship between lumbar flexibility and low back pain has not been proven, most agree that athletes with poor flexibility are at higher risk for lumbar strain injuries. In regards to prevention of lumbar strain injuries during competition, it is likely that the timing of the pregame warm-up is important. Warm-up exercises are designed to increase core body temperature, improve extremity blood flow, and improve flexibility in an effort to prevent injury. Muscular strain injuries in the extremities have been linked to inadequate warm-up, weakness, decreased flexibility and muscle fatigue. Recently, it has been shown that the improved lumbar flexibility gained from pregame warm-up exercises is lost after 30 minutes of rest prior to game time. Although the link between the observed degree of increased stiffness and the subsequent risk of lumbar injury remains unclear, keeping athletes active immediately prior to the game and during rest periods on the sidelines should help decrease the risk of muscle strain injuries.

Ultimately, the best predictor of future occurrences of back pain in athletes is a history of low back pain. The risk of future episodes of low back pain is three times higher in athletes with a history of back pain than in athletes who do not have such a history. Core-strengthening paradigms have been proposed, however, there is no conclusive evidence that these programs decrease the incidence of back pain in athletes. It is likely that emphasis on form and technique combined with appropriate conditioning is the best preventive medicine.

Clinical Findings

A. SYMPTOMS

Lumbar strains are defined as disruption of muscle fibers at various locations within the muscle belly or musculotendinous junction from excessive eccentric loading of the muscle–tendon unit. Lumbar sprains occur by subcatastrophic stretch of one or more of the spinal ligaments. Athletes with lumbar strains can present with either acute or chronic symptoms. In acute lumbar strain, athletes typically report an inciting injury with back pain beginning soon after, becoming most painful about 24–48 hours postinjury. The mechanism is often a twisting injury but can occur from a direct blow as well. Frequently, the intensity of the pain has diminished considerably by the time of presentation to the clinician's office. Athletes with chronic lumbar strains generally report fatigue-related back pain, worsening toward the end of a hard training week or cycle. The clinician should inquire about any recent or sudden increases in training frequency or intensity. It is important to ask the athlete about any previous episodes of back pain and previous treatments. The athlete should also be questioned about neurologic symptoms and variations in the intensity of the pain with coughing, sneezing, or changes in position.

In lumbar strain injuries, radicular symptoms (radiating pain in the lower extremities) are absent and pain is limited to the back and paraspinal muscles. Increased pain intensity with a valsalva maneuver may indicate a herniated nucleus pulposus. Although cauda equina syndrome is extremely rare in the athletic population, the athlete should be asked about the presence of any difficulty with bowel or bladder function.

B. SIGNS

Typically, most athletes will have limitations in range of motion, predominantly from muscle spasm. Muscle spasms occur as the body's response to injury. Although the mechanism is not completely understood, it is thought that local inflammatory mediators trigger muscular contraction in an attempt to stabilize the injured segment. When muscle spasms are severe, a painful trigger point may develop after several days. Trigger points typically are palpated in the paraspinal musculature away from the midline. Lumbar sprains are thought to be due to injury to the interspinous process ligaments so midline tenderness may be present as well.

A full neurologic examination of the lower extremities should be performed and is normal in lumbar strain injuries. Nerve root tension signs such as the supine and seated straight leg raise and Laseques maneuver should also be negative. Pain worsening with lumbar extension in a young athlete raises concern for spondylolysis. The sacroiliac joints should also be palpated and stressed. Abnormalities in strength, reflex, or sensory testing are not consistent with lumbar strains and sprains and should prompt further work-up. It is important to assess all lower extremity joints for range of motion and pain as primary joint pathology may cause back pain. An examination of the athlete's gait and overall spinal balance concludes the physical examination.

C. IMAGING STUDIES

Imaging is not necessary in the vast majority of lumbar strain injuries as 80–90% of these injuries resolve spontaneously. Imaging tests should be considered for the athlete whose pain is severe, was caused by an acute traumatic event, or whose symptoms have not responded to several weeks of conservative treatment. Any neurologic findings warrant radiographic evaluation. Teenage or younger athletes may benefit from earlier imaging as earlier identification of acute spondylolysis may influence outcomes. Plain radiographs including an anteroposterior, lateral, left and right oblique, and coned down lateral view of the lumbosacral junction should be obtained. These radiographs may reveal mild degenerative changes in older athletes but should otherwise be negative.

D. SPECIAL TESTS

When considering the role of advanced imaging for spinal disorders, the high rate of false positive radiographic abnormalities (normal aging degenerative changes) should prompt the clinician to carefully consider what clinical question needs to be answered from the imaging study. Many athletes undergo unnecessary imaging studies for low back pain. These studies may reveal radiographic abnormalities not consistent with their current symptoms that unduly influence treatment. Degenerative changes are more frequent in the athletes, however, the incidence of low back pain is similar to the general population. Degenerative changes seen on MRI have not been shown to be predictive of the development or duration of low back pain. The main indication for obtaining an MRI scan is the presence of neurologic symptoms and signs. Occasionally, a bursal cavity may be seen between the spinous processes in athletes with chronic lumbar strain injuries, although the clinical significance of this finding is unknown.

Treatment

REHABILITATION

Lumbar strains and sprains are generally self-limited processes that respond very well to conservative treatments. A common sense approach to rehabilitation, including a short period of bed rest (no longer than 1–2 days to prevent deconditioning), ice for muscle spasms, nonsteroidal antiinflammatory medication, and physical therapy to strengthen the spinal musculature, is important. A three-cycle rehabilitation program for the treatment of nonradicular low back pain in athletes emphasizes differing degrees of rest, physical therapy, and time to return to play. Essentially, when symptoms are moderate to severe, the athlete is restricted from contact and emphasis is primarily on pain control and cardiovascular conditioning. As symptoms subside, the athlete is allowed to progress to limited practice sessions of increasing duration over time. Recently, motion-specific rehabilitation protocols have gained popularity. In a motion-specific protocol, athletes are placed into categories depending on which range of motion is least tolerated or exacerbates the athlete's symptoms. Treatment is directed first toward improving range of motion in the pain-free arc, then progressively improving motion in the opposite direction. For example, if an athlete's symptoms become worse with extension, flexion-based exercises are initiated and extension exercises are restricted.

Prognosis

Overall, the prognosis from lumbar strain and sprain injuries is quite favorable with resolution in 80–90% of patients. A history of low back pain is the best predictor of future occurrences. Although many athletes experience lumbar strain during their careers, rarely are symptoms debilitating enough to lead the athlete to early retirement. Multiple studies of collegiate wrestlers, rowers, and football players have shown that retirement from sport due to lumbar strain is rare.

Return to Play

Most athletes who experience an episode of lumbar strain or sprain will require a period of reduced activity and perhaps removal from competition for a short period. Return to competition is allowed once the athlete's pain is tolerable, flexibility is restored, and muscle spasms have diminished.

Aure OF et al: Manual therapy and exercise therapy in patients with chronic low back pain: a randomized, controlled trial with 1-year follow-up. Spine 2003;28:525.

Bono CM: Low-back pain in athletes. J Bone Joint Surg Am 2004;86A(2):382.

Fujiwara A et al: The interspinous ligament of the lumbar spine: magnetic resonance images and their clinical significance [Diagnostics]. Spine 2000;25(3):358.

George SZ, Delitto A: Management of the athlete with low back pain. Clinics Sports Med 2002;21:105.

Green JP et al: Low-back stiffness is altered with warm-up and bench rest: implications for athletes. Med Sci Sports Exerc 2002;34:1076.

Greene HS et al: A history of low back injury is a risk factor for recurrent back injuries in varsity athletes. Am J Sports Med 2001;29:795.

Nadler SF et al: The relationship between lower extremity injury, low back pain, and hip muscle strength in male and female collegiate athletes. Clin J Sports Med 2000;10:89.

Trainor TJ, Wiesel SW: Epidemiology of back pain in the athlete. Clinics Sports Med 2002;21:93.

LUMBAR FRACTURES

An extensive discussion of all lumbar spine fractures is beyond the scope of this chapter, however, the sports medicine clinician may be called upon to treat minor fractures of the lumbar spine. These injuries include anterior compression fractures, spinous process and transverse process fractures, adolescent vertebral end plate injuries, and pedicle or sacral stress fractures. Anterior compression fractures generally result from a mechanism involving forced flexion. Spinous process and transverse process fractures generally result from a direct blow or torsional injury. Adolescent athletes may suffer avulsion injuries of the end plates as the spinal ligaments tend to be stronger than the vertebral end plates. Stress fractures of the lower lumbar pedicles have been reported, most commonly in fast bowling cricketers. Sacral stress fractures, although uncommon, are generally overuse injuries that may develop in running athletes.

ESSENTIALS OF DIAGNOSIS

- *Symptoms (history) of significant trauma in acute settings.*
- *Insidious onset of asymmetric low back or gluteal pain.*
- *Recalcitrant back pain after physical therapy.*
- *Back pain or paramedian pain with localized tenderness.*
- *Radiographic studies demonstrating fracture.*

Prevention

Fortunately, fractures of the lumbar spine are rare injuries in sports competition. Prevention of such injuries includes emphasis on sound tackling techniques, adequate protective equipment, and maintaining abdominal and lumbar muscle conditioning.

Clinical Findings

A. SYMPTOMS

The history of a violent or high-energy injury combined with symptoms of acute back pain alert the clinician to the possibility of a lumbar spine fracture. Pain that is worse when sitting up and is relieved by lying supine may indicate a compression fracture. The athlete should be carefully questioned for neurologic symptoms and for difficulties with bowel or bladder function. A history of the mechanism of injury and the energy associated with that injury should be obtained. Falls from significant height, violent collisions, and diving injuries raise the suspicion of fracture. Chronic low back pain refractory to conservative measures may represent a stress fracture of either the pedicles or sacral spine. In female athletes, a nutritional and menstrual history should be obtained to identify risk factors for osteoporosis. Additionally, positional variations that make such pain worse with extension could indicate a stress fracture of the posterior bony elements. In the chronic setting, it is important to ascertain any recent changes in frequency or intensity of training or competition. The clinician should also ask the athlete to attempt to pinpoint the area of most discomfort as sacral stress fractures may present as low back or buttock pain.

B. SIGNS

In the acute setting, spine precautions with log-rolling should be utilized during the evaluation. Palpation of the posterior spine should be performed looking for step-off, hematoma, and midline versus paraspinal tenderness. A complete neurologic examination including motor, sensory, and reflex testing should follow. A rectal examination should be performed to assess for perianal sensation and rectal tone.

In the chronic setting, active and passive lumbar range of motion should be assessed. Increased pain with extension should alert the clinician to the possibility of a posterior bony element injury. The sacral spine should also be examined because sacral stress fractures are usually tender to palpation. Asking the patient to perform single leg support and single leg hopping maneuvers may provide clues to a sacral stress fracture as well.

C. IMAGING STUDIES

Plain films including anteroposterior, lateral, and oblique radiographs should be obtained. These radiographs should be examined for overall spinal alignment, presence of soft tissue swelling, interspinous process distance, vertebral body height, scoliosis, or evidence of instability. Anterior compression fractures are seen as a fracture of the anterior superior portion of the vertebral body. Anterior and posterior vertebral body height should be measured at the level of injury and compared to adjacent levels. The posterior interspinous process distance should be scrutinized. An increase in this distance indicates that the fracture may potentially be unstable. In simple anterior compression fractures, there is minimal loss of height, no increased interspinous process distance, and no rotational deformity on the anteroposterior radiograph.

Spinous process fractures are best visualized on the lateral radiograph. The interspinous process distance should be carefully evaluated and compared to adjacent levels. Although the fractured portion of the spinous process can be significantly displaced, the remaining portion should maintain its normal relationship with adjacent vertebrae.

Transverse process fractures are best visualized on the anteroposterior radiograph. Single transverse process fractures are considered minor injuries, however, the presence of multiple transverse process fractures raises the suspicion of a more serious injury.

Plain radiographs are usually unrevealing in stress fractures of the pedicles or sacrum. Occasionally, fracture callus or sclerotic lines may be seen as clues to the diagnosis.

D. SPECIAL TESTS

Advanced imaging studies should be obtained in athletes with compression fractures, multiple spinous process or transverse process fractures, or for persistent symptoms despite previous conservative management. CT allows differentiation between compression and more complex (eg, burst or chance-type) fractures. CT will also rule out associated severe spinal fractures in athletes with multiple spinous process or transverse process fractures. Fracture lines with sclerotic margins may be seen in athletes with pedicle or sacral stress fractures. Athletes with multiple spinous process or transverse process fractures or any neurologic symptoms should undergo MRI. MRI allows excellent visualization of the neural elements as well as the integrity of the posterior ligamentous supporting structures.

If plain films and CT fail to provide a diagnosis, single-photon emission computed tomography (SPECT) or MRI may reveal stress reactions of the lumbar pedicles or sacral spine. In female athletes with compression or stress fractures of the lumbar spine, bone densitometry should be performed to assess for the presence of osteoporosis.

Treatment

A. Compression Fractures

Nonsurgical management is the mainstay of treatment for minor fractures of the lumbar spine. Nondisplaced or minimally displaced compression fractures should be supported with either a lumbosacral corset or thoracolumbosacral orthosis (TLSO) for 6–12 weeks. Frequent radiographs should be obtained because progressive collapse or instability can occur. Upright flexion and extension radiographs should be obtained at the conclusion of bracing and approximately 4–6 weeks postbracing to assess final alignment. Once clinical and radiographic healing has been obtained, the athlete may begin a physical therapy program emphasizing range of motion and cardiovascular conditioning. Strengthening exercises should begin after range of motion has been restored.

B. Spinous and Transverse Process Fractures

Spinous process and transverse process fractures should be managed with activity restriction and a lumbosacral corset for comfort. The majority of these fractures heal in approximately 6 weeks. As pain decreases and the athlete is comfortable, physical therapy is started with emphasis on range of motion and cardiovascular conditioning. As the athlete tolerates, therapy may shift toward a strengthening paradigm.

C. Sacral and Pedicle Stress Fractures

Sacral stress fractures are treated nonoperatively with rest and protected or non-weight bearing. As symptoms abate, progressive mobilization and weight bearing are begun and activities are resumed.

Pedicle stress fractures if detected early, prior to establishment of a nonunion, are treated with a TLSO for 6–12 weeks. Follow-up radiographs should be obtained frequently to assess for alignment and stability. CT scans may be necessary to document fracture union prior to discontinuation of brace treatment. Pedicle fractures that are detected late and have evidence of nonunion are managed surgically with bone grafting and instrumented fusion.

D. Apophyseal Ring Injuries

The literature regarding apophyseal ring injuries in the adolescent spine predominantly consists of case reports. There is no general consensus for treatment. Suffice to say, case series of asymptomatic patients treated conservatively have yielded good results. In symptomatic patients, with radicular or claudicatory (pain radiating into the extremities with exertion such as walking) symptoms, surgical decompression of the anterior thecal sac from the posteriorly protruding vertebral end plate has yielded good results.

Prognosis

Although there are no outcome data on minor fractures of the lumbar spine in athletes, extrapolating data from the adult nonathlete population would suggest that the prognosis should be good. Provided overall spinal alignment has been maintained a full recovery with minimal residual symptoms is expected.

Return to Play

Currently, there are no published guidelines regarding return to sports after lumbar fractures. Upon demonstration of clinical and radiographic healing it is appropriate for the athlete to begin functional restoration with physical therapy on a phased continuum. Full, painless range of motion should be achieved prior to engaging in sport-specific training.

Folman Y, Gepstein R: Late outcome of nonoperative management of thoracolumbar vertebral wedge fractures. J Orthop Trauma 2003;17(3):190.

Johnson AW et al: Stress fractures of the sacrum. An atypical cause of low back pain in the female athlete. Am J Sports Med 2001; 29:498.

Parvataneni HK et al: Bilateral pedicle stress fractures in a female athlete: case report and review of the literature. Spine 2004;29(2):19.

SPONDYLOLYSIS

ESSENTIALS OF DIAGNOSIS

- *Athletes may be asymptomatic or report low back and buttock pain.*
- *Symptoms (history) of repetitive lumbar hyperextension.*
- *Demonstration of lytic defect in pars interarticularis.*
- *Spondylolisthesis may or may not be present.*

Spondylolysis, a defect in the posterior neural arch, is seen in both athletic and nonathletic populations. It is most common at the L5 spinal level and is next most common at the L4 level. Although the precise etiology of spondylolysis is not known, it is widely thought that repetitive hyperextension of the lumbar spine leads to a stress fracture within the pars interarticularis. Epidemiologic studies have demonstrated a prevalence of 4–7% in the general population. Although athletes in certain sports (diving, gymnastics, weightlifting, wrestling, football, rowing) demonstrate a higher incidence of spondylolysis, occurrence in the athletic and nonathletic populations is similar. Spondylolysis is twice as common in boys as in girls and longitudinal studies suggest a familial predisposition.

Prevention

Strategies for prevention of spondylolysis are aimed at early detection of the pars at risk. If stress reactions with the pars interarticularis are detected, treatment can prevent progression to a lytic defect. In the future earlier detection of pending pars fractures may decrease the incidence of spondylolysis in athletes.

Clinical Findings

A. Symptoms

Symptoms of spondylolysis may range from a dull, persistent ache present within the low back to severe pain causing an awkward gait or limiting ambulation. The pain is often worse with lumbar extension and improves when leaning forward. Athletes may report difficulty sleeping or laying flat. Pain is usually limited to the low back but may radiate to the buttock or posterior thigh. Patients may also complain of hamstring tightness and loss of lumbar range of motion. Radicular symptoms may occur but are rare in spondylolysis.

B. Signs

Athletes with spondylolysis generally have few abnormalities on physical examination. Typically, lumbar range of motion is limited, predominantly with extension. Gentle passive extension of the lumbar spine often exacerbates symptoms. The single-leg hyperextension test is a provocative maneuver that can aid in the diagnosis of spondylolysis. When performing the test, the patient stands on one leg and extends the lumbar spine. In patients with spondylolysis, symptoms worsen with this maneuver on the side of the defect. Tenderness to palpation can often be elicited on the symptomatic side. If spondylolisthesis is not present, there should not be a palpable step-off. Provocative maneuvers for radiculopathy such as straight leg raising and the Laseques maneuver are negative and the neurologic examination is usually normal.

C. Imaging Studies

If spondylolysis is suspected, imaging should begin with plain radiographs. An initial radiographic series including anteroposterior, lateral, both left and right obliques, and a coned down lateral view of the lumbosacral junction will demonstrate a lytic defect of the pars interarticularis in 85% of cases of spondylolysis (Figure 7–5). The coned down lateral view centers the x-ray beam on the lumbosacral joint, not the lumbar spine. A break in the "neck" of the "Scottie Dog" may be seen. Radiographs should also be assessed for the presence of spondylolisthesis, which is present in 50–75% of initial radiographs when a lytic defect is seen. The older the athlete at the time of presentation, the higher the likelihood that spondylolisthesis is present.

D. Special Tests

If the initial radiographic examination is negative and the athlete has a compelling history and physical examination concerning spondylolysis, advanced imaging is indicated. This may consist of a bone scan, CT, SPECT,

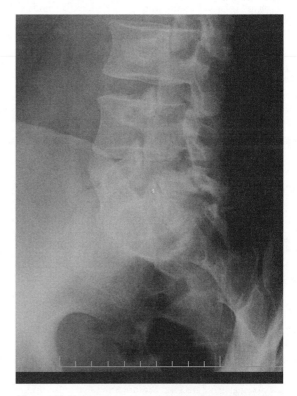

Figure 7–5. Oblique radiograph of the lumbar spine demonstrating a defect in the pars interarticularis of the L5 vertebrae. The defect is seen in the neck of the "Scottie Dog."

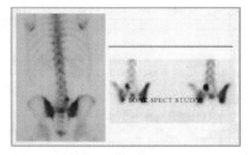

Figure 7–6. SPECT scan of spondylolysis. Notice the area of increased uptake near the left L5 pars interarticularis.

or MRI. Stress reactions in the pars may be detected by radionuclide imaging prior to progression to a lytic defect (Figure 7–6). Athletes with back pain and a pars defect on radiographs should undergo a bone scan to determine if active bone turnover is present. If uptake is not demonstrated on bone scanning, it is unlikely that spondylolysis is the cause of the athlete's symptoms. SPECT scanning is more sensitive and specific than the standard bone scan; it has shown uptake in the pars when bone scans were negative. SPECT has also been shown to be negative in asymptomatic athletes with spondylolysis. Given the high sensitivity and specificity of SPECT scanning for symptomatic spondylolysis, it is the imaging study of choice when initial radiographs are negative and the clinical suspicion is high.

CT is more sensitive than plain radiographs for spondylolysis and the defect in the pars interarticularis is demonstrated well on the axial cuts. The defect may be unilateral or bilateral. The major disadvantages of CT include difficulty in determining the age of the defect as well as the clinical significance if a defect is present. Sclerotic margins and hypertrophic bone ends may indicate a chronic nonhealing defect. Given the prevalence of spondylolysis in the general population, an adjunctive bone scan may be necessary to determine the defect's clinical significance. If a bone scan does not show increased uptake, it is unlikely that the pars defect is the source of the athlete's symptoms.

MRI, which is not as sensitive as a bone scan in symptomatic spondylolysis, is not commonly used in the diagnosis. Additionally, the temporal relationship between clinical healing and reversal of MRI abnormalities has also not been elucidated.

Treatment

A. REHABILITATION

The treatment of spondylolysis depends on several factors including the athlete's age, the severity and duration

of symptoms, and radiographic findings. Asymptomatic athletes with a radiographic finding of a pars defect do not require treatment and should be allowed to participate in sports. If the athlete's symptoms are mild and are limited to low back pain, core strengthening and cardiovascular conditioning should be emphasized. If neurologic symptoms are present or if the athlete's symptoms are severe, play should be restricted and further evaluation should be performed to establish a diagnosis. In athletes with back pain and radiographic findings consistent with spondylolysis, limitations in activity and bracing result in a greater than 90% rate of success.

The need for bracing and the best method of bracing are debatable. In a series of seven athletes with spondylolysis, rest and restriction of activity without bracing allowed clinical healing in all athletes. The results of that study have been challenged and have not been reproduced. A short period of brace treatment is the usual recommendation. Soft and rigid, lordotic and antilordotic braces have all been utilized with good success. An antilordotic brace (0° flexion) is thought to unload the posterior elements and aid the healing process and is our preference. Time spent within the brace has varied among series and does not appear to be linearly correlated with clinical success. We currently recommend continuous bracing during waking hours with sleeping permitted out of the brace. The duration of bracing is generally 6–8 weeks, accompanied by restriction from sports. In adolescent athletes the recommendation is to repeat the radiographs every 6 months until skeletal maturity. In skeletally mature athletes, repeat radiographs are indicated only if symptoms return.

The goal of treatment in athletes with stress reactions (increased uptake on SPECT imaging with negative plain radiographs) or fractures of the pars is bony healing of the defect. In athletes with stress reactions a quantitative reduction in uptake on SPECT imaging can be seen following brace treatment. In athletes with a pars defect and uptake on a bone scan, bony union is possible. The likelihood of osseous union is greatest in unilateral defects and least when a defect is present on one side and a stress reaction is present on the contralateral side. Importantly, the rate of return to sports has not been correlated with the achievement of osseous union. It is postulated that a stable fibrous union occurs at the site of the defect allowing resolution of symptoms. Most clinicians recommend a discontinuation of bracing and a return to sports when the athlete is asymptomatic.

After immobilization, the athlete is advanced to a rehabilitation program emphasizing flexion-type exercises and flexibility. The athlete may resume activities over the next 6–8 weeks.

B. SURGERY

Due to the clinical success of nonoperative management of spondylolysis, surgery is rarely indicated. Athletes with symptoms that persist for more than 6 months despite restriction of activity and bracing are candidates for surgical intervention.

Historically, the gold standard for the treatment of symptomatic spondylolysis in the adolescent athlete at the L5 level has been surgery consisting of in situ uninstrumented posterolateral L5–S1 fusion. Although successful, segmental motion is sacrificed. Over the past two decades there has been considerable interest in direct repair of the pars defect as an alternative to fusion. The major advantage of a direct pars repair versus fusion is preservation of motion. As many athletes with spondylolysis are in their adolescent to early adult years, fusion should not be considered lightly. Several techniques have been described for the direct repair of the pars including the Scott wiring technique, hook-wire constructs, the translaminar interfragmentary screw (ie, Buck) technique, and pedicle screw–rod-hook constructs with bone grafting (Figure 7–7). The pedicle screw–rod-hook technique is theoretically the most rigid construct. Direct repair of pars defects from L3 to L5 have been reported. In several series of competitive athletes, both the interfragmentary technique and wiring techniques have produced good to excellent results and return to sports at the same level of competition in over 90%. Given the good success with multiple techniques, it is likely that the most important aspect of the operation is autogenous bone grafting of the defect.

Athletes treated operatively for symptomatic spondylolysis should show evidence of bony healing prior to beginning a rehabilitation program. Once healing has been achieved, a rehabilitation program stressing flexion-type exercises, flexibility, and trunk strengthening is begun.

Return to Play

Athletes treated nonoperatively for spondylolysis are allowed to return to sports after clinical resolution of symptoms. Athletes may return to play when they are pain free, regardless of radiographic evidence of pars healing. Athletes returning to high-risk sports such at football, soccer, or gymnastics are five times more likely to have a poor clinical outcome compared to athletes returning to low-risk sports such as baseball, track, or swimming.

Timing for return to sports in athletes treated by direct pars repair is controversial. We believe that once healing of the pars has been demonstrated, the athlete may return to sports participation when pain free, range of motion has been established and trunk strength has been regained. This may take between 5 and 12 months.

Eck JC, Riley LH: Return to play after lumbar spine conditions and surgeries. Clinics Sports Med 2004;23:367.

Herman MJ et al: Spondylolysis and spondylolisthesis in the child and adolescent athlete. Orthop Clin North Am 2003;34:461.

Lim MR et al: Symptomatic spondylolysis: diagnosis and treatment. Curr Opin Pediatr 2004;16:37.

Lonstein JE: Spondylolisthesis in children: cause, natural history, and management. Spine 1999;24(24):2640.

Reitman CA, Esses SI: Direct repair of spondylolytic defects in young competitive athletes. Spine J 2002;2(2):142.

Rubery PT: Athletic activity after spine surgery in children and adolescents: results of a survey. Spine 2002;27(4):423.

Standaert CJ, Herring SA: Spondylolysis: a critical review. Br J Sports Med 2000;34:415.

SPONDYLOLISTHESIS

 ESSENTIALS OF DIAGNOSIS

- *Athletes may be asymptomatic or have back or leg pain.*
- *Increased pain with lumbar extension and hamstring tightness are common.*
- *Anterolisthesis (ie, anterior displacement) of the cephalad vertebrae on the caudad vertebrae.*

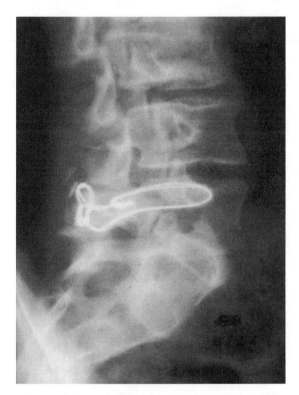

Figure 7–7. Lateral radiograph of the direct repair of the pars interarticularis defect with wiring technique and bone grafting.

Spondylolisthesis is commonly divided into five types based on the Wiltse classification: Type I is dysplastic or congenital. In this type, a congenital deficiency of the L5–S1 facets allows slippage of L5 on S1. Type II is isthmic or spondylotic spondylolisthesis. The defect in the pars interarticularis allows forward slippage of the vertebral body while the posterior elements remain in place. The defect in the pars may be a lytic fracture, an acute pars fracture, or an elongated but intact pars. Type III is degenerative, occurring in older individuals with associated facet arthropathy and spinal stenosis. Type IV, traumatic, is an acute fracture in a vertebrae other than the pars. Type V, pathologic, involves a pedicular or pars lesion because of generalized bone disease or tumor. Isthmic spondylolisthesis is the most common type in athletes and will be the focus of this discussion.

Spondylolysis and spondylotic spondylisthesis appear to have a genetic predisposition and often coexist. Spondylolysis is present in 4–6% of the general population. Spondylolisthesis is present in 50–80% of athletes with a pars defect on initial radiographs. Athletes in high-risk sports (football, gymnastics, soccer) may develop symptoms at a higher rate than the general population, in which the incidence of symptoms is low. Recently, in a large study of high school and college football players, athletes with spondylolysis or spondylolisthesis were twice as likely to report an episode of back pain than athletes without these diagnoses. Natural history studies in young athletes have shown that about 40% of athletes with spondylolisthesis will show evidence of progression over a 5-year period, however, the progression is small (10%) and does not correlate with worsening symptoms.

Clinical Findings

A. SYMPTOMS

The most common presenting symptom in spondylolisthesis is back pain, however, there are a significant number of athletes who will not report symptoms. The association of spondylolisthesis with disability and symptoms is difficult to establish. In studies of young athletes with spondylotic spondylolisthesis, frequent problems related to pain or disability have not been observed. Athletes with L4–5 isthmic spondylolisthesis, greater than a 25% slip, or degenerative disk disease at the level of the slip are more likely to complain of back pain. Athletes may complain of back or leg pain but few patients have associated neurologic complaints. If neurologic symptoms are present, they are usually radicular in nature.

B. SIGNS

The physical examination of athletes with isthmic spondylolisthesis is generally unrevealing. The two most common findings based on physical examination in adolescents are increased pain with lumbar extension and hamstring tightness. Decreased lumbar range of motion and tenderness may be present but are nonspecific findings. In athletes with high-grade slips, III or IV, a palpable step-off between spinous processes may be present. Low-grade slips are very difficult to detect on palpation. Nerve root tension signs are usually negative and the neurologic examination is usually normal. When neurologic deficits are noted, they are frequently seen as weakness of the muscles innervated by the lumbar root exiting at the level of the slip, such as extensor hallucis longus weakness in an L5 pars defect. An awkward gait may be demonstrated if hamstring contracture is present. Severe hamstring contracture or listhetic posturing of hip and knee flexion, anterior pelvic tilt, and lumbar lordosis may indicate spinal instability.

C. IMAGING STUDIES

Spondylolisthesis is demonstrated on plain radiographs as anterolisthesis of the cephalad vertebrae on the caudad vertebrae (Figure 7–8). Isthmic spondylolisthesis may occur at any level in the lumbar spine but is most common at the L5–S1 level. The Meyerding classification system is used to grade the degree of slip: Grade I <25%, Grade II 25–50%, Grade III 50–75%, and Grade IV >75%. Grade V or spondyloptosis rarely occurs. In isthmic spondylolisthesis, the pars defect is more easily seen on plain radiographs. Approximately 75% of patients will be classified as Grade I or II at the time of presentation. Grades III, IV, and V account for only 5% of cases of spondylolisthesis. The slip angle defines the degree of lumbosacral kyphosis and the actual percentage of slip can be calculated by dividing the millimeters of anterolisthesis by the total width of the caudad

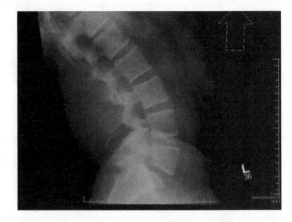

Figure 7–8. Lateral radiograph of the lumbosacral spine demonstrating spondylolysis with Grade I spondylolisthesis.

vertebrae. Radiographic parameters associated with an increased risk of progression of spondylolisthesis include higher degree of slip at initial presentation and increased lumbosacral kyphosis. Although a dome-shaped sacrum and trapezoidal L5 vertebrae may be seen in high-grade slips, these findings are not prognostic for slip progression. Given the differences in interrater reliability with measurements of the degree of slip, documentation of progression requires a 10–15% change in slippage or an increase in subluxation of 4–5 mm. Flexion and extension views of the lumbar spine have not been proven to be useful in isthmic spondylolisthesis.

D. SPECIAL TESTS

CT scans with fine cuts (1–2 mm slice thickness) can demonstrate the lytic defect in the pars interarticularis quite well. Additionally, CT is useful as a preoperative planning tool. Pedicle anatomy, size, and orientation can be easily determined. Associated dysplasia is also demonstrated well.

MRI is useful in evaluating the intervertebral disc at the level of the slip and at adjacent levels. Degenerative discs display less signal on T2-weighted images due to loss of water content. It is thought that spondylolisthesis may progress in adulthood as a result of continued disc degeneration. Additionally, MRI also details nerve root compression associated with spondylolisthesis. Nerve root compression is best visualized on T1-weighted images as loss of fat signal surrounding the nerve root. Importantly, it should be noted whether the root is being pinched from cephalocaudal collapse of the foramen or between the posterolateral aspect of the disc and the remaining pars of the cephalad vertebrae.

In athletes for whom operative intervention is planned, predominant cephalocaudal collapse of the foramen may be an indication for use of an interbody fusion technique to restore foramenal height. In addition, provocative discography may be useful in the selection of fusion levels. Although controversial, exact reproduction of low back pain during discography of an adjacent segment may indicate that the fusion level should be extended to include that segment.

Treatment

A. REHABILITATION

1. Children and adolescents—The goal in the treatment of isthmic spondylolisthesis is symptom reduction, not healing of the pars defect. In asymptomatic athletes with Grade I or II isthmic spondylolisthesis, there is no need for treatment or for restriction from activities or sports. In young athletes, serial radiographs are recommended every 4–6 months until the age of 10, semiannually from age 10 to age 15, and annually after age 15 until skeletal maturity. Asymptomatic athletes with Grade III

or IV spondylolisthesis should not participate in contact sports. Surgical intervention is recommended even in the asymptomatic adolescent athlete with Grade III or IV spondylolisthesis.

In symptomatic athletes with Grade I or II spondylolisthesis, a short period of bracing (6–8 weeks), activity modification, and flexion-based trunk strengthening exercises should be instituted. Bracing is not intended to prevent slip progression but to decrease symptoms. Two-thirds of adolescent athletes with Grade I or II spondylolisthesis will respond to conservative treatment. Serial radiographs are recommended until skeletal maturity.

Less than 10% of symptomatic athletes with Grade III or IV spondylolisthesis respond favorably to bracing, activity modification, and rehabilitation. Most athletes with symptomatic Grade III or IV spondylolisthesis require surgical intervention.

2. Adults—We believe that nonoperative care of isthmic spondylolisthesis in adults should be similar to care for acute low back pain. Avoidance of long periods of bed rest and return to activities are recommended. Symptomatic treatment with ice or cold packs may be beneficial. The use of transcutaneous electroneural stimulation (TENS) units lacks demonstrable efficacy. Additionally, manipulative therapies have not been shown to provide long-term relief in this patient population.

Flexion exercises of pelvic tilts and seated chest-to-thigh maneuvers have shown favorable results in both short- and long-term symptom reduction. Short-term improvements can be seen with aggressive physical therapy and stretching combined with high-intensity resistance training. Recently, programs of cocontraction-specific stabilization exercises involving the deep abdominal and multifidus muscles proximal to the pars defect have shown promise in reducing pain and disability in this population.

B. RISK OF PROGRESSION

Overall, significant progression, defined as a greater than 10% change, is seen in only a minority of patients. Minor progression, less than a 10% change, may be seen in up to 75% of adolescent athletes. The risk of progression is not influenced by the athlete's sport and progression has not been shown to lead to an increase in symptoms. Progression of spondylolisthesis is more common in adolescents during the growth spurt and is unlikely after skeletal maturity. Progression after skeletal maturity is associated with disk degeneration. In general, females and those with dysplastic spondylolisthesis show higher rates of progression.

C. SURGERY

1. Children and adolescents—The indications for surgical intervention in the adolescent athlete include persistent pain despite 6–12 months of conservative treatment, a progressive slip greater than 50%, an ongoing neurologic deficit, or gait changes due to the slippage and associated muscle spasm. High-grade spondylolisthesis is a relative indication for surgical intervention.

The gold standard for Grade I and II isthmic spondylolisthesis is uninstrumented in situ posterolateral fusion with iliac crest bone grafting. Decompressive laminectomy is indicated only if severe neurologic symptoms are present. For high-grade slips when the L5 transverse process is anterior and inferior to the sacral alae, extension of the fusion to L4 is recommended and postoperative spica casting is added. Bone graft that is placed in the lateral gutter between the transverse process of L5 and the sacral alae is under shear forces. Bone graft that is laid in the lateral gutter up to the L4 transverse process is more vertical and under less shear force. Recently, instrumentation in adolescent cases has been utilized to decrease the necessity of extending the fusion (Figure 7–9).

Over 90% of patients will obtain relief from pain and improvement in neurologic symptoms, independent of the grade of spondylolisthesis. Outcomes are improved in uninstrumented fusions for low-grade slips if patients are immobilized for 6 weeks postoperatively. We expect excellent results in more than 90% of cases with no low back pain and unrestricted activity at a minimum of 2-year follow-up.

2. Adults—Surgical intervention for adult athletes with isthmic spondylolisthesis is indicated if after 6–12 months of conservative management symptoms have not been reduced enough to maintain quality of life. Persistent radicular or claudicatory symptoms or ongoing neurologic deficit are also indications.

Low-grade slips are treated with an instrumented L5–S1 posterolateral fusion with iliac crest bone grafting.

If preoperative studies indicate significant degenerative disc disease at the adjacent segment, consideration for extension of the fusion to include that segment should be given. A decompressive procedure should be added if radicular or claudicatory symptoms are present.

High-grade slips are treated with an instrumented L4–S1 posterolateral fusion with iliac crest bone grafting. Improved outcomes of surgery for adult isthmic spondylolisthesis have been associated with the achievement of a solid fusion. Interbody fusion techniques (anterior, posterior, and transforaminal lumbar interbody fusion) have been shown to improve fusion rates in isthmic spondylolisthesis. However, differences in clinical outcome between posterolateral fusion only and posterolateral plus interbody fusion procedures have not been demonstrated.

Return to Play

Few guidelines exist regarding return to play after lumbar fusion surgery in adolescents. A recent survey of surgeons in the Scoliosis Research Society revealed that about 50% do not permit return to noncontact activities for 6 months postoperatively. One-third of surgeons allow return to collision sports at 1 year. Sixteen percent do not allow athletes with low-grade slips to return to collision sports. Twenty-five percent of surgeons do not allow athletes with high-grade slips to return to collision sports. Unrestricted return to sports is possible in athletes with a stable fusion and who are fully rehabilitated without symptoms at 1 year.

There are currently no reports of return to competitive sports after lumbar fusion procedures in adults. Of concern is the risk of adjacent segment degeneration in

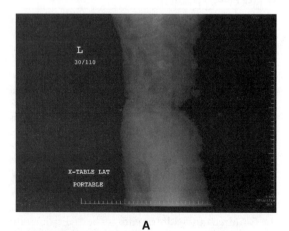
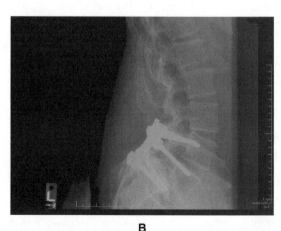

A   B

Figure 7–9. Lateral radiograph of the lumbosacral spine demonstrating Grade III isthmic spondylolisthesis before (***A***) and after (***B***) posterior instrumented fusion with pedicle screw instrumentation.

this population. Adult athletes should be encouraged to participate in exercises for cardiovascular fitness, however, return to contact sports is not recommended.

Hilibrand AS, Silva MT: The surgical management of isthmic (spondylotic) spondylolisthesis. Semin Spine Surg 2003; 15(2):160.

Kuntz K et al: Cost-effectiveness of fusion with and without instrumentation for patients with degenerative spondylolisthesis and spinal stenosis. Spine 2000;25:1132.

Lurie JD et al: Rates of advanced spinal imaging and spine surgery. Spine 2003;28(6):616.

Moller H, Hedlund R: Instrumented and noninstrumented posterolateral fusion in adult spondylolisthesis: a prospective randomized study: Part 2. Spine 2000;25:1716.

Rainville J, Mazzaferro R: Evaluation of outcomes of aggressive spine rehabilitation in patients with back pain and sciatica from previously diagnosed spondylolysis and spondylolisthesis. Arch Phys Med Rehabil 2001;82:1309.

Rainville J et al: Evaluation and conservative management of lumbar spondylolysis and spondylolisthesis. Semin Spine Surg 2003;15(2):125.

Rhee JM, Riew KD: Radiographic assessment of lumbar spondylolisthesis. Semin Spine Surg 2003;15(2):134.

Concussion

8

Michael W. Collins, PhD, & Jamie E. Pardini, PhD

Concussion, or mild traumatic brain injury (MTBI), is a topic that has received much recent attention in the field of sports medicine, both in national and international forums. By early estimates, the reported incidence of concussion in high school football players was approximately 19%, though a recently published study has shown a decreasing trend in concussion in football players, with a 4% reported incidence in 1999. However, given the significant variation in definitions and diagnostic criteria for concussion, the incidence of this injury is likely underestimated. Although most media coverage of the injury as a public health issue has focused on cases of professional athletes, it is high school and collegiate athletes who are at greatest risk and are most commonly seen in sports medicine clinics for evaluation of concussion.

ESSENTIALS OF DIAGNOSIS

- *Trauma-induced alteration in mental status.*
- *May occur with or without loss of consciousness.*
- *Most commonly reported symptoms are headache, problems with balance, lack of coordination, dizziness, and a sensation of feeling "foggy."*
- *High school and collegiate athletes are at greatest risk.*

General Considerations

One of the many problems in managing concussion in athletes is the lack of a universally accepted definition of concussion. Over the past 40 years, the most widely accepted definition has been the one proposed by the Committee on Head Injury Nomenclature of Neurological Surgeons in 1966. That committee defined concussion as "a clinical syndrome characterized

by the immediate and transient post-traumatic impairment of neural function such as alteration of consciousness, disturbance of vision or equilibrium, etc., due to brain stem dysfunction."

More recently, however, other definitions of concussion have been posed. Many clinicians and researchers currently use the definition of concussion proposed by the American Academy of Neurology (AAN): "Any trauma induced alteration in mental status that may or may not include a loss of consciousness."

This definition was prompted by the belief of the AAN that the definition of the Committee on Head Injury Nomenclature may be too limiting, as the injury is not confined to the brain stem and may involve other brain structures (eg, cortical areas). This definition also served to emphasize the fact that concussion may occur with or without a loss of consciousness.

Bailes JE, Cantu RC: Head injury in athletes. Neurosurgery 2001;48:26.

Levy ML et al: Analysis and evolution of head injury in football. Neurosurgery 2004;55:649.

Lovell MR, Collins MW: Neuropsychological assessment of the head-injured professional athlete. In: *Neurological Sports Medicine*. Bailes JE, Day AL (editors). American Association of Neurological Surgeons, 2001.

Pathogenesis

Recent research into the subtle metabolic effects of concussion has led to increased understanding of its acute presentation and implications. Using a rodent concussion model, a process was elucidated whereby significant changes occur in the intracellular and extracellular environment of injured cells. These metabolic changes are the result of excitatory amino acid (EAA)-induced ionic shifts with increased Na/K-ATPase activation and resultant hyperglycolysis. Thus, there is a high demand for energy within the brain shortly after concussive injury. This process is accompanied by a decrease in cerebral blood flow that is not well understood. Decreased cerebral blood flow is hypothesized to be the result of an accumulation of endothelial Ca^{2+}, which is thought to cause widespread cerebral neurovascular constriction. The resulting "metabolic mismatch" between energy demand and energy supply within the brain may propagate a cellular vulnerability that is particularly susceptible to even minor changes in cerebral blood flow, increases in intracranial pressure, and apnea. Animal models have indicated that this dysfunction can last up to 2 weeks or theoretically longer in the human model. Although the generalization of this theory of metabolic dysfunction to humans remains premature, it does raise important questions regarding the threat of vulnerability, how long it lasts, and if it is accompanied by identifiable markers of both injury and recovery.

Bergschneider M et al: Cerebral hyperglycolysis following severe human traumatic brain injury: a positron emission tomography study. J Neurosurg 2003;86:241.

Hovda DA et al: Neurobiology of concussion. In: *Sports Related Concussion*. Bailes JE et al (editors). Quality Medical Publishing, 1999.

Clinical Findings

Given the subtleties and variation in the presentation of a concussive injury, a thorough assessment of *all* signs and symptoms is crucial in making an accurate diagnosis of concussion. Following a concussion, athletes may present with only one symptom or a constellation of many postconcussion symptoms, any and all of which are important from a diagnostic and management standpoint. It should be stressed that sideline presentation

may vary widely from athlete to athlete, depending on the biomechanical forces involved, an athlete's prior history of injury, and numerous other factors. To date, no individual sign or symptom of concern (eg, headache, anterograde amnesia, retrograde amnesia, and balance problems) has been proven to directly correlate with the severity of the concussion. There is speculation, as well as published data, that retrograde amnesia and/or posttraumatic amnesia may be better indicators of poor outcome, though stating this conclusively is premature. Table 8–1 summarizes common on-field signs and symptoms of concussion as presented on a commonly used sideline concussion card provided by the University of Pittsburgh Medical Center.

It is most helpful, though not always possible, to gain information on symptoms from multiple informants (athlete, athletic trainer, coach, teammates, parents) across multiple time points (eg, symptoms immediately following injury, a few hours later, at 24 hours, at 48 hours, etc). Multiple informants are useful, not only because a presenting amnesia and/or loss of consciousness may prevent athletes from accurately describing their own symptoms for a given period of time, but also because athletes may minimize, deny, or mask their symptoms, hoping to return to play more quickly.

A. SYMPTOMS

1. Headache—Headache is the most commonly reported symptom of concussion and has been reported in up to 80% of affected athletes. However, the absence of headache does not preclude a diagnosis of concussion,

Table 8–1. University of Pittsburgh Medical Center's sideline concussion card: signs and symptoms of concussion.

Signs Observed by Staff	Symptoms Reported by Athlete
Appears to be dazed or stunned	Headache
Is confused about assignment	Nausea
Forgets plays	Balance problems or dizziness
Is unsure of game, score, or opponent	Double or fuzzy/blurry vision
Moves clumsily	Sensitivity to light or noise
Answers questions slowly	Feeling sluggish or slowed down
Loses consciousness	Feeling "foggy" or groggy
Shows behavior or personality change	Concentration or memory problems
Forgets events prior to play (retrograde)	Change in sleep pattern (appears later)
Forgets events after hit (posttraumatic)	Feeling Fatigued

highlighting the importance of a thorough assessment of all symptoms. Assessment of postconcussion headache may be complicated by the presence of musculoskeletal headaches and other preexisting headache syndromes (eg, migraine disorder or frequent stress headaches). However, any presentation of headache following a blow to the head or body should be managed with care.

Most frequently, a concussion headache is described as a sensation of pressure in the skull that may be localized to one region of the head or may be more generalized in nature. In some athletes (particularly athletes with a history of migraine), the headache may take the form of a vascular headache, may be unilateral, and is often described as throbbing or pulsing. Most commonly, postconcussion headache becomes worse with physical exertion. Thus, if the athlete's headache becomes worse during provocative exertional testing or return to play, postconcussion headache should be suspected and conservative management is indicated. Headaches due to concussion may not develop immediately after injury, and in fact may not develop until many hours after injury, again underscoring the need to assess symptoms at multiple time points postinjury.

Given the prevalence of headache with a concussive injury, the relation of this symptom to outcome has recently been examined. One study examined concussed high school athletes who reported headache versus those who did not at an assessment occurring approximately 1 week postinjury. Results indicated that athletes with headaches performed significantly worse on reaction time and memory measures on computerized neuropsychological testing, reported significantly more symptoms on the Post-Concussion Symptom Scale, and were more likely to have experienced an on-field anterograde amnesia than athletes without headaches. Another recent project examining headache type and outcome from concussion emphasizes the importance of proper assessment for the presence and type of postconcussion headache. Concussed athletes who present with no headaches (non-HA) or with headaches that do not meet the criteria for posttraumatic migraine (HA), and athletes who present with headaches that include symptoms of posttraumatic migraine (PTM) were compared on various postconcussion outcome measures. Overall, PTM athletes demonstrated the worst outcomes. Specifically, the PTM group (those reporting headache, nausea, and sensitivity to light and/or noise) demonstrated more pronounced cognitive deficits at postinjury testing than did either the HA or the non-HA group. The PTM group also demonstrated a greater departure from baseline neuropsychological testing scores than did either of the other headache groups. Thus, concussed athletes presenting with symptoms of posttraumatic migraines may need to be more conservatively managed than others, and may evidence more significant deficits and perhaps protracted recovery times.

Although headache following a concussion does not necessarily constitute a medical emergency, a severe or progressively worsening severe headache, particularly when accompanied by vomiting or rapidly declining mental status, may signal a life-threatening situation such as a subdural hematoma or intracranial bleed. This should prompt immediate transport to a hospital and imaging of the brain with computed tomography (CT) and/or magnetic resonance imaging (MRI).

2. Other common symptoms—In addition to headache, many other symptoms may emerge as the result of a concussive injury. Balance problems, lack of coordination, or dizziness may also be reported. Moreover, an athlete may report increased fatigue, feeling slowed down (cognitively or physically), or feeling lethargic. Fatigue is especially common in concussed athletes in the days following injury, and from a clinical perspective, seems to occur almost as frequently as headache. Athletes often report brief changes in vision as a result of concussion. These may include blurred vision, changes in peripheral vision, seeing "spots" or "lines," and/or other visual disturbances. They may also report cognitive changes, including problems with attention, concentration, short-term memory, learning, and multitasking. These symptoms typically manifest after an athlete has returned to school or work. Changes in mental status such as confusion may also be reported by athletes, although because it is typically a readily observable phenomenon, it is reported most frequently and in better detail by others.

Another frequently reported symptom that has gained recent research attention is a reported sensation of feeling "foggy" following concussion. Specifically, a sample of concussed high school students who indicated feeling "foggy" on a symptom inventory were compared to concussed high school athletes who did not experience this sensation. Results indicated that the "foggy" group demonstrated significantly slower reaction times, attenuated memory performance, and slower processing speed via computerized neurocognitive testing. In addition, the "foggy" athletes also indicated a significantly higher number of other postconcussion symptoms when compared to the group who did not experience fogginess. The results of this study, like the studies examining posttraumatic migraines and headaches in general, reveal the potential importance of any reported or observed symptom in impacting the diagnosis and recovery time or in indicating the severity of the concussion.

Another commonly reported or observed symptom involves emotional changes. Most often, athletes will report increased irritability, or having a "shorter fuse." However, other emotional changes may occur such as sadness/depression, nervousness/anxiety, or even (much less commonly) silliness or euphoria. Affect may be described by the athlete or parent as flattened or labile.

Emotional changes may be very brief (eg, a linebacker bursts into tears for 30 seconds on the sideline) or may be prolonged in the case of a more significant injury (an athlete reports persistent depression).

B. Signs

Appropriate acute care and management of the concussed athlete begin with a detailed and accurate assessment of the severity of the injury. As with any serious injury, the first priority is always to evaluate the athlete's level of consciousness and ABCs (airway, breathing, and circulation). The attending medical staff must always be prepared with an emergency action plan in the event that the evacuation of a critically head- or neck-injured athlete is necessary. This plan should be familiar to all staff, be well delineated, and be frequently rehearsed.

1. Loss of consciousness—Upon ruling out more severe injury via neurologic and clinical examination, the acute evaluation continues with assessment of concussion. First, the clinician should determine whether a loss of consciousness (LOC) has occurred. By definition, LOC represents a state of brief coma in which the eyes are typically closed and the patient is unresponsive to external stimuli. LOC is relatively rare and occurs in less than 10% of concussive injuries. Moreover, prolonged LOC (>1–2 minutes) in sports-related concussion occurs much less frequently. Athletes with LOC are typically unresponsive for only a brief period of time, sometimes only 1–2 seconds, which may at times make LOC difficult to diagnose, as it often takes medical personnel at least several seconds to reach the injured athlete. Any athlete with documented LOC should be managed conservatively and return to play is contraindicated.

Although many of the concussion grading and management scales rely heavily upon the presence or absence as well as on the duration of loss of consciousness, research has indicated that the *brief* losses of consciousness (less than 1 minute) typically associated with sports-related concussion may be unrelated to outcome, and that other markers, such as amnesia, may be more important in predicting outcome. Recent work with athletes has found no differences in acute recovery from concussion between those experiencing brief LOC and no LOC. Certainly, extended LOC (typically defined as greater than 1 minute) should warrant immediate neurologic evaluation.

2. Confusion—A more common form of mental status change following concussion involves confusion and amnesia. Confusion (ie, disorientation), by definition, represents impaired awareness and orientation to surroundings, though memory systems are not directly affected. An athlete demonstrating postinjury confusion will typically appear stunned, dazed, or "glassy-eyed" on the sideline or playing field. In athletes who do not remove themselves from play confusion is often manifested by difficulty

with appropriate play-calling, failure to correctly execute their positional assignment during play, or difficulty in communicating game information to teammates or coaches. Teammates are often the first to recognize that an athlete has been injured when the athlete begins demonstrating the above signs and has difficulty maintaining the flow of the game. On the sidelines, confused athletes may answer questions slowly or inappropriately, may ask "what is going on" or "what happened," and may repeat things during evaluation. Some may be temporarily disoriented to time or place, and even, very rarely, to person (eg, not knowing coaches or teammates).

To properly assess the presence of confusion, medical personnel can ask the athlete simple orientation questions such as the date or the names of the stadium, city, and opposing team. Table 8–2 contains a list of orientation questions extracted from the University of Pittsburgh Medical Center's Concussion Card.

3. Amnesia—Amnesia is emerging as perhaps the most important sign to carefully assess following concussion (clearly, after more serious injuries have been ruled out). Amnesia due to concussion may present as retrograde amnesia (difficulty remembering events prior to the injury) or posttraumatic/anterograde amnesia (difficulty remembering events following the injury). Both forms of amnesia should be assessed thoroughly and taken very seriously in the evaluation and management of sport-related concussion. Athletes who present with one or both types of amnesia may initially have difficulty recalling large spans of time either before or after the injury (or both), though these larger periods of amnesia will frequently shrink as the injury becomes less acute. The presence of amnesia, even for only a few seconds, has been found to be predictive of postinjury cognitive deficits and postconcussion symptoms.

Posttraumatic amnesia and anterograde amnesia are synonymous terms that represent the duration of time between the head trauma (eg, an ice hockey player's forehead striking the boards) and the point at which the athlete reports a return of normal continuous memory functioning (eg, remembering the athletic trainer asking the athlete orientation questions in the locker room). On-field or sideline anterograde amnesia may be assessed through immediate and delayed (eg, 0, 5, 15 minute) recall for three words (eg, girl, dog, green), as detailed in Table 8–2 (University of Pittsburgh Medical Center Concussion Card Mental Status Testing).

At times, especially during an acute assessment, confusion and anterograde amnesia may be difficult to disentangle. It is important to remember that confusion is not associated with a loss of memory, whereas amnesia is present only with a loss of memory. This memory loss may span a few seconds, hours, and, less frequently in concussion, days. A practitioner may be unable to dissociate confusion and amnesia until the athlete's confusion

Table 8–2. University of Pittsburgh Medical Centers' sideline concussion card: acute (sideline or on-field) mental status testing.

On-Field Cognitive Testing
Orientation (ask the athlete the following questions)
• What stadium is this? • What city is this? • Who is the opposing team? • What month is it? • What day is it?
Posttraumatic amnesia (ask the athlete to repeat the following words)
• Girl, dog, green
Retrograde amnesia (ask the athlete the following questions)
• What happened in the prior quarter or half? • What do you remember just prior to the hit? • What was the score of the game prior to the hit? • Do you remember the hit?
Concentration (ask the athlete to do the following)
• Repeat the days of the week backward, starting with today • Repeat these numbers backward (63)(419)
Word list memory
• Ask the athlete to repeat the three words listed above (girl, dog, green)

has resolved, and he or she is better able to discuss actual memories surrounding the injury. Once the athlete is lucid, the practitioner may gain additional insight into any existing anterograde amnesia by asking the athlete to recall the events that occurred immediately following the trauma (eg, rising from the ground, walking/skating to the sideline, memory for any part of the game played or observed after the injury, memory for the score of the contest, and memory of the ride home). Anterograde amnesia is indicated by failure to remember any of the above (or similar) details.

Retrograde amnesia is the inability to recall events preceding a head trauma. To determine the presence and duration of retrograde amnesia, the patient should be questioned about events that occurred immediately before the concussion. Commonly used questions to assess retrograde amnesia are presented in Table 8–2. Medical personnel may ask the athlete to recall details of the actual injury (eg, seeing a linebacker charge toward him with his helmet down, then falling backward and striking the back of his head on the ground). Then, additional questions can probe events that are increasingly remote from the injury (eg, the score at the beginning of the first quarter, coming onto the field for stretching exercises, getting dressed in the locker room).

The length of retrograde amnesia will typically "shrink" over time. As recovery occurs, the period of retrograde amnesia may contract from hours to several minutes or even seconds. However, by definition, a permanent loss of memory prior to the injury will remain. As with anterograde amnesia, even very brief retrograde amnesia may be considered pathognomonic and possibly linked to outcome in the form of protracted recovery, increased symptoms, etc.

Burgeoning data and studies emphasize that any athletes exhibiting a change in mental status (eg, confusion), posttraumatic/retrograde amnesia, and/or LOC be removed from and not be allowed to return to play, regardless of how long these symptoms take to "clear."

C. IMAGING STUDIES

Given that concussion is a metabolic and not a structural injury, traditional neurodiagnostic techniques such as the CT scan, MRI, or neurologic examination are almost always unremarkable following injury. Despite this fact, these techniques are invaluable in ruling out more serious pathology (eg, cerebral bleed or skull fracture) that may also occur with even seemingly mild head trauma. It is important to remember that a negative finding on a CT scan, MRI, etc does not rule out concussion, and should not be the basis for determining if an athlete is ready to return to play. Clinically, the sports medicine practitioner will likely encounter cases in which an athlete has been mistakenly returned to play based upon a negative CT and the athlete's assertion that he or she "feels fine." These individuals may return days or weeks later with a second concussive injury that has resulted from seemingly minimal force and that typically requires much more time to resolve.

Despite the insensitivity of traditional neuroimaging in detecting concussion, there are many new neurodiagnostic techniques under investigation for their potential utility in identifying and/or managing concussion. Functional imaging and other techniques, though in early stages of development, may provide valuable information regarding concussion in the future. Techniques such as magnetoencephalography (MEG), functional magnetic resonance imaging (fMRI), positron emission tomography (PET), and the monitoring of brain electrophysiological activity through event-related potentials (ERPs) may provide additional insight into the physiology of injury and recovery, and may provide the foundation for the establishment of neurodiagnostic norms against which clinicians may accurately assess the severity of the concussion and the prognosis for recovery.

D. SPECIAL TESTS

Perhaps the most important new development in the management of sports-related concussion is the recognition of neuropsychological or neurocognitive testing (synonymous terms) as a key element of the postconcussion evaluation process. Neurocognitive testing has contributed to the development of a more individualized and data-driven approach to the management of concussion. Neurocognitive testing was first used as a diagnostic tool in sports medicine in the mid-1980s within the context of a large multisite research project undertaken by Barth and his colleagues at the University of Virginia. The study demonstrated the utility of neuropsychological test procedures in documenting cognitive recovery within the first week following concussion. In the 1990s, a series of events shifted the use of neuropsychological testing in sports from the research to the clinical arena. First, concussive injuries in well-known professional athletes raised awareness and resulted in the implementation of baseline neuropsychological testing by a number of National Football League (NFL) teams. Similarly, after career-ending concussive injuries in athletes in the National Hockey League (NHL), the NHL mandated baseline neuropsychological testing for all athletes. In addition to the increased use of neuropsychological testing in professional sports, several large-scale studies of collegiate athletes were undertaken. These studies further demonstrated that neuropsychological testing yielded useful clinical information. Specifically, it allowed a baseline/postinjury analysis of

the subtle aspects of cognitive function likely affected by concussive injury, thus providing objective data that could be used to make more informed decisions regarding return to play.

Neuropsychological testing of athletes participating in contact sport has been accomplished in two ways. In its early phases, and in many settings today, traditional neuropsychological testing (eg, paper and pencil testing) has been used to provide both baseline cognitive functioning levels and postinjury follow-up. However, as an increasing number of sports organizations recognized the utility of neuropsychological testing, many limitations to traditional testing procedures emerged. For example, traditional neuropsychological testing is quite time consuming and costly, making it difficult to implement in amateur (eg, high school) settings. Also, the availability of trained neuropsychologists to administer and interpret the tests is limited. Lastly, the majority of athletes participate in sports at the amateur, high school, and college levels, where traditional testing is often not practical, affordable, or possible. These limitations, as well as a continual increase in the number of sports organizations seeking neuropsychological testing as a key element in concussion management, led to the development and proliferation of computer-based neuropsychological testing procedures.

Computer-based neuropsychological testing procedures have a number of advantages and relatively few disadvantages when compared to more traditional testing procedures. First, the use of computers allows large numbers of student athletes to be evaluated with minimal manpower. For example, an entire football team may be baseline tested in one or two sessions in a school's computer laboratory. Second, data acquired through testing can be easily stored in a specific computer or computer network and can therefore be accessed at a later date (eg, following injury). Third, the use of the computer promotes a more accurate measurement of cognitive processes such as reaction time and information processing speed. In fact, computerized assessment allows response times that are accurate to 1/100 of a second to be evaluated, whereas the accuracy of traditional testing is only 1–2 seconds. This increased accuracy no doubt increases the *validity* of test results in detecting subtle changes in neurocognitive processes. Fourth, the utilization of the computer allows for the randomization of test stimuli, which should improve *reliability* across multiple administration periods, minimizing the "practice effects" that naturally occur with multiple exposures to the stimuli. These practice effects have clouded the interpretation of research studies and have also presented an obstacle for the clinician evaluating the true degree of neurocognitive deficit following injury. Lastly, computer-based approaches allow clinical information to be rapidly disseminated into a coherent clinical report that can be easily interpreted by the sports medicine clinician. In summary, there are many benefits derived from a computer-based approach insofar as the technology has appropriate sensitivity, reliability, and validity in measuring the subtle aspects of concussive injury.

Neurocognitive deficits resulting from concussion have been documented in many studies, and cognitive testing appears to be a highly valuable tool in documenting impairment or incomplete recovery from concussive injury. Neurocognitive deficits associated with concussion have also been documented in studies of collegiate and high school football players, amateur soccer players, and samples of athletes across multiple sports. Neurocognitive evaluation is a sensitive tool that may be utilized to assess the often subtle and potentially debilitating effects of concussive injury. Neurocognitive test data appear to provide objective, quantifiable, and individualized standards to better determine safe return to participation and overall management of the concussed athlete, and should therefore be considered a critical factor in the management of concussion.

E. Special Examinations

Although neuropsychological testing is currently regarded as a gold standard in management of concussion, there are other measures that may be beneficial in the diagnosis and evaluation of concussion. The NeuroCom Smart Balance Master has been used to test for postural instability after mild head injury in an attempt to set the precedence for establishing recovery curves based on objective data. Concussed athletes exhibited increased postural instability for the first 3 days following injury. Balance testing or postural stability has recently been a popular topic among some clinicians, but current research in this area has been conducted with small sample sizes and has yet to be confirmed with larger groups of athletes.

Differential Diagnosis

The diagnosis of cerebral concussion can be a difficult process for many reasons. As previously mentioned, many differences exist in diagnostic criteria/classification, and there is a lack of one unified definition for the injury. In addition, there may be no direct or observed trauma to the head. Also, the concussed athlete often does not lose consciousness as a result of the injury. At times, an athlete may not immediately be aware that he or she has been injured. The injury may be very subtle and the athlete may not show any obvious signs of concussion such as disequilibrium, gross confusion, or obvious personality change. To further complicate the situation, athletes at all levels of competition may minimize or hide symptoms in an attempt to remain in the game, thus creating the potential for exacerbation of their injury. However, a clinical interview and thorough assessment of signs and symptoms will assist in making an accurate diagnosis.

Aubry M et al: Summary of the first international conference on concussion in sport. Clin J Sport Med 2002;12:6.

Collins MW et al: Relationship between post-concussion headache and neuropsychological test performance in high school athletes. Am J Sports Med 2003;31:168.

Collins MW et al: On-field predictors of neuropsychological and symptom deficit following sports-related concussion. Clin J Sport Med 2003;13:222.

Dupuis F et al: Concussions in athletes produce brain dysfunction as revealed by event-related potentials. Neuroreport 2000; 11:4087.

Echemendia RJ et al: Neuropsychological test performance prior to and following sports-related mild traumatic brain injury. Clin J Sport Med 2001;11:23.

Iverson GL et al: Relation between subjective fogginess and neuropsychological testing following concussion. J Int Neuropsychol Soc 2004;10:1.

Johnston KM et al: A contemporary neurosurgical approach to sport-related head injury: The McGill Concussion Protocol. J Am Coll Surg 2001;192:515.

Johnston KM et al: New frontiers in diagnostic imaging in concussive head injuries. Clin J Sport Med 2001;11:166.

Lovell MR: Evaluation of the professional athlete. In: *Sports-Related Concussion*. Bailes JE et al (editors). Quality Medical Publishing, Inc., 1999.

Lovell MR, Burke CJ: Concussion management in professional hockey. In: *Neurologic Athletic Head and Spine Injury*. Cantu RE (editor). Saunders, 2000.

Maroon JC et al: Cerebral concussions in athletes: evaluation and neuropsychological testing. Neurosurgery 2000;47:659.

McAllister TW et al: Brain activation during working memory 1 month after mild traumatic brain injury. Neurology 1999;53:130.

Mihalik JP et al: Post-traumatic migraine characteristics in athletes following sports-related concussion. J Neurosurg 2005;102:850.

Schnirring L: How effective is computerized concussion management? Phys Sportmed 2001;29:11.

Treatment

Presently there are no curative medical treatments for concussion. This emphasizes the importance of early identification, evaluation, and management of a concussion and the resultant symptoms, as well as the prevention of additional injury or the exacerbation of a current injury through early return to physical exertion or early return to play. If a concussion does not resolve after a month or more, and/or postconcussion symptoms become unbearable and interfere with a patient's daily functioning, a physician may elect to treat the symptoms of concussion. For example, a patient with severe post-traumatic migrainous headaches may be treated with preventative (eg, Effexor, Wyeth Pharmaceuticals) or abortive (eg, Imitrex, GlaxoSmithKline) medication (or a combination of both). A patient troubled by significant dizziness, balance problems, or presyncopal symptoms may be referred for evaluation and treatment through a balance clinic or referred to a neurologist for further evaluation. If an athlete remains troubled by extreme fatigue or difficulties with attention, a physician may elect to try a stimulant or similar medication to alleviate those symptoms (eg, Strattera, Eli Lilly and Co.). In more severe cases of unremitting cognitive problems, a patient may be referred for cognitive rehabilitation. Although the treatment modalities described above my alleviate some of the symptoms related to concussion or mild traumatic brain injury, none has been demonstrated to "cure" the metabolic dysfunction of concussion.

Prognosis

As previously detailed, current research has yet to delineate the exact metabolic process of concussion in humans. However, the current model of the pathophysiology of concussion raises important clinical and research questions and considerations when attempting to determine the prognosis of injury. Based upon research findings thus far, it has been postulated that until metabolic dysfunction resulting from concussion is fully resolved, the injured person may be at significantly increased neurologic vulnerability if a second trauma (even minor) is sustained. In theory, sustaining a second head injury during a period of increased vulnerability with unresolved metabolic dysfunction has been linked to second impact syndrome.

Second impact syndrome has been previously reported in the literature and varying reports suggest that as many as 35 or more athletes in the past decade have succumbed to this syndrome. In all cases, athletes sustained an initial concussive injury, returned to sports or other activities, and sustained a second, typically milder, concussive injury. The second blow resulted in dysautoregulation, massive edema, uncal herniation, and coma, which is followed by death shortly after the blow. Morbidity is 100% in the case of second impact syndrome, whereas mortality is reported to occur in up to 50% of cases. To date, all reported cases of second impact syndrome have occurred in younger athletes, typically adolescent high school students. Theory posits that younger athletes may be more vulnerable to the dysautoregulation seen in this syndrome. Regardless, it appears that younger, "immature" brains may be more vulnerable to the devastating effects of this condition. Debate does surround this construct and whether an initial concussion is definitively required for second impact syndrome to occur.

Current clinical experience and research have suggested that proper management of concussion should lead to a good prognosis with minimal or no evidence of chronic or catastrophic brain dysfunction. Long-term deficits in the form of postconcussion syndrome have been observed from a single concussive event, though it is much more common in repetitive occurrences of concussion with poor management and premature return to play following an initial concussion. Postconcussion syndrome typically results in a constellation of somatic (eg, headaches, dizziness, balance deficits), cognitive (eg, deficits with memory, attention, executive dysfunction), personality (eg, depression, anxiety), and/or sleep disturbances (eg, difficulty initiating and maintaining sleep) that, though tacit, may be incapacitating and chronic. The duration of postconcussion syndrome is quite variable, though it has been observed to last months, or even years, in athletes. The true incidence of postconcussion syndrome in athletes remains unknown, though it is experientially relatively frequent, especially at the high school level of sport participation.

Medical professionals agree that allowing an athlete to participate in contact sports prior to *complete* recovery may greatly increase the risk of poor outcome, including chronic postconcussion syndrome or even catastrophic neurologic sequelae (as in cases of second impact syndrome). Thus, the most important step a practitioner can take toward a positive prognosis is proper assessment and management of concussion in the acute and follow-up stages of injury. A management protocol will be presented later in this chapter.

Management Guidelines

More than 20 concussion management guidelines have been published over the past 30 years, all of which were intended to assist physicians in determining both the severity of injury as well as when an athlete may return to play. Most were primarily developed by panels of experts in the field and are based on popular belief or clinical impressions. When using these guidelines, severity of injury was determined by an accompanying grading scale. In general, a Grade 1 concussion involves symptoms lasting 15–20 minutes or less; a Grade 2 concussion involves symptoms lasting longer than 15 or 20 minutes; and a Grade 3 concussion is typically any concussion involving loss of consciousness. However, perusal of the guidelines and grading scales reveals many differences of clinical opinion. The significant variations that can occur between scales, the fact that these scales are often based upon clinical impressions rather than research, as well as the multitude of guidelines that exist create confusion and debate among practitioners. Within this context, grading scales have helped in creating awareness of concussive injury and in establishing a nomenclature for classification. Although "grading scales" are appropriately being replaced with individualized management protocols (see above), they have played an important role in the "evolution" of proper management of concussion.

In 1999, the American Orthopaedic Society for Sports Medicine (AOSSM) published a report detailing the state of the current guidelines and establishing possible practical alternatives to the guideline system. Although the AOSSM guidelines did not differ substantially from prior grading systems and guidelines, this report stressed more individualized management of injury, rather than applying general standards and protocols (eg, grading systems) to all injuries.

In 2001, the Federation Internationale de Football Association (FIFA) in conjunction with the International Olympic Committee (IOC) and the International Ice Hockey Federation (IHF) assembled a group of physicians, neuropsychologists, and sports administrators in Vienna, Austria to explore methods of reducing morbidity and improve outcomes secondary to sports-related concussion. The agreement statement that arose from this meeting was published in 2002. Perhaps the most important agreement to emerge from the meeting was that none of the previously published concussion management guidelines was adequate to ensure proper management of every concussion. In their statement, the group emphasized the more individualized management and implementation of postinjury neuropsychological testing as a "cornerstone" of proper postinjury management and decisions involving return to play. A return-to-play protocol consistent with the Vienna group's recommendations will be elucidated later in this chapter.

In summarizing the evolution and current state of guidelines on the management of concussion, it is clear that these systems cannot be exclusively relied upon to make return to participation decisions. As previously stated, the number and variety of existing grading procedures, many with only subtle differences, can understandably create communication difficulties among medical personnel and others who manage concussed athletes. This lack of uniformity and lack of research reinforce current thinking that concussion is not a unitary phenomenon, and injured athletes must therefore be evaluated and managed on a case-by-case basis.

Return to Play

Once an athlete has sustained a concussion, the clinician must decide when the athlete may safely return to play. There is no simple evidence-based formula available to direct the clinician in this regard. The process may seem more ambiguous than many other decisions clinician may face, given the subtlety of the injury and the lack of research-grounded guidelines. Making the return to play decision is an individualized and dynamic process that should include evaluation of factors such as the severity of the injury (as measured by duration of loss of consciousness, amnesia, and confusion), the athlete's appraisal of the presence and intensity of symptoms (eg, headache, dizziness, visual changes), and, if available, the athlete's performance on neurocognitive testing.

Importantly, a general awareness that symptoms of concussion may evolve over time and are also prone to worsen with exertion (ie, increased cerebral blood flow) is critical in helping to guide the clinician in establishing an assessment strategy. The one uniform agreement among experts is that any athlete known to be exhibiting signs or symptoms of concussive injury should not return to play, given the general issues surrounding increased neurological vulnerability to a second injury and that less biomechanical force may likely result in more severe postconcussion presentation.

In addition to signs and symptoms, there are many other factors that may play a role in an athlete's recovery trajectory, as well as in the decision as to when to return an athlete to participation in sports. Neuropsychological testing and continuing research have made it possible to identify individual factors that may play a role in the incidence, severity, and length of recovery regarding concussion.

A. Age

In recent years, there has been an increase in the number of younger athletes who participate in sports. This influx of younger athletes focused attention on another limitation of grading scales, which is that most guidelines for return to play do not include or mention developmental considerations that are likely to be important when managing concussion, given that brain development continues throughout adolescence. Unfortunately, there has been no published research exploring the potential developmental differences in physiological recovery in the child or adolescent, though current theories are explored below. Recent research on cognitive recovery has demonstrated that high school athletes may recover more slowly than their collegiate counterparts, when recovery is defined as a return to baseline levels of cognitive functioning. Even in cases of very mild concussion or "bell ringers," adolescent athletes were found to exhibit neuropsychological and symptom deficits for at least 7 days postinjury. These results are congruent with earlier studies showing age-based differences in recovery from concussion. Results from these age-specific research studies provide support for stopping all athletes under the age of 18 from participating in the athletic event in which they sustained a concussion, so that further evaluation can be undertaken (symptom inventories, cognitive testing, etc). Similar to this, recommendations from the Vienna meeting state that all athletes in whom concussion is diagnosed be removed from the playing contest. However, it should be noted that no prospective studies have examined the issue of mild concussion in college or professional-aged athletes. In addition, the overall risk/benefit analysis is likely to be different at different levels of competition. For example, professional athletes may be willing to assume greater risk through earlier return to play, given the obvious monetary and other considerations. Conversely, few parents would risk injury in a high school athlete, most of whom are unlikely to continue to compete beyond high school.

In addition to differences in cognitive recovery, age should be regarded as an important issue in management of concussion based on the fact that of the approximately 35 documented deaths related to second impact syndrome, the majority occurred in athletes between the ages of 13 and 18. Although no available research documents an age-based physiological or developmental vulnerability, many clinicians and researchers suspect that individuals who are younger, and therefore developmentally more immature, are at increased risk for second impact syndrome, and perhaps at risk for protracted recovery times following concussion.

One physiological theory exploring age-related differences is that children may undergo more prolonged and diffuse cerebral swelling after MTBI, which suggests that they may be at an increased risk for secondary intracranial hypertension and ischemia. This may also lead to a longer recovery period and could increase the likelihood of permanent or severe neurological deficit should reinjury occur during the recovery period. Another hypothesis is that the immature brain may be potentially 60 times more sensitive to glutamate-mediated N-methyl-D-aspartate (NMDA) excitotoxic brain injury. This hypersensitivity may render the child or adolescent more susceptible to the ischemic and injurious effects of EAA after MTBI.

As an alternative to theories of developmental vulnerability, the popular concept of cortical plasticity suggests that younger athletes should make a more complete recovery than their older counterparts. There has been clinical evidence of marked synaptic excess in children, relative to adults, which allows for neural pathway rerouting during recovery and functional plasticity in the developing brain. As time is not addressed in this theory, it may be assumed that a more complete recovery is possible due to the described plasticity, although it may take a longer period of time. Longitudinal and prospective studies examining the effects of age on outcome of sports concussion are currently underway and, in time, may elucidate this important clinical consideration.

B. Gender

Recent trends in sport participation have also indicated increased participation of girls and women. Thus, the issue of whether there are gender differences in incidence of concussion, recovery, and severity has become quite important. To date, very little research has specifically examined gender differences in MTBI. The majority of the published literature has focused on nonathletic populations (eg, accident victims) and on rodents. A recent meta-analysis of 8 studies and 20 outcome variables revealed that across 85% of those variables, outcome in

women was worse. In studies unrelated to sports, findings have suggested that women with MTBI are more likely to report sleep disturbances and headaches up to a year after injury, may be less likely than men to be employed or in school 1 year after mild head injury, and suffer a significant decrease in grade point average (GPA) as compared to controls; there were no similar findings for men. Even when controlling for other demographic, premorbid, and event-related factors, most research to date has shown that women have worse outcomes than men after MTBI.

Although the literature on gender-based sports concussion is limited, a few studies have emerged. Barnes et al. retrospectively demonstrated that male elite soccer players suffered concussions of greater severity and were subject to a higher incidence of injury than were female elite soccer players. A prospective study involving 15 National Collegiate Athletic Association (NCAA) men's and women's soccer teams over two seasons revealed a similar incidence of concussion in men and women.

Although much of the available literature reveals poorer outcome among women suffering from MTBI, animal models suggest that female sex hormones may actually protect neurons in the brain following concussive injury. Progesterone is thought to reduce cerebral edema and potentially facilitate cognitive recovery, whereas studies of estrogen influence have yielded mixed results. One study has shown that estrogen plays a protective role in males while increasing mortality in females. Other research has demonstrated that estrogen can assist in maintaining normal cerebral blood flow and actually decrease mortality when administered acutely. All of the aforementioned research suggests there may be important gender differences impacting the incidence and severity of MTBI. More research in this area is necessary to accurately delineate the implications of such differences.

C. Learning Disability

Learning disability (LD) refers to a heterogeneous group of disorders characterized by difficulties in the acquisition and use of listening, speaking, writing, reading, reasoning, or mathematical abilities and that is traditionally diagnosed in early childhood. The presence of a learning disability has been linked to lower baseline cognitive performance within a large, multiuniversity sample of football players. Learning-disabled football players who also reported a history of multiple concussions demonstrated reduced overall cognitive functioning when compared to athletes with multiple concussions who did not have a learning disability, and when compared to those with no history of concussion who had a learning disability, suggesting a potential additive effect. Therefore, knowing the educational history of athletes is important, as the presence of a learning disability certainly has the potential to complicate the diagnosis of concussion as well as the decision on return to play.

D. CONCUSSION HISTORY

The potential contributing factor of a history of concussion to vulnerability to injury and to recovery is an often discussed topic in sports medicine, though consensus on this issue is elusive. Several studies suggest there may be cumulative detrimental effects of multiple concussions. These studies have typically examined cognitive impairment and neurological abnormalities in boxers. Lately, however, this topic has been of increasing concern among other athletic populations. In a study of almost 400 college football players, Collins and others discovered long-term subtle neurocognitive deficits in those suffering two or more concussions. Another study conducted by Matser and others similarly suggested that cumulative long-term consequences can be seen from repetitive blows to the head in professional soccer players. In another study Collins and colleagues found that high school and collegiate athletes suffering three or more concussions appear to be more vulnerable to subsequent injury than athletes with no history of injury. A study in 2004 by Iverson and others found baseline and postinjury deficits between amateur athletes with and without histories of concussion. Specifically, athletes with a history of concussion exhibited more symptoms of concussion at baseline (preinjury evaluation), scored lower on memory tests at 2 days postinjury, and were almost eight times more likely to demonstrate a significant drop in memory performance when compared to amateur athletes without a history of concussion. This accumulation of recent research points to likely cumulative effects of concussions; however, no currently reliable data are available to determine the number of concussions that should preclude return to participation or force retirement from sports. In addition, research has yet to determine the potential beneficial impact of properly managing each concussion prior to returning an athlete to play. Allowing a concussion to completely resolve through management according to Vienna conference-type recommendations (see below) may reduce the deleterious effects of multiple concussions.

American Academy of Neurology: Practice parameter: the management of concussion in sports (summary statement). Report of the Quality Standards Subcommittee. Neurology 1997;48:581.

Aubry M et al: Summary of the first international conference on concussion in sport. Clin J Sport Med 2002;12:6.

Bailes JE, Cantu RC: Head injury in athletes. Neurosurgery 2001;48(1):26.

Barnes BC et al: Concussion history in elite male and female soccer players. Am J Sports Med 1998;26:433.

Cantu RC: Posttraumatic retrograde and anterograde amnesia: pathophysiology and implications in grading and safe return to play. J Athletic Train 2001;36:244.

Collins MW et al: Relationship between concussion and neuropsychological performance in college football players. JAMA 1999;282:964.

Collins MW et al: Current issues in managing sports concussion. JAMA 1999;282:2283.

Collins MW et al: Cumulative effects of sports concussion in high school athletes. Neurosurgery 2002;51:1175.

Farace E, Alves W: Do women fare worse: a metaanalysis of gender differences in traumatic brain injury outcome. J Neurosurg 2000;93:539.

Field M et al: Does age play a role in recovery from sports-related concussion? A comparison of high school and collegiate athletes. J Pediatr 2003;142:546.

Grindel SH et al: The assessment of sports-related concussions: the evidence behind neuropsychological testing and management. Clin J Sport Med 2001;11:134.

Iverson GL et al: Cumulative effects of concussion in amateur athletes. Brain Injury 2004;18:433.

Lovell MR et al: Recovery from mild concussion in high school athletes. J Neurosurg 2003;98:296.

Lovell MR et al: Grade 1 or "ding" concussions in high school athletes. Am J Sports Med 2004;32:47.

Matser E et al: Neuropsychological impairment in amateur soccer players. JAMA 1999;282:971.

Roof RL, Hall ED: Estrogen-related gender differences in survival rate and cortical blood flow after impact acceleration head injury in rats. J Neurotrauma 2000;17:367.

Wojtys ED et al: Concussion in sports. Am J Sports Med 1999;27:676.

Concussion Management Model

A. PREINJURY MEASURES

Ideally, and if possible, a concussion management program for athletes should begin with baseline neurocognitive testing of athletes considered at high risk for concussion or mild traumatic brain injury. The definition of a "contact sport" varies from organization to organization, though it usually includes the sports of football, rugby, ice hockey, and soccer. Wrestling, field hockey, and basketball are also sports in which concussions are frequently seen. Even sports that do not seem to involve contact may on occasion lead to a concussive injury. In the sports of cheerleading, swimming, and diving, there have certainly been documented and sometimes severe cases of concussion. Baseline testing may also incorporate a baseline symptom report, such as the Post-Concussion Symptom Scale (see Table 8–3), to gain insight about an athlete's individual tendencies to report symptoms such as headache or attention problems when uninjured. Baseline testing is usually accomplished through the team athletic trainer or other athletic team staff. Once an athlete receives a valid baseline test, that test should serve for the tenure of the athlete's participation at that level of competition (eg, high school, college, professional levels).

It is also useful prior to the beginning of the season to educate athletes about sport-related concussion.

Table 8–3. The postconcussion symptom scale.

Symptom	None	Minor		Moderate		Severe	
Headache	0	1	2	3	4	5	6
Nausea	0	1	2	3	4	5	6
Vomiting	0	1	2	3	4	5	6
Balance problems	0	1	2	3	4	5	6
Dizziness	0	1	2	3	4	5	6
Fatigue	0	1	2	3	4	5	6
Trouble falling asleep	0	1	2	3	4	5	6
Sleeping more than usual	0	1	2	3	4	5	6
Sleeping less than usual	0	1	2	3	4	5	6
Drowsiness	0	1	2	3	4	5	6
Sensitivity to light	0	1	2	3	4	5	6
Sensitivity to noise	0	1	2	3	4	5	6
Irritability	0	1	2	3	4	5	6
Sadness	0	1	2	3	4	5	6
Nervousness	0	1	2	3	4	5	6
Feeling more emotional	0	1	2	3	4	5	6
Numbness or tingling	0	1	2	3	4	5	6
Feeling slowed down	0	1	2	3	4	5	6
Feeling mentally "foggy"	0	1	2	3	4	5	6
Difficulty concentrating	0	1	2	3	4	5	6
Difficulty remembering	0	1	2	3	4	5	6
Visual problems	0	1	2	3	4	5	6

Adapted from Lovell MR, Collins MW: Neuropsychological assessment of the college football player. J Head Trauma Rehabil 1998;13:9.

Athletes at all levels should receive information about the common signs and symptoms of concussion, the variability in injury presentation, and the importance of reporting even a suspected concussion to the on-site medical personnel. In addition, either verbally or through educational materials, common myths about concussion should be dispelled (eg, athletes often believe that a concussion has not occurred if they do not experience loss of consciousness). In cases of child and adolescent athletes, the sports organization should attempt to educate parents and caregivers as well.

B. Acute Postinjury Management

Appropriate acute care of the concussed athlete begins an accurate assessment of the gravity of the situation. As with any assessment of a serious injury, the first priority is always to evaluate the athlete's level of consciousness and ABCs (airway, breathing, and circulation). The attending medical staff must always have an emergency action plan in the event that the evacuation of a critically head or neck-injured athlete is necessary. This plan should be familiar to all staff, be well delineated, and frequently rehearsed.

If concussion, without other brain injury, is suspected, the injured athlete should be administered a simple sideline mental status examination [eg, Standardized Assessment of Concussion (SAC) or University of Pittsburgh Medical Center (UPMC) On-Field Concussion Evaluation, see Table 8–2] to identify cognitive deficits and signs and symptoms of injury.

Through this process, the clinician should document the presence and duration of loss of consciousness, amnesia, and confusion, as well as any other symptoms of concussion. Methods of assessing these symptoms have been described in the sections on "symptoms" and "signs" in this chapter.

A sideline assessment of cognitive functioning, signs, and symptoms should be completed even if the athlete asserts that he or she is "fine." During the on-field examination, any overt neurologic/cognitive deficit or single sign or symptom of injury (eg, headache, confusion, balance problems, personality change) should preclude return of the athlete to participation for that contest, and signal the necessity of a more comprehensive examination. Serial evaluation and assessment of the athlete's status throughout the competition are important, especially as the presentation of concussion sequelae may be an evolving process. If there is resolution of all signs and symptoms (typically within 15 minutes) on a serial sideline examination as well as on exertion, returning the athlete to active participation that day may be a viable option. However, the risk–benefit ratio of returning younger athletes to play on the same day of competition should be carefully considered before a decision is made. Typically younger athletes, especially high school and below, are not returned to play during the same contest.

C. NONACUTE POSTINJURY MANAGEMENT

At present, prevailing standards of care require that an athlete satisfy three conditions before returning to play. From the standpoint of a sports medicine physician, the athlete should be asymptomatic at rest and during noncontact exertion before return to play is indicated. Once asymptomatic at rest, the athlete progresses through increasing noncontact physical exertion until he or she has demonstrated asymptomatic status with heavy noncontact physical exertion and noncontact sport-specific training. If there is access to cognitive/neuropsychological testing, the third Vienna conference criteria may be added whereby the athlete must exhibit intact cognitive functioning (ideally, through baseline-level performance on neurocognitive testing). Assessment of the three steps is reviewed below.

1. Asymptomatic status at rest—Separately or in conjunction with administration of a neurocognitive test battery, the athlete should complete a symptom inventory [such as the Postconcussive Symptom Scale (PCSS), see Table 8–3] or symptom interview both on the sideline (may be brief) and serially throughout recovery. Before progressing to any significant level of physical exertion, the athlete should report being asymptomatic at rest for at least 24 hours. If it is suspected that the athlete's report of asymptomatic status is false, a careful discussion of the importance of reporting all symptoms should be initiated. If there are others who

present for evaluation with the athlete (parents, athletic trainers, teammates), asking these third party informants about the athlete's previous or current symptom complaints or signs of illness may be helpful.

2. Asymptomatic status with physical exertion—An athlete who demonstrates asymptomatic status at rest should begin a graduated return to physical exertion prior to contact participation, as postconcussion difficulties may evolve with increased cerebral blood flow. The Vienna group has suggested a graduated protocol as outlined by Aubry et al. Briefly, an athlete successfully moves through the following exertional steps in 24-hour periods: (1) light aerobic exercise (walking, stationary biking), (2) sport-specific training (ice skating in hockey or running in soccer–typically moderately exertional), and (3) noncontact training drills (usually heavily exertional). Athletes whose previously resolved postconcussion symptoms reappear at any point during the graded return to physical exertion should return to the exertion level at which they were last asymptomatic. Clearly, prior history of concussion, outcome from previous concussion, as well as any suspected deception by the athlete in reporting symptoms may influence return to participation and management directives.

3. Neurocognitive testing—If an athlete has been excluded from competition and severe intracranial pathology has been ruled out, postinjury assessment in the form of neurocognitive evaluation may be used to help determine overall management and return-to-participation issues (even for those athletes who were initially cleared to play). An athlete's cognitive status can be determined by an objective neurocognitive evaluation. Cognitive recovery is achieved when the athlete's performance either returns to baseline levels or, in the absence of return to baseline, is consistent with premorbid estimates of functioning when the test data are compared to normative values (clinicians should utilize test batteries that have readily available athlete-specific norms).

As described above, a preseason or baseline neuropsychological assessment would be helpful in comparing postinjury functioning to "normal" functioning for the injured athlete. Many practitioners prefer to complete serial follow-up using computerized neuropsychological testing to gain insight into the extent and type of cognitive impairment created by the injury. The first test may be performed while the athlete is still symptomatic and then completed once the athlete is asymptomatic to gauge progress and ensure a return to baseline or premorbid expectations of cognitive functioning. Other practitioners prefer to conduct the test when the athlete is asymptomatic both at rest and with heavy noncontact exertion, prior to returning the athlete to any type of contact participation. This may maximize the chance that neuropsychological testing will need to be performed only once at follow-up.

Athletes who are symptom free both at rest and with physical exertion, are within expected levels on cognitive testing (if available), and therefore are medically cleared may return to full-contact training and then to competition. Again, if any symptoms reemerge with return to contact participation, the athlete should return to non-contact physical activity.

Aubry M et al: Summary of the first international conference on concussion in sport. Clin J Sport Med 2002;12:6.

Bailes JE, Cantu RC: Head injury in athletes. Neurosurgery 2001;48(1):26.

Conclusions & Future Directions

The clinical management of concussion remains a topic of interest and of debate in the medical community. Science and theory of concussion management and return-to-play decisions are evolving rapidly, though there remains much to learn about both the short-and long-term consequences of injury. Clearly, the injury can have serious consequences, especially if not properly assessed, diagnosed, and managed. The realization that there is currently no one formula or guideline that can safely manage an injury as complex and multifaceted as concussion is perhaps the greatest breakthrough in research over the past decade.

As research continues to investigate the biomechanics, pathophysiology, and clinical course of sports-related concussion, management strategies will continue to evolve. Although the future of concussion management remains somewhat uncertain, emerging recommendations support individualized management of the injury through baseline testing, serial assessment of signs, symptoms, and cognitive function, and graduated return to exertion. Certainly, the practitioner must establish an absence of any clinical symptomology (at rest and exertion) as well as normal brain function prior to authorizing a return to play.

The Youth Athlete

9

Jan S. Grudziak, MD, PhD, & Volker Musahl, MD

Injuries among the skeletally immature athlete are to some extent unique and specific to this population. Because the biology and physiology of soft tissues and bone are different in the pediatric or adolescent patient, an injury seen in the adult population might require treatment different from one occurring in a growing child. A typical example is an anterior cruciate ligament (ACL) injury in a skeletally immature patient.

Usually, the child is able to heal faster and more predictably than the adult. The growing organism can compensate for and correct residual deformities that are commonly accepted by pediatric orthopedic surgeons familiar with the amazing, restorative powers of the growing organism. Unfortunately, the growing parts are also subject to trauma, damage to the growth plate, and subsequent abnormal development. Surgically caused damage to a growth plate can result in progressive deformity and alter the initially perfect result of otherwise properly executed treatment. In this respect, injuries in the pediatric and adolescent population might be quite challenging to manage, and their results unpredictable. Detailed knowledge of the physiology and pathology of the immature organism is crucial to avoid iatrogenic insult to the growing organism and to improve the end result of treatment.

There is no doubt that the intensity and frequency of sport competition have increased in recent years. More teenagers involved in sports results in fewer problems related to drugs, obesity, teenage pregnancy, and lackluster performance in school. The competition of sport creates a valuable groundwork for the demands of adult life. Being involved in a sport teaches the young athlete how to focus on goals and achieve the highest level of performance. Girls join the rush and since some injuries happen to them at a higher than average rate, they contribute to the overall frequency of sports-related injuries. Some sports, such as soccer, have attracted more young athletes over the past two decades than ever before.

College and professional scouts seemingly infiltrate the earliest levels of competition. At the high school level they offer enticing deals, usually featuring some monetary incentives, such as a "free ride" scholarship.

All these factors mean that competition has become fiercer, as the pressure from peers and parents has increased significantly. Today's young athlete is better prepared to compete, but also faces greater pressure to win. This creates a perfect environment for overuse and repetitive trauma injuries. The increased intensity of sports training and competition is visible, especially at the high school level; although sports-related injuries among students occur in all age groups, they peak in high school students.

Some sports carry a higher risk for specific injuries (Table 9–1). Advances in equipment and technique sometimes totally change the spectrum of sport-specific injuries. Skiing is a typical example; in the past, tibia fractures and ankle fractures were the most common injuries. As a result of technical advancement and changes in equipment (bindings, skis, helmets), the prevalence of skiing-related injuries has decreased in all age groups, and the spectrum of the injuries has shifted from fractures to soft tissue injuries.

GROWTH PLATE

Anatomy & Physiology

The growing human organism shows a unique blend of the ability to repair and to remodel a deformity, and vulnerability to growth problems as a result of an injury (Figure 9–1). The growth plate is most commonly responsible for these problems. The maturing bone, with its adjacent joint cartilage, undergoes a fascinating process that eventually results in a fully mature skeleton and mature hyaline cartilage. The blood supply evolves as well. In some circumstances, a richer blood supply to the growing bone provides advantages over the mature bone: for example, healing is faster and regeneration occurs more quickly. Sometimes, however, the unique patterns of blood supply to the young bone are unfavorable to the function of the skeletal system, potentially causing serious problems (Figure 9–2). Typical examples include a higher risk of avascular necrosis (AVN) of the

194

Table 9–1. Sport-specific injuries and their rate (per year) among high school athletes in the United States.

	Boys	Girls
Football	1.97	
Wrestling	1.82	
Soccer	1.19	1.14
Basketball	0.93	0.80
Track	0.68	0.73
Cross country	0.66	0.65
Cheerleading		0.51
Gymnastics		0.44
Swimming	0.21	0.21

	Risk	Injuries
Ballet dancers	Low	Ankle, metatarsal, spondylolysis
Baseball	Moderate	Little League elbow, ankle
Basketball	Moderate	Ankle, knee sprains, anterior cruciate ligament (ACL), finger fractures
Cycling	High	Closed head injuries, fractures: femur, forearm
Diving	High	Head, C-spine
Football	High	Head, C-spine, knee
Gymnastics	Moderate	Spondylolysis, wrist
Ice hockey	Moderate to high	Head, shoulder, laceration, clavicle fracture, ACL
Horseback riding	Moderate to high	Head, C-spine
Running	Low to moderate	Overuse, lower extremities, pelvis
Skateboarding	High	Head, C-spine, knee, forearm fracture
Skating inline	Low to moderate	Wrist, upper extremities
Skiing	Moderate to high	Tibial fracture, ACL, thumb, shoulder, head, spine
Snowboarding	Moderate to high	Upper extremities (wrist), ankle, calcaneus
Soccer	Moderate	ACL, meniscus, overuse fractures
Swimming	Low	Overuse: shoulder, knee, back
Tennis	Low	Overuse: elbow; Sprains: lower extremities
Trampoline	High	Head, C-spine, upper extremities fractures
Weight lifting	Low to moderate	Overuse, acromioclavicular joint
Wrestling	High	Upper extremities fracture and dislocation

Adapted, with permission, from Staheli LT: *Fundamentals of Pediatric Orthopedics.* Lippincott-Raven, 1998.

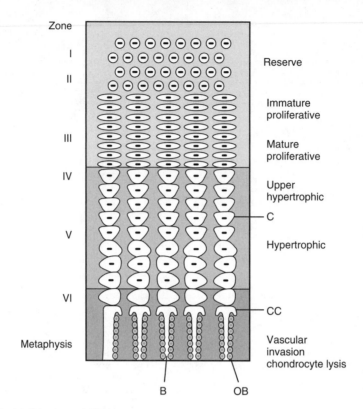

Figure 9–1. Physiology of the growth plate.

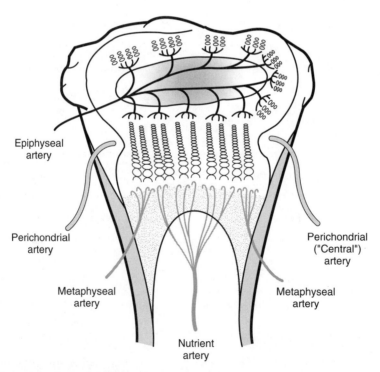

Figure 9–2. Blood supply to the growth plate.

femoral head after a femoral neck fracture, especially a subcapital fracture, and limb length discrepancy as a result of the overgrowth of a femur following its fracture. Bone growth starts at the seventh embryonic week and continues until growth is finished at skeletal maturity. There are two distinct forms of bone formation: the endochondral and the intramembranous.

Endochondral bone formation occurs at the growth plate, and is also responsible for repair of a fracture. Osteoblasts initiate endochondral bone formation; their activity results in the development of an osteoid, and its subsequent maturation into fully differentiated bone tissue. Endochondral bone formation occurs through maturation of the osteoid in the growth plate. Maturation starts from the reserve zone and advances through the proliferative zone, the maturation zone, the degenerative zone, and into the zone of provisional calcification. Bone development from the primary to secondary spongiosa occurs in the metaphysis. As a result, the new bone is deposed at the metaphyseal face of the growth plate.

A different mechanism forms bone on the periosteal surface of the clavicle, pelvis, scapula, and skull (CPSS). This process is called intramembranous bone formation.

The production of a new bone from a growth plate is a highly complicated process. An excellent review by Ballock and O'Keefe discusses the most important elements of the biochemistry and physiology of the growth plate (Table 9–2). The role and function of chondrocytes have been studied extensively. A differentiating chondrocyte of the growth plate undergoes a complex morphologic and biochemical alteration, with precise signaling at the molecular level. The proliferation of chondrocytes, their maturation, and hypertrophy ultimately culminate in precisely programmed chondrocyte death, or apoptosis. The synthesis, secretion, and mineralization of the matrix with resultant osteoid formation are controlled by many factors. Finally, vascular invasion, necessary for the distribution of the local growth factors and hormones, orchestrates endochondral bone formation as well as closure of the growth plate at maturity (Table 9–3).

The blood supply to the growth plate varies with age. The epiphyseal arteries, the metaphyseal network created by the main nutritional artery, and the perichondrial arteries of the perichondrial ring of LaCroix supply blood to the growth plate and secondary center of ossification. The epiphyseal arteries and their terminal branches supply blood to the epiphyses. The main nutritional artery of a long bone enters the metaphysis via a network of terminal vessels, which supply blood to the primary and secondary spongiosa. This artery does not penetrate the hypertrophic zone; instead oxygen and nutrients are transported into the growth plate via diffusion from arcades of the terminal branches of the main nutritional artery. The perichondrial arteries of the perichondrial ring of LaCroix supply the periphery of the growth plate. There is no connection between the epiphyseal and metaphyseal system as long as the growth plate exists. As a result, the blood supply to the epiphysis is limited, and relies exclusively on the network of epiphyseal vessels; thus, the probability of disrupting this system is relatively high. In the absence of additional blood flow from the metaphysis, with torn or kinked epiphyseal vessels, the risk of AVN following fractures increases. AVN of a femoral head following femoral neck fracture in children and teenagers is a prime example of this problem. The differences between adult and skeletally immature bone blood supply also explain the higher rate of AVN of the femoral head in adolescents, associated with intramedullary nailing of a femur fracture with the starting point in the piriformis fossa.

In this chapter we focus on the unique aspects of sports-related injuries suffered by skeletally immature athletes. First we discuss injuries to the growth plate. Subsequently injuries to the lower extremities (hip, knee, and foot and ankle) and upper extremities are discussed.

Injuries

The Hueter–Volkmann law states that compressive forces inhibit, whereas tensile stresses promote, the growth of long bones. This law holds true to a certain extent. An equilibrium of tensile and compression forces across the growth plate is part of the normal kinetics of a growing organism, and is necessary for normal function of the growth plate and growth of the bone. The abnormally high tension or compression can cause growth arrest rather than normal growth, and excessive forces through the growth plate, either acute or chronic, may fracture or permanently injure the growth plate.

The growth plate is quite resistant to mechanical damage, however, in younger children it is often the weakest link in the muscle/tendon/bone or ligament/bone chain. Very frequently an injury that causes sprain or strain in adults results in fracture through the growth plate in the pediatric or adolescent population. The mechanical properties of the growth plate seem to approximate those of articular cartilage, however, the complex, layered anatomy of the growth plate limits the ability to generate exact numbers. Very few studies discuss this subject, and the mechanical properties of the growth plate cartilage and mode of failure are not entirely understood. There are limited data about the compression properties based on animal models: numerical data regarding the shear forces, tensile properties, or model of failure of the growth plate cartilage have not been published.

In clinical settings the hypertrophic zone of the growth plate seems to be its weakest part, since the fracture line usually goes through this zone. The high

Table 9–2. Factors regulating the matrix production, life cycle of the chondrocytes, vascular invasion, and final closure of the growth plate.

Regulation of synthesis of the matrix

Transcription factor Sox 9: required for expression of collagen types II, IX, XI, and aggrecan; might control cell surface protein expression

Transcription factors L-Sox 5, Sox 6: together with Sox 9 activate gene transcription

Regulation of proliferation of the chondrocytes

Parathyroid hormone-related peptide (PTHrP): controls the pace of hypertrophy

Indian hedgehog (Ihh): increases production of PTHrP

Transforming growth factor-β (TGF-β): inhibits cell hypertrophy, inhibits type X collagen expression and alkaline phosphatase activity, acting through Smad 3

Insulin-like growth factor-I (IGF-I): increases rate of cellular division

Fibroblast growth factor (FGF): controls PTHrP feedback with Ihh

Cyclin-dependent kinases (CDKs): stimulates chondrocyte proliferation

CDKs inhibitors: play a role in the termination of chondrocyte differentiation

Maturation and hypertrophy of the chondrocytes

Type X collagen (unique to hypertrophy zone)

Alkaline phosphatase: calcification of the matrix, increases phosphate ions

Bone morphogenic proteins (BMPs): completion of maturation

Thyroxin: induces type X via activation of BMP-2

Retinoid acid: increases Smad 1 and Smad 5, inducing expression of BMP

Core binding factor-1 (CBF-1): induces terminal differentiation

Smad 1,5,8: enhance hypertrophy

Matrix mineralization

Ca^{2+}

Annexin II, V, and VI: part of calcium channels

Collagen types II and X: adhere to vesicles with annexin V, stimulate annexin V calcium channels and deposition of Ca^{2+}

Alkaline phosphatase: hydrolyze the pyrophosphate

Matrix metalloproteinases (MMPs): necessary for angiogenesis and calcification, cleavage of type II

MMP-13: activates TGF-β

MMP-9: angiogenesis

Vitamin D_3: increases activity of MMP and alkaline phosphatase, Ca^{2+} resorption

Chondrocyte apoptosis:

Caspases: cleave proteins

bcl-2 protein: blocks caspases

BAX: stimulates caspases

Phosphate ions: stimulate apoptosis, release of cytochrome *c*

FGF-2: binds to FGFR-3 increasing apoptosis

PTHrP: inhibits apoptosis

Vascular invasion

Vascular endothelial growth factor (VEGF): stimulates capillary invasion into growth plate

Core binding factor-1 (CBFA-1): stimulates angiogenesis

Basic fibroblast growth factor (BFGF): stimulates angiogenesis

PTHrP: slows angiogenesis

Physeal closure

Estrogen: closure of the growth plate in both females and males

---

Based on Ballock RT, O'Keefe RJ: The biology of the growth Plate. J Bone Joint Surg Am 2003;85-A:715.

Table 9–3. Patterns of growth rate and fusion of different growth plates.

	Epiphyses and Apophyses	
	Appearance	*Fusion*
Femoral head	3–8 months	14–20 years
Greater trochanter	5–7 years	13–22 years
Lesser trochanter	6–11 years	12–20 years
Iliac crest	12–15 years	13–20 years
	Proportions of the Growth of the Long Bones	
	Proximal Growth Plate	*Distal Growth Plate*
Femur	30%	70%
Tibia	55%	45%
Humerus	80%	20%
Radius	25%	75%

content of cells, with a relatively low matrix component is the probable reason for this relative weakness. As the bone and growth plate mature, the matrix content augments the cartilage, the growth plate becomes thinner and more irregular, rather then smooth and linear, and resistance to damaging forces increases, especially to shear injuries.

Salter & Harris Classification

The classification system of growth plate fractures is based on the classic work of Salter and Harris. They categorized growth plate injuries into five types (Figure 9–3):

Type 1 is a shear injury through the hypertrophic zone, which separates the epiphysis from the metaphysis. A classic type 1 is visible on a radiograph as displacement of the epiphysis in respect to the remaining part of a long bone. Often, however, injury forces are not strong enough to displace the epiphysis, and radiographs of such an injury might show no abnormalities except for soft tissue swelling. In this situation, a diagnosis of nondisplaced Salter–Harris 1 fracture is based on the mechanism of injury, combined with clinically discovered tenderness exactly at the level of the involved growth plate.

Type 2 fracture extends through the growth plate and exits into the metaphysis, creating a Thurston–Holland fragment. Type 2 is an extraarticular fracture and often happens at the distal radius and distal femur. It should be easily appreciated on routine radiographs.

Type 3 traverses the epiphysis. It extends into the joint surface and splits the articular cartilage. The displaced fragment separates from the metaphysis through the hypertrophic zone of the growth plate. Because type 3 is an intraarticular fracture, it needs to be anatomically reduced and stabilized, and often requires surgery.

Type 4 is intraarticular as well, splits the epiphysis, crosses the growth plate instead of curving into it, and extends into the metaphysis, creating a free epiphyseal/metaphyseal fragment. This type bears a high risk for permanent growth plate damage. It requires anatomic reduction as often as type 3.

Type 5 is a compression type, often unrecognized at first, as radiographs usually fail to show an injury. It is commonly diagnosed retrospectively, when a growth arrest causes growth problems as a result of a preceding compression injury.

The original Salter–Harris classification includes types 1 through 5. Type 6, added by some authors, is an injury to the periphery of a growth plate, and carries a relatively high risk for growth problems.

The growth plate injury can cause a deformation or abnormal growth of a bone with shortening or angulation. Generally, type 1 carries a low risk for physeal damage, type 2 higher, etc. More violent trauma increases the possibility of developing permanent growth plate problems. Displaced fractures more commonly end up with physeal bar formation; however, Salter–Harris types 1 and 2 can be left slightly displaced. The intraarticular

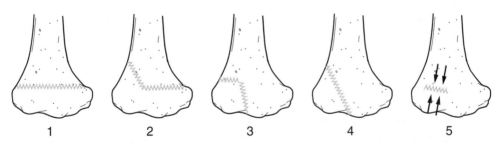

Figure 9–3. Salter–Harris classification (1–5) of physeal injuries.

types (types 3 and 4) might predispose a joint to osteoarthritis. Those types need anatomic reduction and stabilization, with the major factor being a reduction of the articular surface, not a reduction of the fracture line at the growth plate. The final outcome of a growth plate injury depends on several factors: the magnitude of forces causing the injury, type of growth plate fracture, age at the time of the initial trauma, and location of a fracture. The most important prognostic factor is the location of the fracture. For example, a Salter–Harris 2 fracture of the distal femur bears a much higher risk of growth arrest than a type 2 fracture of the distal radius.

ALIGNMENT OF THE LOWER EXTREMITIES

Mechanical alignment of the lower extremities changes as a child grows. Usually the newborn presents with varus of the lower extremities. This "bowlegged" period lasts up to 18 and sometimes 24 months of age, after which the mechanics of the lower extremities changes into valgus or "knock-knees" (Figure 9–4). An examination of the mechanical axis of the lower extremities is not complicated, although radiographs are sometimes required in case of asymmetry, progressive deformities, pain, or lack of regression. Changes in the angular alignment at adolescence may be caused by trauma to the growth plate, metabolic diseases, endocrinologic problems, or other conditions such as an adolescent form of Blount's disease. Deformities that result in serious deviation of the mechanical axis must be corrected. Currently, asymmetric stapling of the growing physis seems to be the logical choice for slow correction of excessive valgus/varus deformity. The surgery requires a relatively small incision. The staples are removed after a slight overcorrection is achieved. Theoretically, the possibility of permanent growth plate closure and overcorrection does exist, but this situation is not a problem in clinical practice. After growth has ceased, or if the remaining growth potential is low, an osteotomy to acutely correct a deformity would be a better choice.

Torsional alignment of the lower extremities rarely causes long lasting problems and rarely requires surgical correction. To evaluate the rotational alignment of a child it is helpful to follow a certain order to assess the rotational profile:

- Internal/external rotation of the hip.
- Thigh–foot angle.
- Tibial torsion.
- Foot morphology.
- Foot progression angle as a dynamic assessment.

Femoral anteversion and tibial torsion vary greatly as a child grows. The initially elevated femoral anteversion

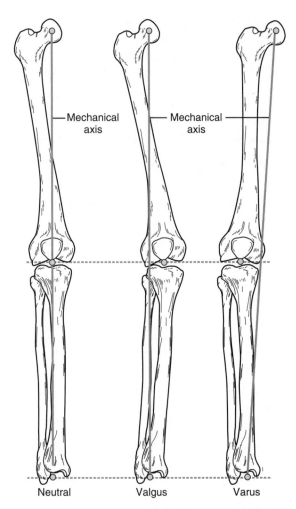

Figure 9–4. Alignment of the lower extremity and rotational elements. (Grudziak JS and Bosch P: Angular Deformities of the Lower Extremities. In: Tometta, P and Einhorn TA, ed. *Orthopedic Surgery Essentials.* LWW, 2004.)

reduces to the adult level of 8–20° by the early school years, and the very common decreased tibial torsion, or internal tibial torsion, resolves spontaneously without intervention in the vast majority of children. Although a variety of orthopedic shoes and braces had been used to "speed up" the remodeling process, current research does not support the use of any orthopedic devices to treat rotational and angular "deformities" as the majority resolve spontaneously.

Final anatomic alignment of the lower extremities is established around the age of 7–9 years. Therefore correction of a rotational deformity should be postponed until this age. Sometimes, an isolated rotational deformity may need to be corrected at this age if it creates functional or cosmetic problems. There is a strong belief, especially in the German speaking world, that decreased femoral anteversion is associated with arthritis of the hip joint, however, according to most researchers, arthritis of the hips, knees, and ankle joints does not seem to be related to increased anteversion of the femur or internal or external tibial torsion. A combination of increased femoral anteversion and increased external tibial torsion is a known risk factor for patella maltracking and anterior knee pain.

Ballock RT, O'Keefe RJ: The biology of the growth plate. J Bone Joint Surg Am 2003;85-A(4):715.

Garrick JG, Requa RK: Sports and fitness activities: the negative consequences. J Am Acad Orthop Surg 2003;11(6):439.

Kocher MS, Newton PO: What's new in pediatric orthopaedics. J Bone Joint Surg Am 2005;87(5):1171.

Purvis JM, Burke RG: Recreational injuries in children: incidence and prevention. J Am Acad Orthop Surg 2001;9(6):365.

■ HIP & PELVIS

Pathogenesis

In the adult population the pelvic ring consists of two innominate bones, connected by the symphysis pubis. Posteriorly, the ring is closed via the sacroiliac joints and the body of the sacrum. The general shape of the pelvis resembles the adult type with typical gender differences. In growing children the innominate bone is a combination of three separate bones: the ilium, ischium, and pubis. The central connecting point for the bones is the triradiate cartilage, made up of anterior and posterior horizontal limbs and a vertical limb. A connection between the ilium and ischium posteriorly and the os pubis anteriorly builds up the horizontal limb of the triradiate cartilage. The vertical limb connects the ischium and pubis. Apophyses are located over the top ridge of the iliac wind, along the ischial tuberosity, adjacent to the symphysis pubis, around the acetabulum, and at the anterior inferior iliac spine (Figure 9–5).

The femoral head articulates with the acetabulum, creating the hip joint. Growth of the acetabulum occurs at the triradiate cartilage apophyses, with adjacent parts of those three bones creating the cavity of the acetabulum. Additional growth centers at the superior brim of the acetabulum contribute to its depth and breadth. The acetabulum is more plastic, enlarging as a result of appositional growth from the ilium, ischium, and pubis.

The proximal femur grows from the proximal femoral physis. The femoral head is a secondary center of ossification, separated from the neck by a growth plate. In addition to this main growth plate, the proximal femur has two apophyses: at the lesser and greater trochanters.

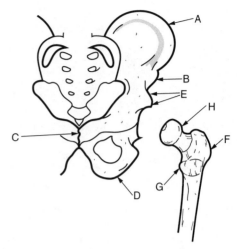

Figure 9–5. Growth zones of the pelvis and femur. **A:** Iliac apophysis. **B:** Anterior inferior iliac spine (AIIS). **C:** Symphysis pubis. **D:** Ischial tuberosity. **E:** Acetabulum. **F:** Greater trochanter. **G:** Lesser trochanter. **H:** Femoral head.

The hip joint is fully formed at the moment of birth; the acetabulum will develop as a child grows but the structure is essentially similar to the adult joint. Contact surfaces include the semilunate cartilage of the acetabulum and the cartilage of the femoral head. The transverse ligament connects the distal horns of the semilunate cartilage. The acetabular labrum increases the depth of the acetabulum. The ligamentum teres connects the femoral head to the cavity of the acetabulum and supplies blood to a limited part (less then 5%) of the femoral head.

The orientation of the acetabulum, measured by inclination and anteversion, seems to change little, if at all, as a child grows. The acetabulum becomes more horizontal during development, thus covering more of the femoral head. The neck-shaft angle is usually around 120–135°. Femoral anteversion measures 35–45° at birth, gradually reducing to the adult value of 8–20°.

Clinical Findings

Pain in the groin or around the pelvis is usually the main reason to seek medical attention (Figure 9–6). A careful history will greatly aid the physician in establishing a proper diagnosis. A history of trauma or lack thereof, the presence of fever, malaise, or mechanical symptoms, and participation in sports with a higher incidence of pelvic and hip injuries should be ascertained. Acute onset of discomfort will be typical for an avulsion fracture, acute slipped capital femoris epiphysis, torn

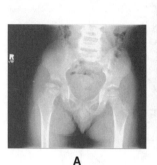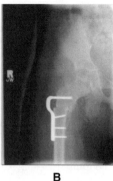

A	B

Figure 9–6. Seven-year-old soccer player with prolonged vague right hip pain and limp. **A:** Perthes disease of the right hip: Herring type B. **B:** Varus subtrochanteric osteotomy has increased the coverage of the femoral head.

labrum, or fracture of the bony structure of the pelvis or femur. The inability to bear weight is also common. A dysplastic acetabulum, as a result of developmental dysplasia of the hip, may manifest with slowly progressing pain. Pain slowly increasing with activity will be common for stress fractures, overuse syndromes, and hip dysplasia. Fever and pain without previous injury might indicate septic arthritis (gonococcal arthritis in adolescents). Self-limiting pain lasting a few days, especially with a preceding upper respiratory infection, is characteristic of transient synovitis. Snapping and clicking around the hip or groin might point toward intraarticular pathology or coxa saltans. Bursitis usually presents as a localized pain. A malignant process might manifest as a diffuse discomfort, with prolonged duration. Radiation of pain into the groin could be the result of disk herniation. Retroperitoneal pathologic processes have been reported to cause radiating pain at the hip and knee region. Any knee pain might indicate hip pathology.

SPECIAL TESTS

FABER or Patrick's: *F*lexion, *ab*duction, and *e*xternal *r*otation: pain of the sacroiliac joint.

Whitman: Flexion of the hip causes simultaneous external rotation: slipped capital femoral epiphysis.

Trendelenburg: Insufficiency of the gluteus medius/minimus muscles causing a drop of the contralateral pelvis while standing on the involved leg. It is caused by weakness due to paralysis, myelomeningocele, muscular dysplasia, or disc herniation; incorrect resting length due to hip dislocation, epiphyseal dysplasia (Fairbank), coxa vara, or slipped capital femoral epiphysis; and pain due to fracture, idiopathic chondrolysis, or AVN.

Duchenne: Lateral tilt of the trunk toward the involved side while testing the Trendelenburg. The causes are similar to Trendelenburg.

Thomas: Flexion of the nontested hip until the lumbar spine touches a hand placed under it. Flexion of the contralateral (tested) hip equals flexion contracture. It is also used to test for a labral tear: a snap with extension of the uninvolved hip.

Staheli: Prone over the edge of a table and extension of the involved hip: elevation of the pelvis equals flexion contraction.

Pace's sign: With the hip extended, forced internal rotation causes pain of the piriformis (piriformis syndrome).

Ober: In the side decubitus position, with the contralateral leg resting against the table, the tested leg is held abducted, with the knee flexed 90° and the hip slightly flexed. Holding the hip in abduction, the examiner extends the hip and then adducts the hip. With no iliotibial (ITB) contracture the leg could be adducted 20–30°.

SLIPPED CAPITAL FEMORAL EPIPHYSIS, HIP DYSPLASIA, & LEGG–CALVE–PERTHES DISEASE

General Considerations

The classic triad of hip problems includes slipped capital femoral epiphysis (SCFE), developmental hip dysplasia (DDH), and Legg–Calve–Perthes (LCP) disease. Age at presentation, symptoms, classification, differential diagnosis, treatment, and return to sport guidance are shown in Table 9–4.

Clinical Findings

The age of onset of DDH varies: an early diagnosis provides the best chance to end up with an essentially normal hip. Late discovered DDH carries a less favorable prognosis. DDH is not a very common cause of hip/groin pain in adolescent patients, but should be kept on the differential diagnosis list (Figure 9–7).

SCFE, a disease that manifests from the preteen age to maturity, requires urgent surgical stabilization. Bilateral involvement might be as high as 60–70%. Early onset, short body stature, and delayed bony age raise suspicion of underlying endocrinologic disorders such as hypothyroidism and renal osteodystrophy. It is possible to attain an almost normal looking hip joint as a result of early treatment of early discovered, mild SCFE. However, asymptomatic SCFEs are a common cause of arthritis, with 30% of "idiopathic arthritis" showing typical changes of preexisting slippage (Figure 9–8).

Table 9–4. Characteristics of DDH, SCFE, and LCP.[1]

	DDH	SCFE	LCP
	0–adulthood	*7–8 to 14–15 years old*	*4–8 years old*
Symptoms	Early: limited abduction, sonograph, X-ray Walking age: none or limp Late (teenage): pain, limp	Chronic or acute pain, groin or knee Limp Inability to bear weight External rotation of the leg Whitman Trendelenburg Slight shortening	Mild pain, discomfort Limp Decreased ROM Trendelenburg
Classification	Dysplasia Subluxation Dislocation	Stable/unstable Chronic/acute or acute on chronic Mild, moderate, severe	Lateral pillar (Herring) Types: A B C
Differential diagnosis	Usually radiographs are enough to establish diagnosis	Arthritis DDH Septic hip Labral pathology Neurogenic problems Malignancy Fracture Knee problems	Septic hip Transient synovitis Dysplasias Renal causes Thyroid related Trauma
Laboratory tests	Not necessary	Renal Endocrine Thyroid	None; if necessary renal, thyroid
Treatment	Age dependent	Urgent stabilization of the femoral head (usually single screw) Osteotomy for persistent deformity	Very controversial Benign neglect Petrie cast Femoral or pelvic osteotomy or combined
Complications	OA, pain	Persistent abnormal ROM AVN Reslip OA Chondrolysis Progressive slippage	OA Decreased ROM Slight shortening
Return to sport/ limitation	In cases treated early, with normal X-ray: no limits	Limited activities with no high impact activities until fusion of the physis	In active phases modification of activities Long term: avoid high-impact activities

[1] DDH, developmental dysplasia of the hip; SCFE, slipped capital femoral epiphysis; LCP, Legg–Calve–Perthes disease; ROM, range of motion; OA, osteoarthritis; AVN, avascular necrosis.

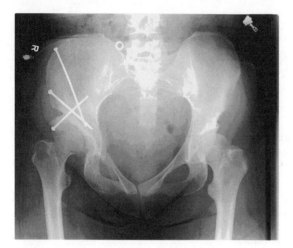

Figure 9–7. Nineteen-year-old female with a 2-year history of groin pain. Bilateral dysplasia of the hip. Extreme reorientation of the acatabulum using Ganz osteotomy has addressed the dysplasia of the right hip. The patient is awaiting a similar procedure to improve the coverage of the femoral head and or ientation of the acetabulum.

LCP is a disease of the femoral head, occurring as early as 2 years of age and up to 12 years of age. Current classification in based on Hering's work, with the denominator being a flattening of the lateral pillar as seen on anteroposterior (AP) radiographs:

- Type A: minimal.
- Type B: up to 50%.
- Type C: more then 50%.

Treatment

Nonoperative treatment has consisted of bracing, range of motion (ROM) exercises, casting, and prolonged non-weight bearing. Currently treatment includes modification of activity and sometimes a limited period of Petrie's cast for synovitis. Indications for surgical treatment vary. Children who are 8 years of age or older at the onset of LCP with type C and B/C hips might achieve a better outcome with surgical treatment. Patients younger than 8 years of age with type A and B hips do well regardless of the treatment. Patients with type C hips do poorly with or without treatment in all age groups. Girls have a poorer prognosis.

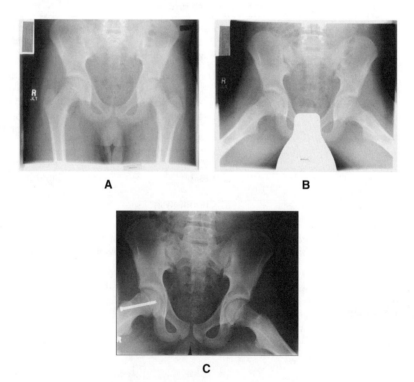

A

B

C

Figure 9–8. A 12-year-old male with 5 days history of right knee pain. ***A:*** Mild slipped capital femoral epiphysis of the right hip. ***B:*** Lateral radiograph shows the slipped capital femoral epiphysis (SCFE) much better then the anteroposterior view. ***C:*** SCFE treated with single screw fixation.

Rehabilitation & Return to Play

SCFE, DDH, and LCP influence the growth and anatomy of one of the most important joints in the lower extremities. A patient with early detected and successfully treated DDH will form a normal hip joint and should be allowed to participate in all activities. Patients with suboptimal results of DDH treatment and patients with LCP and SCFE should be advised to concentrate on low-impact activities. A significant percentage of theses patients will require total hip arthroplasty. Daily exercises, proper nutrition to maintain low body weight, diet, and selection of appropriate sports will be very important.

AVULSION FRACTURES

Pathogenesis

In growing individuals most avulsion fractures involve the muscles originating from the pelvis. The connection between the pelvis and the muscles usually occurs through an apophysis. Because this is commonly the weakest link of the working unit of bone, apophysis, tendon, and muscle, the fragment usually separates from the pelvis through the apophysis.

Clinical Findings

A. SYMPTOMS AND SIGNS

Symptoms include pain and limitation of active motion of the injured muscle, especially with resistance. The patient might not recall any sudden onset of pain, but many young athletes report a painful "pop" and shot of pain with sudden acceleration or deceleration. The most common avulsion fracture sites include the following:

- Anterior superior iliac spine (ASIS): origin of the sartorius.
- Anterior inferior iliac spine (AIIS): origin of the straight head of the rectus.
- Lesser trochanter: iliopsoas muscle.
- Ischial tuberosity: hamstrings.
- Posterior/superior brim of the acetabulum: origin of the reflected head of the rectus femoris.
- Greater trochanter: gluteus medius and minimus.

Imaging Studies

Radiographs are taken to recognize the displaced and unstable avulsion fractures. The majority of the avulsion fractures are stable and minimally displaced.

Differential Diagnosis

- Fractures, especially the hip/pelvis.
- Stress fractures.
- Any problem listed in Table 9–5 (groin pains).
- SCFE.

Treatment

In rare occasions a severely displaced and unstable fracture might need an open reduction with internal fixation (ORIF) of the avulsed fragment, but the majority of avulsion fractures will be minimally displaced and stable. Those fractures may require an initial short period of immobilization, with the RICE (rest, ice, compression, and elevation) protocol employed.

Rehabilitation & Return to Play

As soon as symptoms are under control and the fracture remains undisplaced, walking with touchdown weight bearing is permitted. Gentle, active assisted and passive

Table 9–5. Differential diagnosis of hip/pelvis problems.

Slipped capital femoral epiphysis
Legg–Calve–Perthes disease
Osteoarthritis
Septic arthritis
Transient synovitis
Gonococcal arthritis
Stress fractures
Overuse syndromes
Avulsion fractures
Lyme disease
Intraarticular pathology
Sacroiliac joint problems
Osteitis pubis
Snapping hip
Tumor
Pathologic fracture (through a cyst)
Osteoid osteoma
Osteomyelitis
Abdominal strain
Hernia
Radicular symptoms

ROM exercise will be the next step, and once the patient is able to walk without pain, active ROM with increasing resistance might begin. Stretching should follow. Because the total time required to recover from an avulsion fracture might easily exceed 3 months, the parents and the patient should be informed about the prolonged recovery time as soon as diagnosis is established.

SNAPPING HIP

Pathogenesis

Traditionally, the term "snapping hip" referred to symptoms of external and internal snapping hip. The traditional term, "internal snapping hip," is very imprecise, as the symptoms could be caused by many factors. This term should therefore be abandoned, given that hip arthroscopy and magnetic resonance imaging (MRI) arthrographs have broadened our knowledge of the intraarticular pathology. The entire spectrum of the "internal snapping hip" will be discussed in the section on groin pain. This section will focus on the "external snapping hip" (ESH).

Clinical Findings

A. CLASSIFICATION

- Classic coxa saltans: tight iliotibial band.
- Greater trochanteric bursitis.
- Fibrosis of the gluteus maximus muscle.

B. SYMPTOMS AND SIGNS

- Painful snapping.
- Pain at the greater trochanter.
- Sudden snap and jerk with internal/external rotation.
- Snap while getting up from squatting.
- Tightness of the ITB as detected by the Ober test.

ESH often results in a quite frustrating experience. The tight ITB snaps over the greater trochanter with a hard jerk, possibly interfering with physical activities or even with activities of daily life. Usually the patient will easily demonstrate the snapping. Symptoms occur in early teenage years and are more frequent among girls. Runners and cyclists suffer ESH very frequently.

C. IMAGING STUDIES

Diagnosis of ESH is made based on clinical symptoms, but radiographs help to rule out other causes of hip pain. In cases when differentiation from internal snapping is necessary, MRI, computed tomography (CT) scan, bone scan, or bursography should be considered.

Differential Diagnosis

Differential diagnosis includes internal snapping, alignment problems of the lower extremity, and referred pain from the lumbar region.

Treatment

A. NONSURGICAL

Patients with symptoms of the classic coxa saltans might benefit from an extended ITB stretching program. Initially, the mechanical hard snap, characteristic of coxa saltans, may be the only reason why patients seek medical attention. However, with prolonged symptoms, the bursa between the lateral aspect of the greater trochanter and ITB becomes inflamed, causing pain with snapping. In this phase oral nonsteroidal antiinflammatory drugs (NSAIDs) and injection of long-acting steroids directly into the bursa may help reduce inflammation.

In the rare occasions when snapping is caused be a fibrotic gluteus maximus, proper stretching of the muscle should help in controlling the pain.

B. SURGICAL

Surgical treatment of coxa saltans is occasionally necessary. Partial resection or Z-lengthening has been employed with overall good results. Surgery can be combined with stabilization of the ITB into the greater trochanter, using heavy stitches or suture anchors. Excision of the inflamed bursa is optional. Osteotomy of the greater trochanter or proximal femur has been tried; however, this should not be utilized as a primary surgical treatment. It might appear excessive to an adolescent patient to be placed in a half-spica cast, but some type of immobilization will increase the chance of eliminating the pain. A half-spica cast should be seriously considered for revision surgery, with a hip, knee, ankle, and foot orthosis (HKAFO) possibly serving the same purpose.

Return to Play

After surgery, with or without immobilization, the tissues will need time to heal. Stretching should begin 3–4 weeks later, but the return to sport requires restoration of muscle strength through physical therapy. Therapy should focus on strengthening the gluteus medius as well as other muscles around the hip joint.

Byrd JW, Jones KS: Hip arthroscopy in the presence of dysplasia. Arthroscopy 2003;19(10):1055.

Dobbs MB et al: Surgical correction of the snapping iliopsoas tendon in adolescents. J Bone Joint Surg Am 2002;84-A(3):420.

Herring JA et al: Legg-Calve-Perthes disease. Part II: Prospective multicenter study of the effect of treatment on outcome. J Bone Joint Surg Am 2004;86-A(10):2121.

Kuklo TR et al: Hip arthroscopy in Legg-Calve-Perthes disease. Arthroscopy 1999;15(1):88.

GROIN PAIN

Pathogenesis

Various extraarticular or intraarticular factors can trigger groin pain (Table 9–5). Pain related to intraarticular pathology might be caused by loose intraarticular bodies, a labral tear, a torn ligamentum teres, an osteochondral fracture, Perthes disease, an SCFE, hip dysplasia, AVN, septic arthritis, hemophiliac arthropathy, Lyme disease, or a rare pathology such as synovial chondromatosis (Figure 9–9). Extraarticular causes include stress fracture, overuse, osteoid osteoma, avulsion fracture, apophysitis, iliopectineal bursitis, iliopsoas strain, piriformis syndrome, hamstring syndrome, adductor strain, athletic pubalgia, osteitis or osteomyelitis of the os pubis, cysts such as an aneurismal bone cyst of the os pubis, ilioinguinal nerve entrapment, abdominal hernia, and abdominal muscle strain. Some of these pathologies might present as snapping hip, which usually accompanies the intraarticular problems or inflammation of the iliopsoas muscle or iliopectineal bursa. In the last case, hip snapping occurs when the hip moves from flexion and external rotation into extension and internal rotation. This maneuver helps to determine the source of groin pain.

Clinical Findings

A. SYMPTOMS AND SIGNS

The groin pain could be referred from the lumbar spine or retroperitoneal structures.

1. Labral tear injuries—

   a. Etiology—

- Traumatic.
- Degenerative.
- Idiopathic.
- Congenital.

   b. Morphology—

- Radial flap.
- Radial fibrillated.
- Longitudinal peripheral.
- Unstable.
- Bucket handle.

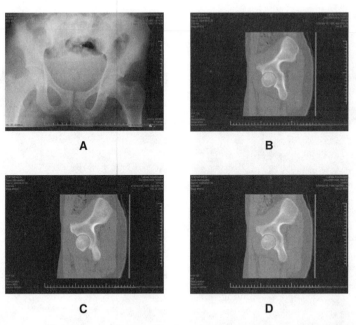

A   **B**

C   **D**

Figure 9–9. Seventeen-year-old male complaining of groin pain while walking. No history of trauma. ***A:*** Radiograph showing a lytic, round defect of the right femoral head. The lesion was removed. The defect was filled with a single-cylinder 10-mm osteochondral autograft, harvested from a non-weight-bearing part of the ipsilateral knee lateral femoral condyle, using the Osteochondral Autograft Transfer System (OATS) (Arthrex, Naples, FL). Pathology examination showed a chondroblastoma. ***B–D:*** One year after the lesion was removed. The follow-up CT scan shows very firm healing of the graft into the femoral head. There are no signs of recurrence of the tumor. The patient has been asymptomatic and has resumed full activity.

2. Ligamentum teres injuries—

- Complete rupture.
- Partial tear
- Degenerative tear

B. IMAGING STUDIES

Radiographs of both hips in two projections are mandatory. Special views such as Judett's, inlet, outlet, or false profile might be necessary for particular patients, depending on the working diagnosis. A bone scan might facilitate diagnosis of stress fractures, inflammation, or infection. An ultrasound of the hip joint might show an accumulation of fluid, but will not narrow down the differential diagnosis. When a fluid distends the hip joint, aspiration of the joint under an image intensifier can provide more specific information about the inflammatory process. A fine cut CT scan with possible three-dimensional reconstruction permits a better understanding of the geometry and morphology of the hip. The intraarticular loose body may show up better on CT images than on MRI because the time needed to generate CT images is shorter. A CT also shows the detailed anatomy of a dysplastic hip.

MRI and MRI arthrography have improved and widened the understanding of hip pathology, especially if caused by intraarticular factors. Detailed images of the labrum, ligamentum teres, transverse ligament, and cartilage are useful, and will also aid in the differential diagnosis of benign and malignant processes, infection, and stress fracture (Figure 9–10).

Differential Diagnosis

- Genitourinary problems.
- Thrombosis.
- Phlebitis.
- Femoral neuropathy.
- Endometriosis and other gynecologic issues.
- Pain related to previous hernia surgery.
- Pain referred from the lumbar region.

Treatment

The varieties of problems that manifest as groin pain deserve thorough analysis (Figure 9–11). The final diagnosis guides the treatment. Modification of activity, a strengthening program, physical therapy, changing the posture and biomechanics of the gait, changing

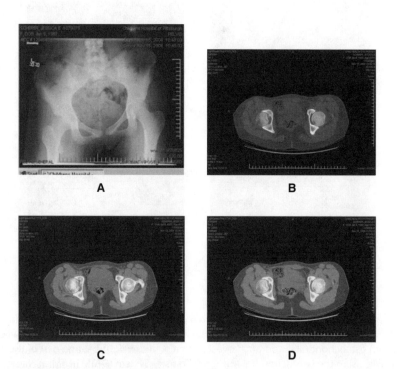

Figure 9–10. Sixteen-year-old female cross-country runner with right groin pain and no obvious trauma. **A:** Radiograph showing fuzzy, narrow joint space. **B–D:** A CT scan shows a type 3 tear of ligamentum teres. The patient underwent arthroscopic resection of the fragment.

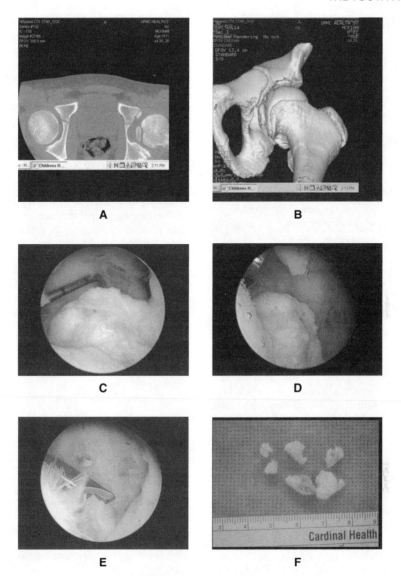

Figure 9–11. Hemophiliac arthropathy, left hip. *A, B:* A CT with three-dimensional reconstruction shows a semi-loose fragment of the femoral head. *C, D:* The fragment visualized during arthroscopy, measuring 2.5% 2.0 cm. *E:* The fragment is partially removed. *F:* Parts of the loose body.

sport-specific techniques, NSAIDs, ice, stretching and massage, or surgery will be employed depending on the diagnosis. Hip arthroscopy emerges as a valuable diagnostic and therapeutic tool. In the pediatric population, hip arthroscopy is an excellent technique to treat the loose intraarticular body, problems related to Legg–Calve–Perthes disease, hip dysplasia and SCFE, ligamentum teres injuries, labral tears, and other rare illnesses.

Rehabilitation & Return to Play

Advances in diagnosis and treatment have made return to sports possible for greater numbers of patients. A properly guided rehabilitation program of the young patient should result in full recovery. In the rare cases of severe Perthes disease, AVN, arthropathy, and rheumatoid diseases, long-lasting limitation may be advocated.

SEPTIC ARTHRITIS & TRANSIENT SYNOVITIS

General Considerations

There are two very common causes of an acute hip/groin pain, which commonly are very challenging to diagnose: septic arthritis and transient synovitis.

Clinical Findings

A. SYMPTOMS AND SIGNS

Septic arthritis and transient synovitis are completely unrelated, although both might manifest with refusal to walk or bear weight, pain of the groin, restricted ROM of the hip, limp, and joint effusion. Differentiating between these two syndromes is vital, because potential damage to hip cartilage and serious sequelae are very likely for untreated septic hip arthritis.

Treatment for septic arthritis and for transient synovitis is entirely different, and a decision about treatment must be made within a short period of time. Within the past 5 years three excellent papers have been published that help differentiate between benign, transient synovitis and the potentially dangerous septic arthritis. In the two studies by Kocher et al a history of fever, together with non-weight bearing, an erythrocyte sedimentation rate (ESR) higher then 40 mm, and a serum white blood cell (WBC) count higher then 12,000 cells/mm^3 all pointed clearly toward septic arthritis. The probability of having septic arthritis with all four predictors was 99.6%. However, in a study by Luhmann et al the probability was only 59% with all four predictors. They found that a history of fever, a WBC >12,000, and a previous health care visit yielded a 71% probability of septic arthritis.

B. IMAGING STUDIES

Radiographs are taken in two standard views. They might show distention of the joint or another reason for the hip pain. An MRI will help to distinguish between osteomyelitis, iliopsoas abscess, pathology of the sacroiliac (SI) point, or other soft tissue problems.

Differential Diagnosis

- Septic arthritis versus transient synovitis.
- Gonococcal arthritis.
- Iliopsoas abscess.
- Osteomyelitis of the pelvis.
- Avulsion fractures.
- Apophysitis.
- SI joint problems.

Treatment

Treatment is based on differentiation between septic arthritis and transient synovitis. Hip aspiration is mandatory in questionable cases. Unfortunately, because about 50% of culture from the fluid joint will be negative, even in the presence of a septic joint, the decision-making process will still depend on clinical symptoms and results of additional studies.

In cases in which the clinical level of suspicion for septic arthritis is high, a formal debridement of the hip joint will be necessary with 6 weeks of intravenous antibiotics. Transient synovitis does not need treatment.

Rehabilitation & Return to Play

In cases of transient synovitis patients will be able to return to sport as soon as the symptoms subside, with no limitations. Proper treatment of septic arthritis diagnosed within 72 hours of the onset of symptoms should yield excellent results with full recovery and return to full activity. In contrast, the results of neglected septic arthritis can be catastrophic. Total destruction of the femoral head, stiffness of the hip, chronic pain, limb length discrepancy, limping, and fast deterioration of the joint are the rule. These patients need either an osteotomy of the femur/pelvis with unpredictable results, fusion of the joint, or early arthroplasty.

Kocher MS et al: A clinical practice guideline for treatment of septic arthritis in children: efficacy in improving process of care and effect on outcome of septic arthritis of the hip. J Bone Joint Surg Am 2003;85-A(6):994.

Kocher MS, et al: Hip arthroscopy in children and adolescents. J Pediatr Orthop 2005;25(5):680.

Kocher MS et al: Validation of a clinical prediction rule for the differentiation between septic arthritis and transient synovitis of the hip in children. J Bone Joint Surg Am 2004;86-A(8):1629.

Luhmann SJ et al: Differentiation between septic arthritis and transient synovitis of the hip in children with clinical prediction algorithms. J Bone Joint Surg Am 2004;86-A(5):956.

Santori N, Villar RN: Acetabular labral tears: result of arthroscopic partial limbectomy. Arthroscopy 2000;16(1):11.

■ KNEE

Anatomy

The knee of a growing athlete is a changing complex driven by growth of the epiphyses, ligaments, muscles, and cartilage. The overall mechanics and function are similar to those of the adult knee; one of the major differences is the presence of growth plates. The distal femoral growth plate looks like two reversed, shallow parachutes, which span each femoral condyle, and connect at the center of the femur. The periphery is slightly more proximal then the "tips" of each parachute. The central "tip" creates the most distal point of the physis. The connection between the lateral and medial part of the growth plate occurs at the roof of the intercondylar notch, and extends through the entire width of the distal femur in the AP direction. The growth plate is about 2–3 mm thick. The ACL originates at the medial aspect of the lateral condyle epiphysis, with its origin adjacent to the physis of the lateral condyle, especially posteriorly.

The growth plate of the tibia more closely resembles a flat disk. It is neither concave nor convex. The center of this growth plate lies at the same level as its periphery. In younger individuals, the anterior part confluences into the growth plate, or apophysis, of the tibial tubercle. Later in skeletal maturity, the tibial growth plate creates a separated layer across the proximal tibia, as the tibial tubercle apophysis separates from it.

The ligaments, menisci, and articular cartilage of the condyles, tibial plateau, and patella are similar to those of the matured knee. In an immature knee the footplate of the ACL insertion is entirely within the articular aspect of the epiphysis. The connection with the tibia is via the epiphysis and physis of the upper tibia.

Clinical Findings

A. SYMPTOMS AND SIGNS

A detailed history is the most important element in the decision-making process. The history should include the circumstances of the injury, direction and magnitude of injury forces, position of the leg at the time of injury, and description of the offending factors. A history of noncontact injury is characteristic of the ACL tear, especially with a "pop" felt at the time of injury. A "pop" might also be associated with patella dislocation. Contact injury with a "pop" more likely points toward a meniscal injury, a collateral ligament tear, or a fracture rather than an ACL tear (Figure 9–12). ACL injury, meniscal tear, and osteochondral fracture typically present with an acute swelling. Locking and catching will be most common with a meniscal injury and a loose intraarticular body. A "giving way" sensation correlates with a ligamentous injury, including ACL, and with patellar instability; a grinding sensation from the knee points to patellofemoral pathology or loose body versus a meniscal injury.

Inspection allows assessment of the color, appearance, and defects of the skin, the amount and distribution of swelling, position of the knee (flexion contraction), fullness/puffiness of the joint line, effusion, appearance of the tibial tuberosity, atrophy of the quadriceps, position of the patella (alta, baja), and camelback sign of the skin (prominent fat pad with patella subluxation). The overall mechanical alignment of the lower extremity should be noted as well. During palpation, it is important to look for warmth of the skin, for grinding, especially from the patellofemoral joint, for the point of maximum tenderness, and for details of an effusion, if present. A dynamic examination will include testing of ROM, stability, and dynamic

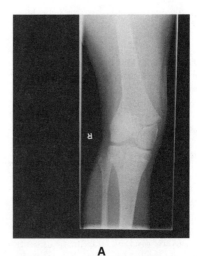

A

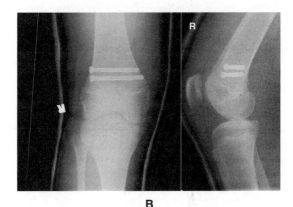

B

Figure 9–12. Fifteen-year-old soccer player, after being tackled down, with acute onset of right knee pain. ***A:*** Salter 2 fracture of the distal femur. ***B:*** The fracture is anatomically reduced and secured with two titanium 7.3-mm screws. Titanium screws will allow an MRI of the knee to be obtained to assess for possible ligamentous injury to the joint.

anatomy of the knee as well as an evaluation of quadriceps and hamstrings strength. ROM of the knee should be unrestricted and there should be no catching or locking. Patella tracking should be undistorted and the Q angle should be less than 10. The J sign is positive when the patella subluxes laterally with the knee approaching its full extension. The apprehension test indicates patellar tracking problems as well as possible previous patella dislocation. The patella relocation test is similar to the relocation test for a shoulder: with a positive apprehension test the patient feels much more comfortable when direct pressure is exerted to stabilize the patella within the femoral groove. Pain of the middle facet of the patella as well as pain over the medial retinaculum and crepitation are closely associated with dislocation of the patella. Other causes of knee pain and locking are medial plica and displaced meniscal tear. Clinical symptoms of medial plica consist of a hard snapping usually over the medial condyle. The plica might be palpated over the medial condyle as a fold of fibrous tissue, and while inflamed and irritated, might cause pain with direct pressure over it. The majority of plicas are clinically silent.

B. IMAGING STUDIES

After the clinical part of the examination is completed, four radiographs of the knee should be obtained. The AP, lateral, Merchant, and tunnel views are the most critical radiographs in the adolescent population. They may show pathognomonic findings, making proper diagnosis easy or obvious (fractures, dislocation of the patella, tumor, osteochondroma) (Figure 9–13). A bone scan, CT scan, or MRI will help to further narrow down the diagnosis.

C. SPECIAL TESTS

Direct palpation of the patella and femoral condyles or the Wilson test can be used when testing for cartilage injuries. The Wilson test indicates a typical osteochondritis dissecans (OCD) of the medial part of the lateral condyle. For this test the knee is internally rotated, flexed, and extended. With internal rotation the tibial spine engages into the OCD defect thus creating pain. External rotation relieves the pain. A positive Wilson test in 30° of flexion, resulting in pain, is highly correlated with an OCD. Direct palpation of femoral condyles localizes a cartilage defect, as the patella does not cover a significant portion of the femoral condyles.

Meticulous palpation shows very precisely the location of an OCD or osteochondral fracture (OCF). Pain with direct palpation may be positive in the presence of a cartilage/bone bruise as well. Anterior knee pain with active hyperextension and direct pressure at the patella signifies the possibility of patellofemoral arthritis or osteochondral changes, whereas tenderness of the distal pole of the patella is characteristic of Sinding–Larsen–Johansson syndrome. Pain at the midsubstance of the patellar ligament might indicate a jumper's knee. Pain and enlargement of the tibial tuberosity is are pathognomonic for Osgood–Schlatter disease.

The McMurray test and Apley test are commonly used to assess a knee for potential meniscal problems. The McMurray test involves extending the knee from full flexion while rotating the foot internally or externally. The Apley test (grinding test) requires a prone position. The knee is flexed 90° and the tibia is compressed against the femur. The tibia is rotated externally and then internally. Pain with both tests as well as joint line tenderness indicate meniscal pathology.

To test medial collateral ligament (MCL) and lateral collateral ligament (LCL) instability the examiner should exert valgus/varus stress forces on a knee that is flexed 30°. Laxity might indicate an MCL or LCL tear or physeal fracture. A positive valgus/varus test in full extension is indicative of a cruciate ligament or growth plate injury.

The anterior drawer, Lachman, and posterior drawer tests check the stability of the knee in the sagittal plane. The anterior drawer and Lachman tests can be graded from 0 to 3, with either a soft or solid end point. Comparison with the contralateral side improves the precision of the examination, especially while testing patients

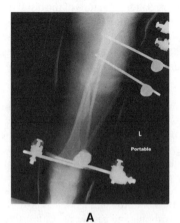

A

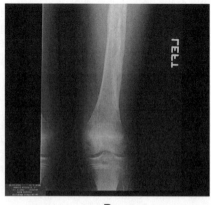

B

Figure 9–13. A 9–year-old female with a severely comminuted femoral shaft fracture as a result of a skiing accident. The fracture could not be treated with a flexible intramedullary nail because of comminution. **A:** The fracture is stabilized by a complex External Fixateur and temporary half-spica cast **B:** Full recovery after 8 months.

with generalized laxity. Pivot shift starts with the knee held in internal rotation and flexed: as the knee straightens into full extension, the tibia subluxates anteriorly; with flexion, the tibia reduces with an audible clunk.

Sagittal, valgus/varus instability and laxity while testing for a posterolateral corner might be observed in patients with Down, Marfan, or Morquio syndromes, osteogenesis imperfecta type 1, and pseudochondrodysplasia. Various symptoms, relatively common in syndromic patients, might be related to the underlying disease rather than to orthopedic problems. For example, anterior knee pain is very common in congenital patella dislocation and nail-patella syndrome (hypoplasia/splitting of the nail, hypoplasia or an absent patella with a hypoplastic lateral condyle and hypoplastic fibular head, iliac spurs, flexion contracture of the elbow with a small capitellum and radial head). Patients with Marfan syndrome show increased laxity as well. Knee hyperextension with laxity and patella and hip dislocation are common in trisomy 21. Diminished ROM with "dimpling" and occasional striae in arthrogryposis are pathognomonic features of the disease. Sometimes, fixed hyperextension of the knee is visible in spina bifida patients and congenital dislocation of the knee. Genu valgum is common in Morquio and Ellis van Creveld syndrome. Rickets usually results in genu varum; however genu valgum could also be seen in this condition.

Faraj AA et al: Arthroscopic findings in the knees of preadolescent children: report of 23 cases. Arthroscopy 2000;16(8):793.

Post WR: Clinical evaluation of patients with patellofemoral disorders. Arthroscopy 1999;15(8):841.

ANTERIOR CRUCIATE LIGAMENT TEAR

Skeletally immature athletes are experiencing more ACL injuries than ever before. The injury is occurring in an increasingly larger number of very young children, with the average age of occurrence declining. The majority of these injuries (about 70%) are the result of a noncontact activity. Usually, the injured knee is close to full extension just prior to a sudden change of direction, during sudden deceleration, or at the time of landing. At the moment of injury, the athlete's center of gravity is low and behind the knee, and the foot is planted flat or in pronation. The contact mode of ACL injuries usually involves flexion and valgus-producing impact. Sports in which there is a high risk of incurring an ACL injury are football, soccer, basketball, volleyball, lacrosse, and skiing.

Prevention

Guided prevention may help to lower the prevalence of ACL injuries. Because the injury is now more common, athletic trainers and coaches should offer specifically designed ACL prevention programs to all students involved in competitive sports. The University of Pittsburgh Sport Medicine Center Program is an excellent example of an ACL prevention curriculum. A significant reduction in ACL injuries could be achieved, especially among girls. Specifically designed training can help to improve reaction time, muscle preparedness, muscle mobilization, proprioception, and general conditioning. It will also teach proper sport-specific techniques. The program should include weight lifting, proprioception, and plyometric and balance training. The Internet offers a good source of information on this topic. Sites such as www.girlscanjump.com provide an excellent overview and links to other pages related to ACL prevention problems.

Clinical Findings

A. Symptoms and Signs

- Sudden "pop."
- Effusion.
- History of giving way.
- Anterior drawer.
- Lachman test.
- Finacetto: severe subluxation of the tibia.
- Anterior drawer with external or internal rotation of the foot.
- Restricted ROM with an impinging tear.
- Pivot shift.
- Pivot jerk.

The last two tests should be performed with the patient under anesthesia as they can result in significant discomfort.

Clinical symptoms of an ACL tear in the pediatric population seem to be identical to those in adults. A typical mechanism of injury, subsequent swelling and effusion, and a subjective sensation of instability are the hallmarks of this injury. With a chronic injury, patients frequently report the knee giving way and collapsing. Pain is not a part of an ACL injury; however, very often it is reported as one of the symptoms. This could be related to a meniscal tear or a bony bruise of the lateral compartment. Pain can also indicate a growth plate injury of the distal femur and proximal tibia. Careful palpation and radiographic assessment help to establish the proper diagnosis. Stress radiographs may be necessary as well.

B. Imaging Studies

- Radiographs: mainly to rule out skeletal injuries.
- MRI: the gold standard for an ACL tear; the classification system is similar to adults (Figure 9–14).

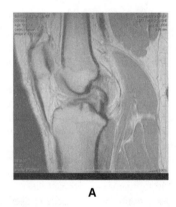

A

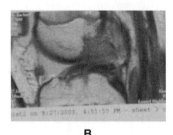

B

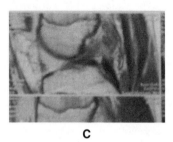

C

Figure 9–14. A: A 14-year-old female basketball player with an anterior cruciate ligament (ACL) tear. *B, C:* An 8-year-old male with a torn ACL.

Differential Diagnosis

- Physeal fracture.
- Tibial spine fracture.
- Meniscal injury.
- Tear of other ligaments.
- Osteochondral injury.
- Patella dislocation.

Treatment

Several options are available when caring for an immature athlete. The first is to reconstruct the ACL surgically as described for the adult athlete with an ACL rupture (see Chapter 3, this volume) or to use physeal sparing techniques. The second option is to wait until the child reaches skeletal maturity and then reconstruct the ACL. The next option is to allow the child to play sports after a decision has been made as to whether to brace or not to brace the knee, hoping to protect it from further damage. The last option is to allow some activities while limiting others.

A. NONOPERATIVE

Nonoperative treatments with bracing, a proprioception program, and strengthening exercises do not prevent a child from incurring subsequent, additional injuries. Braces do not guard against additional trauma. Unlimited activity, with or without a brace, will increase the risk for further injuries and should be discouraged. Sports such as rowing, light weight training, bicycling, or running on an elliptical training track carry a relatively low risk for additional injuries. Swimming is safe as well, except for the breaststroke.

B. OPERATIVE

Theoretically, all children with an ACL injury not willing to change their level of activity should have the ACL reconstructed. On the other hand, results of ACL reconstruction in skeletally immature children are still not as good as in the adult population, and the failure rate and subsequent revision rate are higher.

The consensus now is to either reconstruct the ACL or to limit activity, eliminating all possible movements that may increase the risk of added injury to the ACL-deficient knee. If a family wants a child to continue playing sports requiring cutting, pivoting, changing direction, twisting, and a stop-and-go type of activity, it is advisable to have the torn ACL reconstructed. Prior to the surgery, a thorough discussion with the family about the pros and cons of the procedure is mandatory.

In addition to the usual surgical risks, reconstructing a torn ACL in a skeletally immature patient increases the possibility of growth disturbances such as shortening or angulation, failure of the graft, and persistent symptoms if a nonisometric reconstruction is performed.

C. THE GROWTH PLATE

The development of problems following reconstruction of an ACL in a skeletally immature athlete is related to factors such as drilling tunnels across the growth plate, choices of graft, method of fixation, tension across the growth plate, and placement of the tunnels through the periphery or center of the growth plate. Just drilling a tunnel across a growth plate might itself result in growth arrest and physeal bridge formation. In an experimental study drilling a hole through a physis up to 10% of the growth plate diameter seems to be safe. Reaming the tunnel through a periphery of the growth plate carries a higher risk for physeal bony bridge formation than reaming it through the center part of the physis. Therefore the risk of significant growth problems caused by the femoral tunnel is greater than the risk caused by the tibial tunnel. Passing a soft tissue graft is safer than crossing a growth plate with a bony block. Adding an interference screw across a physis may result in growth arrest. Even tensioning a graft passed just adjacent to the periphery of a growth plate might slow down the growth of the physis. In one study a tensioned graft placed outside a physis caused an angular deformity of the extremity, without physeal bone bridge formation. Another study reported on genu valgum formation with over-the-top passage of the graft and extraphyseal graft placement. All the potential problems should be discussed with the patients and the family prior to the surgery.

Once the decision to go ahead with surgery is made, the type of ACL reconstruction should be carefully selected to diminish the risks of graft failure and growth problems. The graft should be placed in a biomechanically optimal position. Any given procedure should be individually tailored to each child or adolescent to minimize the risks and provide the patient with the best possible reconstruction of the ACL. Biological age, maturity, and growth plate function are the most important factors to consider. Each child develops at an individual pace. To determine a particular child's stage of development, it is necessary to consider age, gender, height, Tanner stage, onset of menarche, height of parents and older siblings, bony age, late versus early boomers in the family, and general distribution of height in the family (Table 9–6). Wide-open physes signify that considerable growth remains. The appearance of the proximal tibial and distal femoral physes is very important. The morphology of the proximal tibial physis is quite unique and the shape of the physis provides additional information about the maturity process. Initially, the physis blends with the tibial tuberosity growth plate, smoothly sloping anteriorly and distally. As a child matures, the proximal tibial physis becomes more horizontal and separates from the tibial tubercle. The tibial tubercle growth plate separates from the main proximal tibial growth plate usually 1–2 years prior to skeletal maturity, and fuses earlier than the tibial growth plate.

Table 9–6. Tanner's staging for boys and girls.

Stage for Girls	Pubic Hair	Breast	
1	None	Preadolescent	
2	Scarce, light, straight	Elevated by small amount	
3	More hair, darker, starting to curl	Breast and areola bigger	
4	Coarse, curly, still less than the adult	Areola, papilla form secondary mound	
5	Adult triangle, spreads to thighs	Mature. Nipple projects, areola part of breast contour	
Stage for Boys	**Pubic Hair**	**Penis**	**Testes**
1	None	Preadolescent	Preadolescent
2	Scanty, long, light	Slight enlargement	Larger, pink, texture changed
3	Darker, curling	Longer	Larger
4	Adult type but less	Glans and breath increase	Larger, scrotum dark
5	Adult, spread to thighs	Adult size	Adult size

Adapted, with permission, from Tanner JM: *Growth at Adolescence,* 2nd ed. Blackwell Scientific Publications, 1962.

The magnitude of potential permanent growth problems associated with an ACL reconstruction is proportional to the growth remaining. Generally 1–2 cm of remaining growth should not pose a danger of creating a significant deformity. The Green and Anderson graft, the Moseley straight-line graph method, or the Multiplier Method by Paley and colleagues will help calculate the exact remaining growth of each individual patient. In a clinical setting, the most practical way to predict the remaining growth is the method of Menelaus and Westh. It is based on a few facts:

- The proximal tibia grows 6 mm/year.
- The distal femur grows 10 mm/year.
- Girls stop growing at age 14 years.
- Boys stop growing at age 16 years.

For example, an average 13-year-old boy will grow about 3 cm from the distal femur and 1.8 cm from the proximal tibia.

D. Tunnel Placement

The adult, transphyseal type of ACL reconstruction requires drilling of tunnels across the distal femoral and proximal tibial metaphysis and physis. This method can be used in older adolescents, but in individuals with significant growth remaining, this type of reconstruction poses a high risk of injury to the growth plates. The graft should not interfere with the development of the physis. Extraarticular reconstruction, extraphyseal methods, or total or partial transepiphyseal graft placement all offer "physis-friendly" routes for the graft.

Extraarticular methods have been largely abandoned, as they do not allow isometric placement of the ACL graft. In addition, the extraarticular positioning of the graft can still result in growth disturbances without the benefit of isometric reconstruction. Extraphyseal and partial or total transepiphyseal methods of reconstruction offer better biomechanics and appear to be safe for the growing extremity. In Tanner's stage 1 and 2, with significant growth remaining and a high risk for shortening of the limb or/and an angular deformity, extraphyseal or transepiphyseal reconstructions seem to lower the risk (Figure 9–15). During extraphyseal ACL reconstruction, a graft is passed into the joint usually through a shallow groove under the intermeniscal ligament and is then stabilized in an over-the-top position at the femoral side. This method is relatively safe but is not entirely isometric, and the position of the graft is not very secure, especially over the brim of the tibia.

A total transepiphyseal reconstruction requires drilling the tibial tunnel within the tibial tubercle epiphysis and through the epiphysis of the lateral femoral condyle (Figure 9–16). This is currently the method of choice if both the distal femoral and proximal tibial growth plates are wide open and there is significant

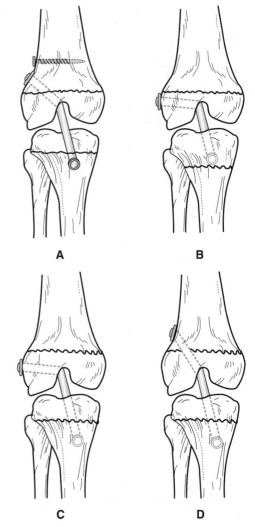

Figure 9–15. Different types of anterior cruciate ligament reconstruction. *A:* Extraphyseal. *B:* Transepiphyseal. *C:* Partial transepiphyseal. *D:* Transphyseal.

growth remaining. This method is technically very demanding. The tunnels should be drilled under the guidance of an image intensifier. The femoral tunnel starts laterally at the center of the lateral condyle and exits as close to the ten thirty or eleven o'clock position for the right knee and one to one thirty position for the left knee. The tunnel must enter the joint just distal to the femoral physis. The tibial tunnel starts between the joint line and the distal extension of the growth plate of the tibial tubercle. It exits about 5 mm at the front of the anterior margin of the posterior cruciate ligament (PCL). The size of the tunnel may limit the diameter of

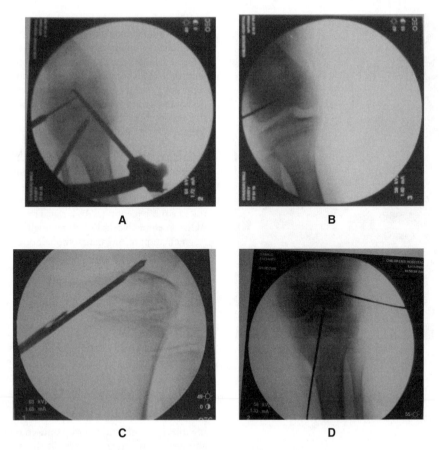

A   B

C   D

Figure 9–16. Intraoperative, image intensifier radiographs, showing the position of the transepiphyseal tunnels. **A:** The guide pin is positioned using the Femoral Retrograde Marking Hook (Arthrex, Naples, FL). **B:** Position of the femoral guide pin. **C:** Tibial guide pin traversing the apophysis of the tibia. **D:** Anteroposterior radiographs showing both guide pins in place. The pins avoid violating the growth plates.

the graft, since the tibial tubercle epiphysis is quite narrow and thin. Especially in younger children, drilling a tunnel larger then 6–7 mm might violate the growth plate of the tubercle, thus increasing the risk for genu recurvatum. On the femoral side, the epiphysis can accommodate essentially any tunnel, even up to 12 mm. The transepiphyseal technique places the graft into an isometric position. The reconstructed knee regains excellent stability, and safety appears to be satisfactory based on early results. There have been no reports of growth problems using this method, but the lack of long-term studies is a potential drawback.

In older adolescents, with still open growth plates and 1–2 cm of remaining growth, the partial transepiphyseal method may be an excellent option. In this method the tibial tunnel is placed transphyseally. Because the tibial tunnel is more vertical and goes through the center of the physis, the transphyseal tibial

tunnel carries less risk for the development of significant growth disturbances. Proximally, the graft is routed either over the top or using the transepiphyseal method.

For girls 14 years and older and boys 16 years and older, in Tanner's stage 4, with minimal growth remaining, it is generally safe to proceed with the transphyseal type of reconstruction. The surgeon, however, should be aware of the skeletal maturity of the patient, family history, Tanner's staging, and height patterns in the family. This will help in the decision-making process.

E. GRAFTS AND FIXATION

Currently, most of the transepiphyseal, extraphyseal, and partial transepiphyseal reconstructions of the ACL in growing patients are accomplished using soft tissue grafts (Figure 9–17). Most surgeons performing ACL reconstruction in skeletally immature patients use hamstring autografts. Double or quadruple grafts have been

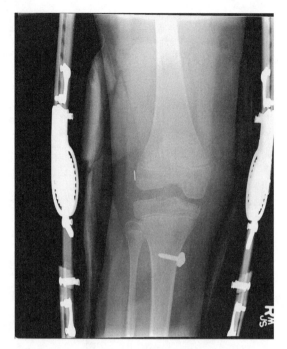

Figure 9–17. An 8-year-old female soccer player. Reconstruction of the torn anterior cruciate ligament using hamstring autografts. Proximal fixation is achieved using a Drummond button. Distal over-the-post fixation with a large fragment AO screw.

used, and the hamstrings are usually used as a free graft. However, for an extraphyseal repair, the distal attachment of the hamstrings to the tibia can be left intact, and the free proximal end of the tendon rerouted into the joint. In younger children, however, the tendinous portion of the hamstrings might be quite tenuous. In this situation other sources of grafts may need to be considered. The bone patella tendon bone grafts can be used safely only if the bone plugs do not contact the growth plate. The routine, adult-type placement of the bony plugs will result in a premature closure of the physis. In the skeletally immature patient the tibial plug is usually partially cartilaginous, thus potentially leading to poor fixation.

ITB autografts can also be considered and used safely. In cases of insufficient quality of an autograft, to diminish graft-related morbidity, or if cosmetics is an important issue, posterior or anterior tibial tendon allografts or Achilles tendon allografts might be considered. Fixation devices should not violate the growth plates. Femoral fixation can be accomplished by a staple over the post, by a transfixion pin, or by using EndoButton with or without a washer. Intraarticular staples for ACL graft fixation have not been recommended.

The tibial end of the graft can be secured over the post or over a staple(s) or can be sown into the periosteum, or the distal attachment of the hamstrings to the tibia can be preserved. Interference screws, routinely employed for both tunnels in adults, can be used safely in older adolescents for fixation of the tibial end of the graft when a partial transepiphyseal method is chosen. Except for one case report there are no reports to date about using interference screws for femoral fixation in growing children.

F. Partial Anterior Cruciate Ligament Tear

A partially torn ACL can be left alone, with the nonreconstructive approach being suitable, if the knee is stable. However, the family should be informed that there is a 30% risk of a subsequent total ACL tear. The torn portion of the ACL sometimes blocks ROM and might need to be excised. Augmentation of AM (anteromedial) or PL (posterolateral) bundle might be considered.

Rehabilitation & Return to Play

After ACL surgery the patient undergoes 5–9 months of rehabilitation. A specially designed postoperative protocol should facilitate the communication with a physical therapist. Generally, during the first days, the patient is allowed to perform heel slides, straight leg rises, and isometric exercises of the quadriceps muscles. Weight bearing can start as soon as tolerated by the patient. With a simultaneous meniscal repair, non-weight bearing is recommended for about 6 weeks. Cutting, pivoting, changing direction, and sudden stop-and-go movements begin about 4 months after surgery. At this time the physical therapist can start sport-specific exercises. After successful treatment the patient is usually released to full activity within 5–9 months. To date, except for the generally accepted belief in a higher failure rate after ACL reconstruction, the exact rate of reinjury among skeletally immature patients is not known.

Meniscal injuries discovered during surgery should be treated concurrently. They will be discussed later in this chapter.

FRACTURE OF THE TIBIAL SPINE/EMINENCE

Pathogenesis

The same forces that cause an ACL tear might result in a tibial spine/eminence fracture; the pain, however, is usually more pronounced. This fracture extends through the epiphysis of the proximal tibia. A large part of the tibial plateau is avulsed from the tibia and might be elevated, displaced, or comminuted. Very often it does extend into the physis. A large, sanguinous effusion with fatty droplets is typical of this fracture.

The tibial eminence fracture is a typical avulsion fracture. The ACL is prestretched before avulsing the tibial spine. For this reason even an anatomically reduced fracture might result in persistent laxity of the knee. This, however, does not seem to cause significant problems.

Clinicial Findings

A.SYMPTOMS AND SIGNS

- Pain.
- Inability to bear weight.
- Effusion.
- Laxity.
- ACL-specific tests are positive.

B. CLASSIFICATION

- Type 1: nondisplaced.
- Type 2: hinged, open trap door.
- Type 3A: displaced.
- Type 3B: comminuted or rotated.

C. IMAGING STUDIES

Lateral and AP radiographs are essential in recognizing the fracture and its displacement (Figure 9–18). They also help in monitoring the position of the eminence following a closed reduction by hyperextension. In cases of irreducible, displaced tibial spine fractures additional studies such as CT scan and MRI might be necessary. In cases of displaced or comminuted fractures, the exact extent of the injury is appreciated only during arthroscopy.

Differential Diagnosis

This is the same as for an ACL injury.

Complications

Late laxity is very common following tibial eminence fractures but rarely causes clinical problems. Abnormal function of the growth plate is rare. Sometimes it takes a long time to recover full ROM, and the patient may require a prolonged course of physical therapy.

Treatment

A cylinder cast applied in hyperextension can reduce and stabilize a tibial spine fracture. If the radiographs show a satisfactory position of the avulsed fragment, the cast is kept on for 6–8 weeks. An arthroscopically assisted reduction and internal fixation are a better option for nonreducible type 2 and type 3 fractures. Visualization can be difficult secondary to a large hematoma in the joint. Additional problems may arise: comminution of the fragment, entrapment of the medial or lateral meniscus with or without a tear, and abutment of the avulsed fragment against the intermeniscal ligament, which might render the accurate reduction of the fragment quite difficult. Fixation accomplished by a metal or bioabsorbable screw will be most appropriate for a solid one-piece fragment.

Heavy stitch, lasso stitch, and wires are a good option for a noncomminuted fracture as well. Fixation of a comminuted fracture is done by weaving a heavy stitch or wire through the distal end of the ACL and through the footprint of the ACL. A lasso technique might be used as well. The stitches or wires used for fixation are passed through very small tunnels in the tibia, and secured over a bony bridge between the tunnels.

Whether a nonoperative or surgical treatment was chosen, a period of non-weight bearing for 6 weeks is

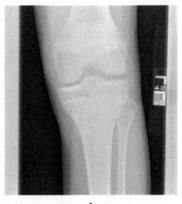

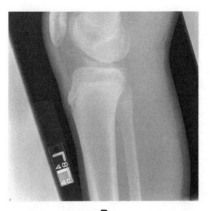

A   **B**

Figure 9–18. Type 3 tibial spine fracture of a 14-year-old basketball player. ***A:*** The anteroposterior view: this view certainly underestimates the amount of displacement. ***B:*** Lateral radiograph showing the exact displacement of the tibial eminence.

mandatory. The cast is then removed and the leg protected in a long, postoperative, hinged knee brace. The brace should permit a gradual increase of the ROM of the knee. A drop lock will lock the brace in full extension for walking and overnight.

Rehabilitation & Return to Play

As soon as the brace is applied, the patient can start gentle exercises of the quadriceps and hamstrings. ROM should be increased gradually, for example, 10–15° every 5 days. Weight bearing increases gradually as well. Before discharge from the office, the patient must demonstrate full strength of the hamstrings and quadriceps, as well as full ROM. Total recovery usually takes 3–4 months.

Anderson AF: Transepiphyseal replacement of the anterior cruciate ligament in skeletally immature patients. A preliminary report. J Bone Joint Surg Am 2003;85-A(7):1255.

Anderson AF: Transepiphyseal replacement of the anterior cruciate ligament using quadruple hamstring grafts in skeletally immature patients. J Bone Joint Surg Am 2004;86-A(suppl 1, pt 2):201.

Andrish JT: Anterior cruciate ligament injuries in the skeletally immature patient. Am J Orthop 2001;30(2):103.

Barber FA: Anterior cruciate ligament reconstruction in the skeletally immature high-performance athlete: what to do and when to do it? Arthroscopy 2000;16(4):391.

Edwards TB et al: The effect of placing a tensioned graft across open growth plates. A gross and histologic analysis. J Bone Joint Surg Am 2001;83-A(5):725.

Fuchs R et al: Intra-articular anterior cruciate ligament reconstruction using patellar tendon allograft in the skeletally immature patient. Arthroscopy 2002;18(8):824.

Guzzanti V et al: Physeal-sparing intraarticular anterior cruciate ligament reconstruction in preadolescents. Am J Sports Med 2003;31(6):949.

Johnson DH: Complex issues in anterior cruciate ligament surgery: open physes, graft selection, and revision surgery. Arthroscopy 2002;18(9 suppl 2):26.

Kocher MS et al: Management and complications of anterior cruciate ligament injuries in skeletally immature patients: survey of the Herodicus Society and The ACL Study Group. J Pediatr Orthop 2002;22(4):452.

Kocher MS, et al: Physeal sparing reconstruction of the anterior cruciate ligament in skeletally immature prepubescent children and adolescents. J Bone Joint Surg Am 2005;87(11):2371.

Millett PJ et al: Associated injuries in pediatric and adolescent anterior cruciate ligament tears: does a delay in treatment increase the risk of meniscal tear? Arthroscopy 2002;18(9):955.

Senekovic V, Veselko M: Anterograde arthroscopic fixation of avulsion fractures of the tibial eminence with a cannulated screw: five-year results. Arthroscopy 2003;19(1):54.

MENISCAL INJURIES

Pathogenesis

The crescent-shaped fibrocartilaginous menisci transform forces between femoral condyles and the tibial plateau. The medial meniscus is more C-shaped; the lateral one is more rounded and more mobile. In the pediatric population the proportion of menisci to knee is essentially the same as in the adult population. The blood supply comes from the periphery, and in early childhood as much as 60% of the peripheral meniscus is supplied by the arteries. This proportion changes as a child grows, and ultimately only the peripheral 30% of the menisci receives a blood supply. The menisci, especially the medial meniscus, serve as a secondary restraint to anterior translation of the tibia. The majority of meniscal tears result from an indirect, twisting injury of the knee with simultaneous flexion. Sometimes the patient recalls a "snap" or "pop," and a sudden onset of pain. Usually there is a well-defined moment of trauma. Pain after injury and swelling with effusion are typical, and the patient may experience difficulties with weight bearing.

Clinical Findings

A. Symptoms and Signs

- Effusion.
- Swelling.
- Decreased ROM.
- Lack of full extension.
- Hard block of motion with a displaced meniscal tear.
- Joint line tenderness.
- McMurray: the knee is passively extended from a fully flexed position with external and internal rotation.
- Apley (grinding): prone, 90° of flexion, compression against the femur with internal and external rotation.
- Quadriceps atrophy with chronic injury.

A diagnosis of a meniscal injury in the pediatric population can be difficult for several reasons: the classic McMurray and Apley test results commonly might not be present, and an examination in an acute setting could be quite unreliable. Joint line tenderness and pain seem to be the most common clinical symptoms in this age group. The tenderness is more sensitive and specific for a lateral meniscus injury and less so for a medial meniscus injury.

Meniscal tears in adolescent patients usually result from abnormal forces applied to normal meniscal tissue; in other words, the degenerative tears, very common among adults, are quite rare. Very commonly, the meniscal tears in this age group occur at the periphery of the meniscus. The classification of meniscal injuries is described in Chapter 3 of this volume (Figure 9–19).

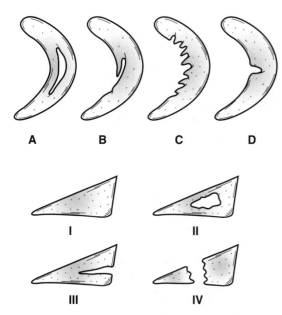

Figure 9–19. ***A–D:*** Types of meniscal tears. ***I–IV:*** MRI classification of meniscal images.

B. Imaging Studies

Radiographs in four views help establish a diagnosis of simultaneous bony injuries. The MRI has become the gold standard in the evaluation of the menisci, PCL, medial collateral ligament (MCL), lateral collateral ligament (LCL), and ACL, with an accuracy in assessing meniscal injuries among adults close to 95%. In the pediatric population, however, MRI is not as accurate.

A meniscal tear can be divided into four grades, with only type III pathognomonic for a tear. Typically, a type III injury is seen as a high signal density across the entire meniscus. In the pediatric population the MRI is commonly overread, and interpretation of type I and II tears might be very difficult. The different blood supply in the pediatric population is one of the sources of mistakes. Because the positive and negative predictive values are lower for the pediatric population than for adults, the MRI reading should be used exclusively as an additional study. The final diagnosis should be based on a detailed history, a physical examination, and additional tests, not exclusively on MRI images.

Differential Diagnosis

- Patella dislocation.
- Intraarticular loose body.
- Osteochondral fracture.
- Osteochondrosis dissecans.
- Ligament or capsular strain.
- Unusual pathology (pigmented villonodular synovitis, osteochondroma, foreign body).

Treatment

A patient going into the operating room usually carries an established diagnosis. Sometimes, however, even after an extensive work-up, arthroscopy is the only way to confirm the diagnosis. This is particularly true in the pediatric or adolescent population. In this age group, the probability of finding some unexpected injuries, or not finding the expected damage, is significant.

In cases in which a diagnosis of a meniscal tear is established, a surgeon can leave the tear alone, repair it, or remove part of or the whole meniscus. In young patients a majority of meniscal injuries are reparable, and preservation is the key. Debridement of the meniscus might be necessary in some cases, but even then, it should be very conservative. Treatment of meniscal injuries is described in Chapter 3 of this volume. In no patient is it more important, if possible, to save or repair the meniscus than in the pediatric athlete.

Rehabilitation & Return to Play

After meniscal repair the patient is not allowed to bear weight for about 6 weeks. ROM can be started as soon as the patient's pain is under control. Formal physical therapy typically starts 2–3 weeks after surgery and includes active, passive, and active assisted ROM and strengthening exercises. Patients return to full activities 3 months after surgery

Bloome DM et al: Meniscal repair in very young children. Arthroscopy 2000;16(5):545.

Klimkiewicz JJ, Shaffer B: Meniscal surgery 2002 update: indications and techniques for resection, repair, regeneration, and replacement. Arthroscopy 2002;18(9 Suppl 2):14.

DISCOID MENISCUS

Pathogenesis

A majority of discoid menisci (DM) occur in the lateral compartment. The prevalence among Asians is much higher (up to 17%) than in whites (5%).

The lateral DM have been divided into three types: complete, incomplete, and the Wrisberg type. A complete DM obliterates the entire lateral compartment of the knee. It is thicker than the normal meniscus, which could be up to 14 mm thick. The middle zone of the meniscus is the thickest one, and the peripheral zone is usually of normal height. The partial DM is enlarged and thicker compared to normal size. Its shape resembles a sausage (Figure 9–20).

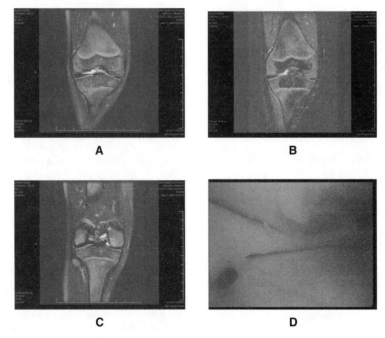

Figure 9–20. Partial, lateral discoid meniscus in a 6- year-old male. *A–C:* An MRI showing the abnormal size of the lateral meniscus. *D:* Intraoperative view of the lateral compartment.

The Wrisberg type is missing the meniscotibial coronary ligaments of the posterior horn and is by definition unstable. Currently the most popular theory concerning the formation of the DM points to an abnormal motion of the initially unstable meniscus as an impulse preventing the meniscus from maintaining its normal shape. The abnormal motion propels enlargement of the meniscus into its abnormal shape and size. The previous theory about lack of involution from a discoid form into a normal crescent shape has not been supported by anatomical studies.

Clinical Findings

A. Symptoms and Signs

- Snapping knee.
- Pain.
- Locking.
- Lack of extension.
- Bulging of the lateral joint line.

Clinical symptoms include locking, catching, snapping of the knee, and an audible clunk. Other symptoms include pain, which might be a late symptom, usually associated with a tear, or the appearance of a "cyst" at the lateral joint line. Sometimes the enlarged meniscus might cause the knee to lock up. Initial symptoms usually occur at school age, however, 2- or 3-year-old children might already be diagnosed with a DM. A high level of suspicion is necessary to make a proper diagnosis.

Many findings have been linked to DM: cupping of the lateral tibial plateau, high riding fibular head, hypoplasia of the lateral femoral condyle and lateral tibial spine, abnormal shape of the lateral malleolus, widening of the lateral joint space, and hypoplasia of the peroneal muscles. An abnormally high position of the fibular head and widening of the joint space are the only features significantly associated with the DM.

B. Imaging Studies

The most accurate imaging for DM is an MRI, which has a high positive predictive value of 92% (Figure 9–21). The diagnosis of DM is established if three or more, 5-mm-wide, contiguous sagittal sections show an uninterrupted meniscus from the anterior to the posterior tibial plateau. Two cuts showing equal height of the midsubstance of the meniscus indicate a high probability of DM. The "bow tie" sign helps establish the diagnosis. Diagnosis of the Wrisberg type could be difficult, as the meniscus may not be enlarged.

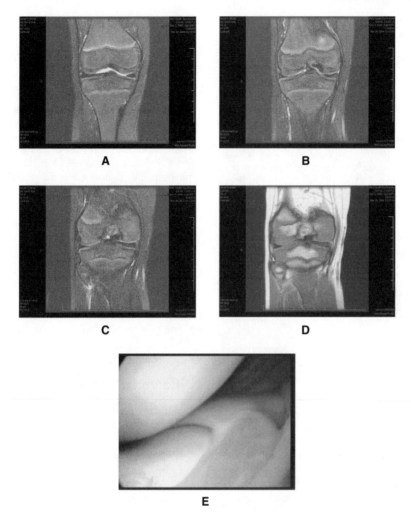

Figure 9–21. Partial, medial discoid meniscus, right knee. **A–D:** MRI images showing the abnormal size of the medial meniscus. **E:** Direct view of the meniscus: the meniscus was unstable and was repaired by the inside-out method.

Treatment

The move toward saving and stabilizing a DM is similar to the trend in meniscal surgery. The total meniscectomy commonly used in the past to "treat" DM should be abandoned, as removal of the entire meniscus can speed up development of osteoarthritis of the knee. An OCD of the femoral condyle following total excision of the DM has been reported.

The goal of surgical treatment is to preserve the meniscus, stabilize it, and reshape it to as close to its normal contour as possible. Saucerization of the meniscus and repair of the instability are probably the best option. Reshaping of the DM is not easy, and requires a lot of time and patience. The abnormal structure of the DM, especially of a complete one, creates problems with visualization during surgery. The cartilage of the DM is also more sturdy and difficult to reshape.

Return to Play

Recovery from DM surgery usually takes 3 months and is similar to recovery from repair of a "normal" meniscus. The patient resumes normal activity after physical therapy.

Ahn JH et al: Discoid lateral meniscus in children: clinical manifestations and morphology. J Pediatr Orthop 2001;21(6):812.

Kim SJ et al: Radiographic knee dimensions in discoid lateral meniscus: comparison with normal control. Arthroscopy 2000;16(5):511.

Klingele KE et al: Discoid lateral meniscus: prevalence of peripheral rim instability. J Pediatr Orthop 2004;24(1):79.

OSTEOCHONDROSIS DISSECANS (OCD) AND OSTEOCHONDRAL FRACTURES (OCF)

Pathogenesis

OCD is a disease of the cartilage and the subchondral bone that results in isolation and sometimes sequestration of an osteochondral fragment without significant trauma. The "classic" OCD typically involves the lateral aspect of the medial condyle (51–85% of all OCDs). An OCD can involve the weight-bearing surface of the medial condyle, the lateral condyle, and the patella (Figure 9–22).

The juvenile form of OCD occurs in younger teenagers with wide-open physes; the adolescent form is seen when a patient nears skeletal maturity. The lesion happens more commonly in boys (about twice as often as among girls). Bilateral involvement is observed in about 25% of cases, which usually show different patterns and different times of onset.

The etiology of OCD is still uncertain. Initially it was thought to be an inflammatory process of the osteochondral layer of the cartilage. For this reason, the suffix "itis" has been used. The inflammatory theory has never been proven. At present all of the possible etiologies include the following:

- Microtrauma: repetitive injury to the lateral aspect of the medial condyle by contact with the tibial eminence.
- Engagement of the odd facet of the patella against the femoral condyle in full flexion.
- Diminished blood supply to the subchondral bone.
- Localized epiphyseal dysplasia.

Hereditary influence is slight, although several members of one family have been reported to have OCD problems. The OCF is related to acute trauma. It can involve the medial and lateral condyle as well as the patella. OCF of the lateral femoral condyle is correlated with patella dislocation.

Clinical Findings

A. SYMPTOMS AND SIGNS

- No history of trauma.
- Usually vague symptoms, activity-related.
- Pain.
- Swelling.
- Locking.
- Loose body symptoms.
- Tenderness of the femoral condyle.
- Wilson test.

B. CLASSIFICATION

- Grade 1: depressed osteochondral fracture.
- Grade 2: osteochondral fragment attached by an osseous bridge (trap door).
- Grade 3: detached nondisplaced fragment.
- Grade 4: displaced fragment (loose body).

C. IMAGING STUDIES

Radiographs may show the exact extension of the OCD or OCF. For a typical OCD of the knee, the best and most sensitive radiograph is the tunnel view. AP, lateral, and Merchant views can help to visualize the defect and the position of loose fragments.

An MRI is especially helpful in distinguishing between stable and unstable lesions. The value of MRI at follow-up is limited. Signs of instability based on a T2 image include the following:

- High signal beneath the OCD.
- High signal line traversing the subchondral bone into the lesion.
- Focal osteochondral defect of the articular cartilage >5 mm.
- 5-mm fluid-filled cyst beneath the lesion (Figure 9–23).

Differential Diagnosis

- Osteochondrosis dissecans versus osteochondral fracture.
- Accessory centers of ossification.
- Osteonecrosis.
- Epiphyseal dysplasia.

Treatment

A. NONSURGICAL

Treatment of OCD is as controversial as its etiology. A consistent, universally accepted treatment protocol does not exist. Elimination of high-impact activities seems to be logical, and protected weight bearing forms the foundation of nonoperative treatment. Non-weight bearing usually lasts several weeks until the symptoms subside; however, the real question is how long the patient should avoid high-impact activities. Moving the knee is recommended. A brace or even a brief period of casting may be necessary for very active students, but the period of immobilization should be limited.

The length of nonoperative treatment and restriction of activities varies, depending on the treating physician's preferences and experience. About 50% of OCD will heal spontaneously following a nonoperative protocol, a fact commonly cited in the literature. In one study, however, 10 OCDs, which were assessed arthroscopically, were reported to be stable. During a second look arthroscopy, at an average of 7.5 years later, 7 of 10 were unstable.

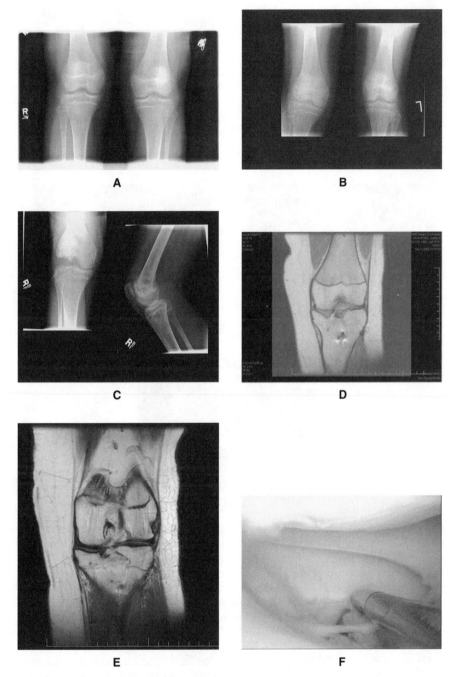

Figure 9–22. Avascular necrosis of the femoral condyle in a 13-year-old female following steroid therapy for dermatomyositis. **A:** Two years ago. **B:** One year ago. **C:** Current radiographs. Osteochondral defect of the tibia plateau after resection of an adamantinoma, at age 10, 6 years ago. **D, E:** MRI images of the tibia. **F:** Arthroscopic pictures of the lateral tibial plateau. The crater-like defect occupies about 50% of the lateral plateau.

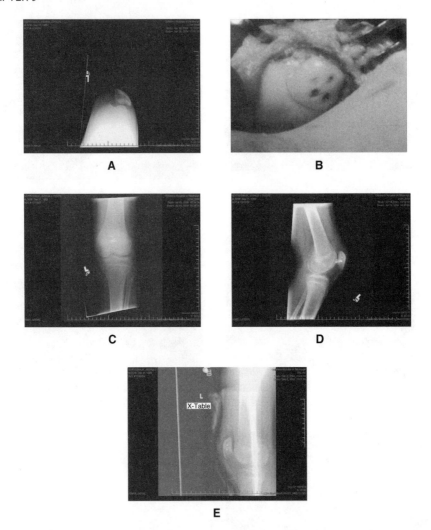

Figure 9–23. Fourteen-year-old male who fell while skateboarding. **A:** Free, osteochondral fragment next to the lateral femoral condyle, in the lateral gutter of the knee. **B:** The fragment is reattached via open reduction with internal fixation, using microscrews from a maxillofacial set and osteochondral darts (Arthrex, Naples, FL). **C, D:** Postoperative radiographs in anteroposterior and lateral views: despite being countersunk, the screws look very prominent on the lateral radiograph. **E:** The screws are removed: part of a broken microdrill bit is left in place. Repair of the retinaculum was accomplished using suture anchors.

Risk factors for failure of nonoperative treatment of the OCD include:

- Older age.
- Larger lesions (determined by medial–lateral diameter, not anteroposterior).
- Lesions of the weight-bearing area (Cahill Zone 2 on an AP radiograph).
- Lesions between 30 and 60°: between Blumensat's line and the posterior femoral line (Cahill Zone B on a lateral radiograph).

B. SURGICAL

Indications for surgical treatment include the following:

- A juvenile OCD that is symptomatic despite 6–12 months of nonoperative treatment.
- Detachment of the previously stable OCD.
- Symptomatic loose body.
- Predicted growth plate closure within 12 months.
- Symptomatic nonunion confirmed by bone scan or MRI.

Surgical options include the following:

- Simple excision or removal of the loose body (not recommended except for a very small lesion of the non-weight-bearing surface).
- "Refreshment" and drilling of the crater.
- Microfracture.
- Reattachment with metal pins (weak); screws (countersunk microscrews from maxillofacial set, cannulated 3.5-mm or 2.4-mm screws, Herbert screw); bioabsorbable OCD darts, arrows, and screws; bone pegs.
- Subchondral, retrograde bone grafting.
- Osteochondral transport (mosaicplasty).
- Osteochondral allografts.
- Autologous chondrocyte transplantation (Figure 9–24).

C. SLEEVE FRACTURES

Sleeve fractures are unique to the patella and involve the proximal or distal pole of the patella or its midsubstance. They can occur at the attachment of the patella tendon into the tibia; in this case, a sort of a slide of the sleeve of soft tissue overlying the patella occurs, rather than a classic bony fracture.

Clinically these fractures manifest with weakness of the quadriceps mechanism, a history of hyperflexion trauma, and minimal abnormalities on radiographs. Sometimes a deficit is palpable at the fracture side, and

an MRI usually shows fracture patterns and the anatomy of the patella tendon.

Treatment of patients with an intact extension mechanism consists of immobilization in a cylinder cast in extension for about 6 weeks, followed by a hinged, long knee brace with gradually increasing ROM and weight bearing.

For patients with a deficit of extension, an open reduction with internal fixation will be necessary to restore full function of the knee. Because the majority of fractures involve soft tissue, heavy sutures passed trough bony tunnels drilled in the patella, or suture anchors, will help restore the continuity of the extensor mechanism.

Rehabilitation & Return to Play

Return to play is a decision very difficult to categorize. Generally, because OCF occurs through "normal" bone, the patient should have no problem returning to full activities 3–4 months after surgery.

The decision regarding patients after OCD surgery, however, is much more complex. The fact that OCD occurs in a clearly pathologic environment worsens the prognosis. The detached OCD, reattached into the "crater" of a potentially abnormal bone, might not heal. A lesion that has been "silent" and stable until skeletal maturity might break off from the femur after skeletal maturity is reached. Presently we lack a reliable tool to follow the OCD and provide predictable information

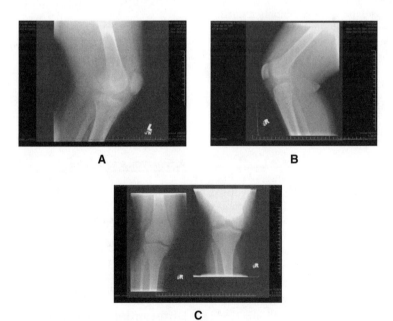

Figure 9–24. Atypical, bilateral osteochondritis dissecans (OCDs) in a 14-year-old female baseball player. **A:** Left knee, atypical OCD dissecting the entire posterior part of the lateral femoral condyle. **B, C:** Displaced OCD of the contralateral knee, lateral condyle.

about healing. For all these reasons, there is no universal consensus as to whether and when high-impact activities should be allowed. Return to sports after symptoms subside, or 4–6 months after surgery, can be considered. It has been proposed that high-impact activities be limited until the patient reaches skeletal maturity.

After surgery for sleeve fractures, casting and rehabilitation are similar to the nonoperative approach. Patients return to sports at an average of 4 months following the injury.

Aglietti P et al: Results of arthroscopic excision of the fragment in the treatment of osteochondritis dissecans of the knee. Arthroscopy 2001;17(7):741.

Brittberg M, Winalski CS: Evaluation of cartilage injuries and repair. J Bone Joint Surg Am 2003;85-A(suppl 2):58.

Mizuta H et al: Osteochondritis dissecans of the lateral femoral condyle following total resection of the discoid lateral meniscus. Arthroscopy 2001;17(6):608.

Pill SG et al: Role of magnetic resonance imaging and clinical criteria in predicting successful nonoperative treatment of osteochondritis dissecans in children. J Pediatr Orthop 2003;23(1):102.

OSGOOD–SCHLATTER DISEASE

Pathogenesis

Osgood–Schlatter disease (OSD) is a painful swelling of the growing tibial tuberosity, categorized as a traction apophysitis. Pain occurs at the growth plate of the tibial tuberosity. The patellar tendon connects to the tibial tuberosity via a growth plate, and similar to other locations, this type of anatomic setup commonly results in pain in growing children. Typically, OSD occurs among active girls and boys; however, even a classic couch potato might suffer from this condition.

Clinical Findings

A. SYMPTOMS AND SIGNS

Symptoms occur during a growth spurt, and sometimes last up to 2 years. Bilateral prevalence is not uncommon.

B. IMAGING STUDIES

Radiographs help to rule out all other causes of pain of the proximal tibia. A diagnosis of OSD is strictly based on history and clinical symptoms. The commonly observed fragmentation of the apophysis of the tibial tuberosity is *not* a sign of OSD.

Treatment

OSD is a self-limiting condition. Treatment, which targets the symptoms and aims to alleviate the severity of pain, consists of icing, ice massage, and stretching of quadriceps, hamstrings, and calf muscles. NSAIDs help to alleviate the pain; modification of activity might be necessary. A cylinder cast applied for 2–3 weeks is sometimes necessary to reduce the inflammation and to decrease the pain. Strengthening of the hamstrings and quadriceps is a valuable addition to the treatment plan. In sports necessitating frequent contact of the knee with hard objects (volleyball), kneepads will protect the tibial tuberosity from direct injuries.

Prognosis

OSD is not a recognized risk factor for osteoarthritis. Fractures through the tibial tubercle in patients with preexisting OSD have been reported; however, no statistical correlation between OSD and subsequent fracture of the tibial tuberosity has been confirmed. The risk of fracture does not increase with OSD, and there is no reason to limit the level of activity because of OSD.

In very rare cases, the fragmentation of the tibial tuberosity does not unite, and a small ossicle within the patella tendon causes constant irritation of the tendon. In these circumstances excision of the offending ossicle may be recommended.

Return to Play

Pain will be the only factor limiting the patient's activities. OSD, as a self-limiting condition, should not prevent students from participating in sports. Continuous participation in sports despite suffering from OSD has not been linked to detrimental long-term effects.

SINDING–LARSEN–JOHANSSON SYNDROME & JUMPER'S KNEE

Pathogenesis

Sinding–Larsen–Johansson syndrome is similar to Osgood—Schlatter disease. It affects the distal pole of the patella instead of the tibial tuberosity.

Jumper's knee manifests as a pain at the midsubstance of the patellar tendon and is considered a form of overuse tendinitis.

Clinical Findings

A. SYMPTOMS AND SIGNS

- Pain at the distal pole of the patella or midsubstance of the patellar tendon.
- Pain related to activity.

B. IMAGING STUDIES

The reported fragmentation of the distal pole of the patella represents a normal variation of the radiographic appearance of the patella.

Differential Diagnosis

- Type 1 of the symptomatic bipartite patella.
- Sleeve fracture.

- Osgood–Schlatter symptoms.
- Tibial tuberosity fracture.

Treatment, Rehabilitation, & Return to Play

Treatment, prognosis, and physical therapy programs are identical to the Osgood–Schlatter protocol.

CONGENITAL DISLOCATION OF THE PATELLA

Pathogenesis

The likelihood that a patient with congenital dislocation of the patella will become involved in sports is rather low. Usually, the condition is recognized and treated in early childhood.

Clinical Findings

A. SYMPTOMS AND SIGNS

Typically, the patella is palpated lying against the lateral femoral condyle. Flexion contraction of the knee, which is normal at an early age, persists beyond the age of walking, and valgus alignment develops as a child grows.

B. IMAGING STUDIES

Radiographs fail to show the nonossified patella and its position. MRI is the best modality to show the entire joint and the patella. It might show dysplasia of the lateral femoral condyle as well. Ultrasonography does not require anesthesia, and may visualize the patella well enough to confirm the diagnosis.

Treatment

Early treatment is the rule. Results are much better with early intervention and restoration of proper alignment and position of the patella. Several surgical options have been discussed in the literature, and generally proximal and distal realignment is required to stabilize the patella. A medial transfer of the lateral part of the patella tendon can augment extensile lateral release with medial plication and transfers of the vastus medialis obliquus (VMO). With early treatment results have been excellent (Figure 9–25).

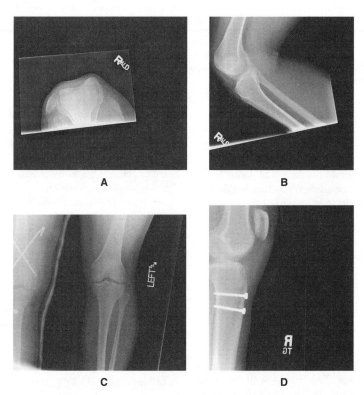

Figure 9–25. A–C: Congenital dislocation of the patella in a 7-year-old female with trisomy 21. ***C:*** Proximal and distal realignments were performed. Distal derotation of the femur was necessary to correct the abnormal torsion of the femur. ***D:*** Fulkerson osteotomy and proximal realignment, performed in a different patient for habitual subluxation of the patella.

PATELLA INSTABILITY & DISLOCATION IN ADOLESCENTS

Pathogenesis

Patella dislocation among teenagers is an entirely different problem, occurring more frequently in girls than in boys. The first occurrence usually results from violent trauma. In girls this is typically a twisting-valgus injury to the knee. Boys are more likely to sustain a direct blow to the patella, which causes the patella to dislocate. The acutely dislocated patella reduces spontaneously in the majority of cases.

Clinical Findings

A. Symptoms and Signs

- Direct or indirect injury to the knee.
- Knee "going out."
- "Pop" at the time of injury.
- Effusion.
- Apprehension and relocation tests are positive.

Risk factors include the following:

- Patella alta.
- Abnormal femoral and tibial torsion.
- Excessive genus valgum.
- Hypoplasia of the lateral condyle.
- VMO hypoplasia.
- Vastus lateralis contracture.
- Hypoplasia of the femoral sulcus.
- Generalized laxity.

Imaging Studies

Regular radiographs in four positions are necessary, and sometimes reveal an obvious fracture or loose body. A CT scan will further localize a potential loose body. MRI is more specific in revealing osteochondral defects and position of the patella in extension of the knee.

Differential Diagnosis

- Meniscal injury.
- ACL tear.
- Physeal fractures.
- Fractures of the patella.

Treatment

A. Nonsurgical

Initial studies should rule out any concomitant fracture or osteochondral fractures. The treatment of first time dislocators without associated osteochondral injury consists of 2–3 weeks of immobilization with protected weight bearing. Prolonged VMO and quadriceps strengthening are necessary to change the dynamic vector of the extensor mechanism. Patella tracking orthosis (PTO) can be a valuable addition to the treatment, and can initially be used for sports activities as well.

Nonoperative treatment has been effective in 80–85% of cases. The remaining patients will experience recurrent dislocations. The greater the number of risk factors present, the more likely the patient will experience two or more episodes of dislocation.

B. Surgical

Indications for surgery include the presence of an osteochondral fracture requiring ORIF, recurrent dislocation, and patella fracture. In an acute setting surgery is targeted toward repairing the fractures. Acute rupture of the medial retinaculum is a relative indication.

In a chronic setting, lateral release, proximal and distal soft tissue realignment, and tibial tubercle osteotomy should be considered.

Rehabilitation & Return to Play

After the first traumatic dislocation, return to sport could take as long as 3–4 months, especially if a surgical procedure was necessary to repair a bony or osteochondral defect. Two to three months of nonoperative treatment, consisting of immobilization and physical therapy, is usually enough to allow the patient to return safely to full activity. Chronic dislocators may need more time before returning to sports.

SYMPTOMATIC PLICA

Pathogenesis

An asymptomatic plica may be discovered in about 50% of the population; symptomatic plicas have of the knee joint have probably been overdiagnosed. Patients report a history of popping, snapping, and giving way. The mediopatellar plica is most commonly discovered during a physical examination. Other problems of the knee have symptoms that mimic the painful plica and vice versa: plica might imitate meniscal injuries, osteochondral problems, and patella symptoms (Figure 9–26).

Clinical Findings

A. Symptoms and Signs

The inflammation of a previously silent plica might be triggered by a direct injury or by repetitive trauma. Once inflamed or irritated it will begin to cause activity-related knee pain.

B. Classification

- Suprapatellar.
- Mediopatellar.
- Infrapatellar (ligamentum mucosum).
- Lateral patellar.

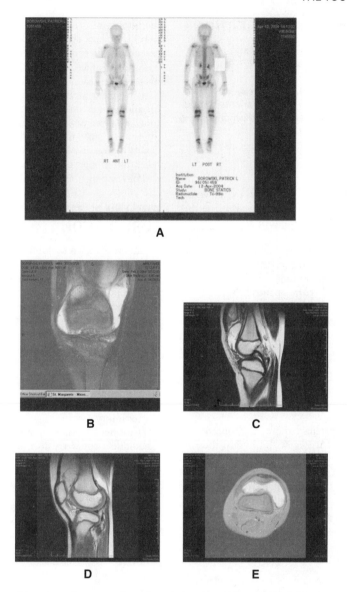

Figure 9–26. An 8-year-old male with pain and swelling following a fall on the left knee while biking. *A:* A bone scan shows a mild increase in uptake around the left knee. *B–F:* MRI showing hypertrophic synovium. Final diagnosis: pigmented villonodular synovitis.

C. IMAGING STUDIES

MRI is the only modality that might show a plica.

Treatment

A. NONSURGICAL

Initial treatment is always focused on stretching, icing, modification of activity, rest, and a patellofemoral program. It sometimes takes several months to relieve pain related to symptomatic plica.

B. SURGICAL

Arthroscopic excision of recalcitrant symptomatic plica is a relatively simple procedure, with a success rate between 70 and 90%. A significant percentage of plicas will regrow and become symptomatic again; scar tissue created during surgery may contribute to recurring symptoms as well.

Rehabilitation & Return to Play

Recovery from surgical treatment is relatively short, and should not last more than 4–6 weeks. Patients should continue the stretching and strengthening program.

BIPARTITE PATELLA

Pathogenesis

The bipartite patella represents a failure to unite two or more centers of ossification into one bone. Because the bipartite patella is generally asymptomatic, it is most frequently discovered on radiographs taken for other reasons. Sometimes, however, the fibrocartilagenous connection between the fragments is disrupted as a result of trauma or repetitive trauma, and the previously nonproblematic patella becomes painful.

Classification (Saupe)

- Type 1: inferior pole of the patella (5%).
- Type 2: lateral patellar margin (20%).
- Type 3: superior-lateral quadrant of the patella (75%).

Treatment

Symptomatic bipartite patella requires immobilization in a cylinder cast for 4–6 weeks, with physical therapy to start soon after. If pain persists, several surgical options are available. A symptomatic, small bipartite patella can be excised. "Refreshment" of the connection between the two parts of the patella, with fixation using screws or wires and supplementary bone grafting, will be a better option for large, painful fragments.

Rehabilitation & Return to Play

Return to sport after 2–3 months of treatment is a realistic expectation. The student will enjoy unrestricted activities after recovery is completed.

MEDIAL COLLATERAL LIGAMENT SYNDROME: BREASTSTROKE KNEE

About 50% of sports-related complaints are associated with problems of overuse, and a typical example is the breaststroke knee (BK). Its repetitive microtrauma to medial structures of the knee causes prolonged pain and discomfort over the medial knee. The MCL appears to be the most affected structure, but the inferomedial margin of the patella may be painful as well.

Poor technique, especially during the initial phase of the rearward throughst and the whip kick, will intensify the symptoms. The amount of hip abduction at initiation of the kick should ideally be between 35 and 45°, and changes in this angle increase the likelihood of developing BK. Athletes with general laxity are at higher risk of suffering BK.

Pain and inflammation over the medial knee may last for a long time, and can mimic medial meniscus symptoms. Pain increases with activity.

Acute symptoms need to be treated by icing, modification of activity, NSAIDs, and stretching. Prevention relies on proper conditioning, general strengthening, and developing a mechanically sound technique.

PROXIMAL TIBIOFIBULAR JOINT SUBLUXATION

A patient with lateral joint pain and catching could be suffering from symptoms originating at the proximal tibiofibular joint. The joint might be acutely dislocated, with rupture of the posterior tibiofibular ligament, LCL, and biceps femoris. An acute dislocation might occur after a twisting and landing injury (snowboarding) or with fracture of the tibia.

Chronic instability has been seen among teenagers with increased general laxity or as a part of Marfan syndrome.

The differential diagnosis includes a torn lateral meniscus, an LCL sprain, a joint cyst, and posterolateral corner injury.

Treatment consists of strengthening and stretching. The athlete could try to use an elastic knee sleeve. In resistant cases, surgical reconstruction of the joint capsule, arthrodesis of the joint, or resection of the fibular head may be necessary.

Canizares GH, Selesnick FH: Bipartite patella fracture. Arthroscopy 2003;19(2):215.

Grelsamer RP: Patellar malalignment. J Bone Joint Surg Am 2000;82-A(11):1639.

Rodeo SA: Knee pain in competitive swimming. Clinics Sports Med 1999;18(2):379.

■ FOOT & ANKLE

LATERAL ANKLE SPRAIN & SALTER-TYPE FRACTURES OF THE DISTAL FIBULA

Pathogenesis

A typical inversion injury that causes a tear of the lateral ankle ligaments very often disrupts the open growth plate of the distal fibula. Caution should be exercised and it is necessary to be aware of the possibility of an injury to the physis to establish the proper diagnosis. Radiographs are useful in cases in which the epiphysis of the fibula has been displaced. Unfortunately, this is seldom the case, and the majority of Salter 1 injuries to the distal fibula present with negative radiographic findings except for soft tissue swelling. In this situation an appropriate diagnosis can be established based on the location of the point of maximum tenderness. Tenderness over the distal growth plate of the fibula and a history of inversion trauma to the ankle are enough to diagnose a Salter 1 fracture of the distal fibula, despite negative findings on radiographs.

Tenderness indicative of injury to the lateral ankle ligaments [anterior talofibular (ATF) and calcaneofibular (CF)] is anterior and slightly distal compared to the tenderness of the growth plate. As an adolescent approaches skeletal maturity, the rate of Salter type injuries declines, and the probability of a classic lateral ankle sprain increases. Just before the physis of the distal fibula closes, it is possible to observe a concomitant Salter 1 fracture together with a tear of the lateral ankle ligaments.

Clinical Findings

A. SYMPTOMS AND SIGNS

- Inversion injury to the ankle.
- Inability to bear weight.
- Point of maximum tenderness.
- Delay in seeking medical attention (especially true with Salter 1 injuries: "They called me from the ED and said there is no fracture visible on the X-ray.").

B. IMAGING STUDIES

With all the limitations discussed above, radiographs are mandatory, as additional injuries may be discovered, such as OCD of the talus. A CT scan may be necessary to evaluate for a possible Tillaux or triplane fracture of the distal tibia. An MRI is recommended for long-lasting problems or for symptoms indicative of osteochondral injury.

Differential Diagnosis

- Salter 1 fracture versus ankle sprain.
- Other fractures of the distal fibula.
- Fractures of the distal tibia.
- Osteochondral fracture or OCD.
- Syndesmotic injury.

Treatment

Treatment of a Salter 1 fracture of the fibula consists of 4–6 weeks of a short leg cast. The patient is asked not to bear weight for about 2 weeks, after which weight bearing can be gradually increased. A persistent pain when trying to bear weight will increase the non-weight-bearing time. After the cast is removed, a solid or hinged brace-boot might be used for added protection. The patient returns to full activities usually after 2–3 months.

A Salter 1 fracture of the distal fibula can reoccur several times in the same ankle. Fortunately, this physis is very resistant to potential growth arrest, and very rarely causes abnormal growth, even after multiple episodes.

Treatment of the ankle sprain depends on its severity. Initial RICE is mandatory. Details will be discussed in Chapter 4, this volume.

TARSAL COALITION

General Considerations

Multiple ankle sprains in a teenager should raise suspicions of the existence of a tarsal coalition. A tarsal coalition remains asymptomatic until the early teenage years. It is caused by a failure to differentiate the primitive mesenchymal tissue into separate hindfoot bones, which results in an abnormal connection between the bones. The coalition could be bony, cartilaginous, or fibrous.

Pathogenesis

Pain in patients with tarsal coalition is frequently at the level of the sinus tarsi or over the medial aspect of the subtalar joint. It is typically dull and aching and activity related; a limp is common after activities.

The most common coalitions are the calcaneonavicular and talocalcaneal. The incidence of coalition is estimated at about 1% of the population. Bilateral coalition occurs in about 50–80% of cases; many tarsal coalitions do not cause pain and go unrecognized, sometimes for life. Family occurrence has been reported.

There is an association between tarsal coalition and fibular hemimelia, syndactyly, Apert syndrome, Nievergelt syndrome, and carpal coalition. Tarsal coalition might be found during surgery for congenital clubfoot. In this case the coalition involves the subtalar joint.

Clinical Findings

A. SYMPTOMS AND SIGNS

- Multiple sprains.
- Activity-related pain.
- Pain at the sinus tarsi or ankle.
- Limited or no subtalar motion.
- Pain with inversion and eversion.
- Peroneal spastic foot.

Classification:

- Bony.
- Cartilaginous.
- Fibrous.

Anatomic:

- Subtalar: talocalcaneal.
- Calcaneonavicular.
- Other rare types: talonavicular, calcaneocuboid, cubonavicular, and naviculocuneiform.

B. IMAGING STUDIES

The classic radiographs in AP, lateral, oblique, and Harris heel views might show some common signs of tarsal coalition (Figure 9–27). The easiest coalition to see is the calcaneonavicular on the oblique view, seen as a bony connection between the anterior process of the calcaneus and the lateral horn of the navicular. On a lateral view, the anteater sign is pathognomonic for calcaneonavicular coalition. At the presence of the coalition, the anterior process of the calcaneus resembles the nose of an anteater. The C-sign on a lateral radiograph refers to a line drawn over the superior dome of the talus, down and posteriorly into the inferior outline of the sustentaculum tali. It is characteristic of subtalar coalition. A dorsal beaking of the anterior process of the talus suggests restricted ROM through the subtalar or Chopart joint. It might be found in tarsal coalition or as a result of clubfoot surgery with limited motion across those joints.

A Harris heel view may show abnormalities of the middle facet of the subtalar joint.

A fine cut CT scan is by far the most important examination confirming tarsal coalition, showing beautifully the location and extent of a coalition. The CT-based three-dimensional reconstruction better indicates the location of the bar, especially the subtalar bar and its relationship to the subtalar joint.

A nonbony coalition may not be directly visualized by CT images. Sometimes, an irregularity of the middle facet suggests its presence, and an MRI is necessary to reveal fibrous or cartilaginous coalition.

Differential Diagnosis

- Fracture.
- Infection.
- Bone cyst.
- Painful flatfoot.
- Painful accessory navicular.
- Complex regional pain syndrome.
- Stress fracture.
- Kohler disease.

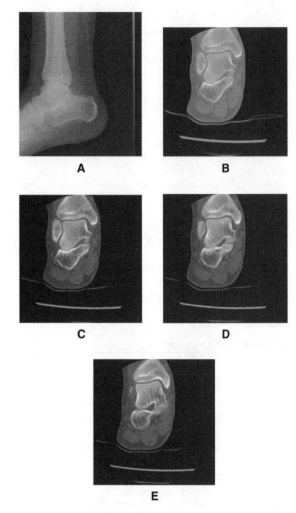

Figure 9–27. Sixteen-year-old football player presenting with several months of dull ankle pain and a history of multiple sprains. Clinical examination reveals severely limited inversion and eversion and a flattening of the longitudinal arch of the foot. **A:** Lateral radiograph shows the classic C-sign: the imaginary C-line follows the dome of the talus, goes down over the posterior wall of the talus, and curves anteriorly under the sustentaculum tali. **B–E:** Four images of a CT scan with deformity of the medial facet and a bony bar between the talus and calcaneus.

Treatment

A. NONSURGICAL

Initially, cast treatment might be tried. A short leg cast worn for 4–6 weeks with protected weight bearing might alleviate the pain. Immobilization should be followed by physical therapy and a gradual return to activities. The success rate of nonoperative treatment is unpredictable, but is usually low.

B. SURGICAL

When the cast does not work, an excision of the bar, with or without interposition of a biologically inert material, is the preferred treatment. Before surgery it is wise to carefully review all available studies looking for a possible second coalition in the same foot, as two tarsal coalitions in one foot can occur.

Excision of a calcaneonavicular coalition is done through a relatively small incision centered over the bar. Lambott osteotomes are the best tools to remove a tarsal bar. The entire coalition should be removed, leaving at least 1.0–1.5 cm of free space between the anterior process of the calcaneus and the navicular. The gap might be filled with an extensor digitorum brevis muscle.

An excision of the subtalar bar is more difficult, requiring a longer posteromedial incision. The flexor hallucis longus (FHL) is a hallmark of the sustentaculum tali; the FHL tendon crosses the ankle joint and curves anteriorly, coursing under the sustentaculum. This helps identify the middle facet. Before excision of the bar it is helpful to visualize the anterior and posterior subtalar facets. Following the orientation of the facets might further help to navigate into the middle facet, which is usually obscured by the coalition. The coalition is then excised using an osteotome, a high-speed bur, and Rongeur or Carsson incisors. The area of the excised middle facet may then be filled with surrounding soft tissues, such as a split flexor digitorum longus (FDL) tendon, or fat tissue, or it may be left alone. Bone wax can be applied to the area of excision, thus lowering the risk of forming a local hematoma, which might propagate bone formation.

Because feet with tarsal coalition are usually flat, other surgical procedures may be directed toward improving the mechanics of the foot; lateral column lengthening, medial closing wedge osteotomy of the calcaneus, or sliding osteotomy of the heel can improve stress distribution across the foot and ease the pain. Excision of the tarsal bar, however, is the preferred initial treatment.

After surgery a short leg cast is applied and worn for 4–6 weeks. ROM and strengthening exercises start as soon as the cast is removed.

Rehabilitation, Complications, & Return to Play

The calcaneonavicular coalition is an extraarticular structure, whereas the subtalar coalition is an intraarticular formation, taking away part of the normal cartilage of the subtalar joint. For this reason, the major prognostic factor for recovery and successful treatment is the location of the bar. The excision of the calcaneonavicular bar

is usually easier, with a higher success rate and faster recovery. After surgery, the patient can return to sport within 2–3 months, assuming there are no symptoms.

Even after a careful excision of the subtalar coalition, the patient may still experience long-lasting pain of the foot, especially if more than 50% of the articular surface was occupied by the bar. In this situation the painful subtalar joint may need to be fused. The subtalar fusion might be done separately, or as part of a triple arthrodesis, especially if the Chopart joint is painful as well.

SEVER DISEASE

Pathogenesis

The most common cause of heel pain in the pediatric or adolescent population is Sever disease, a self-limiting condition characterized by pain of the heel in growing individuals. The pain is activity related, is not the result of trauma, and is more intense the morning after strenuous physical activity. It usually occurs in active and sports-minded individuals, but can be observed among computer games players as well. The symptoms can last for a long time, sometimes even until growth of the foot is completed. Bilateral involvement is common.

Clinical Findings

A. SYMPTOMS AND SIGNS

- Pain at the posterior extent of the heel.
- No swelling or effusion.
- Pain frequently during intense exercise, or the morning after.
- No night pain and no pain at rest.

B. IMAGING STUDIES

Radiographs are mandatory to rule out other causes of the heel pain rather than to confirm the diagnosis. An irregularity of the calcaneal apophysis is a normal finding and is not necessarily a sign of Sever disease.

Differential Diagnosis

- Salter–Harris 1 fracture of the apophysis.
- Achilles tendinitis.
- Plantar fasciitis.
- Stress fracture of the calcaneus.
- Tarsal tunnel syndrome.
- Subtalar coalition.
- Osteomyelitis.
- Bone cyst of the calcaneus.
- Accessory navicular.
- Tumor (Figure 9–28).

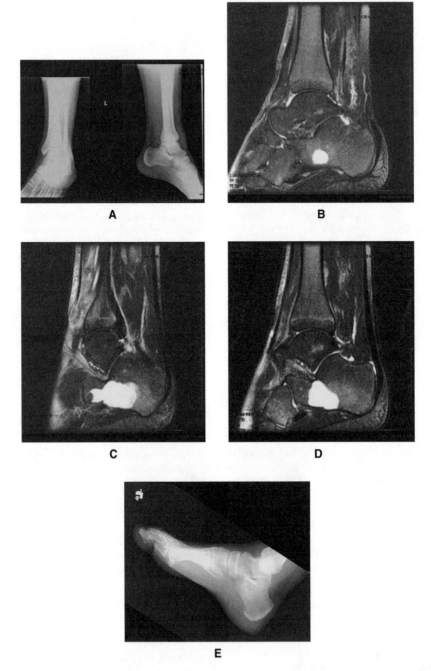

Figure 9–28. Calcaneal cyst barely visible on a lateral radiograph of the foot (*A*). The image was obtained after the patient sprained his ankle playing football. High frequency signal on an MRI (*B–D*), most likely consistent with a bony cyst. The cyst was subsequently curretaged and bone grafted (*E*). The final report shows lining of a unicameral bone cyst.

Treatment

Treatment consists of modification of activity, rest as needed, ice, ice massage, and stretching of the gastrocnemius complex as well as the quadriceps and hamstrings. NSAIDs help to relieve symptoms. A gel heel pad can be used as well as arch supporting insets. If the symptoms do not resolve after a period of rest and stretching, cast immobilization for a brief period of time may be necessary.

Return to Play

Patients with symptoms of Sever disease do not need to stop playing sports. No study links Sever disease to arthritis or subsequent fracture of the heel. Playing through the pain is an acceptable option, as long as the patient and the parents are willing to accept it. However, the symptoms may be difficult to control and modification of activity may be necessary. Symptoms will fade when the apophysis closes up.

ISELIN DISEASE

Pathogenesis

Iselin disease is an apophysitis of the growth plate of the base of the fifth metatarsal.

Clinical Findings

A. SYMPTOMS AND SIGNS

Iselin disease manifests with activity-related pain localized at the base of the fifth metatarsal. Symptoms might last a long time, sometimes up to a year and a half. Patients complain of localized pain over the proximal part of the fifth metatarsal bone. They may try to avoid putting pressure over the fifth metatarsal and keep the involved foot in pronation or extreme supination.

B. IMAGING STUDIES

Similar to other "traction apophysitis," radiographs may rule out other causes of lateral foot pain rather than confirm the diagnosis. The normal separation of the apophysis from the base of the fifth metatarsal should not be read as a fracture.

Differential Diagnosis

- Salter-type fracture.
- Jones fracture.
- Osteomyelitis.
- Tendinitis of the peroneus brevis.

Treatment

In an acute phase, the RICE treatment is usually most effective. In most cases, a few weeks of cast immobilization should alleviate the symptoms.

Rehabilitation & Return to Play

A careful and slow rehabilitation program offers patients the best chance to recover. Physical therapy with slowly advancing exercises of gradually increasing intensity will be the most important element in returning to sport. Very often, however, the treatment lasts for months, and prolonged pain with inactivity can be very discouraging to a young athlete.

ACCESSORY NAVICULAR

Pathogenesis

Multiple centers of ossification contribute to the formation of the navicular bone. The accessory navicular (AN), the most common accessory bone of the foot, is present in about 20–25% of the population. The unfused, accessory, medial part of the navicular bone forms a prominent bony mass, which sometimes becomes painful. Symptoms start in the preteen years.

Classification includes three types:

- Type 1: a small ossicle within the tibialis posterior tendon, commonly termed the os tibiale externum.
- Type 2: larger than type 1; connected to the navicular through a dense synchondrosis.
- Type 3: enlarged navicular; the medial, prominent part of the navicular is the accessory ossicle fused to the navicular bone.

Clinical Findings

A. SYMPTOMS AND SIGNS

A symptomatic AN causes redness, swelling, pain, and sometimes blisters and calluses over the most prominent part of the midfoot. Type 2 is the most commonly painful type. Pain is frequent in skiers, figure skaters, and hockey players, because direct pressure from tight footwear contributes to the discomfort. Commercially available shoes also cause symptoms, if the medial border of the shoe hits the level of the AN. Most likely, fracture through the dense, syndesmotic connection between the AN and the main navicular bone is responsible for the symptoms.

B. IMAGING STUDIES

The navicular bone becomes visible on radiographs after the first year of life, but sometimes does not appear until 5 years of age. Radiographs taken in AP, lateral, and oblique views confirm the diagnosis and help in differentiating the condition from other sources of pain.

Differential Diagnosis

- Painful pes planus.
- Tarsal coalition.
- Koehler disease.

Treatment

A. Nonsurgical

The majority of AN patients will do fine with nonoperative treatment. Doughnut-type pads, which unload the most prominent part of the AN, will be sufficient to decrease pressure and to alleviate pain. A similar effect will be achieved by modification of the shoe or the boot, or by changing the brand of the shoes or boots worn. For example, skiers should be aware of various "last" in different ski boots. The boots vary in the "volume" of the heel, midfoot, and forefoot sections. Athletes should seek help in choosing optimal types of boots and customizing them with appropriate insets. Figure skating and hockey boots can be altered by punching out the part of the boot over the accessory bone.

B. Surgical

Surgical excision is recommended after the nonoperative approach has failed. Simple excision of the offending bone is the standard of care. The previously popular Kidner procedure is rarely utilized today.

Rehabilitation & Return to Play

Usually 3–4 weeks of short leg cast after the surgery followed by another 3–4 weeks of physical therapy is sufficient. After completing treatment, the patient gradually returns to full activity.

OSTEOCHONDROSES

1. Koehler Disease

Pathogenesis

Koehler disease manifests with pain of the tarsal navicular and fragmentation of the bone, visible on radiographs. There is no history of trauma.

Clinical Findings

A. Symptoms and Signs

Symptoms are more common in boys, typically under age 6 years. Pain occurs with activity and is relieved with rest. Weight bearing increases the pain. Point tenderness over the navicular is a pathognomonic finding.

B. Imaging Studies

Radiographs will show fragmentation of the navicular and patchy increased density. As the symptoms subside, follow-up radiographs show reconstitution of the proper shape and structure of the bone.

Differential Diagnosis

- Trauma.
- Painful accessory navicular.
- Infection.

Treatment

Koehler disease is a self-limiting condition, but a difference in duration of symptoms has been noted in children treated with a cast, as compared to no-cast treatment. Symptoms lasted less time in the casted group than in children without casting.

Other options such as arch-supporting insets may also be considered. Surgical treatment is unnecessary.

2. Freiberg Infraction

Clinical Findings

A. Symptoms and Signs

Freiberg disease is a painful infraction of the head of the second metatarsal that occurs predominantly among teenagers. Its etiology is unknown. A possible stress fracture or failure of proper development may cause this condition. The second metatarsal head may be fragile and therefore prone to develop microfractures during the second decade of life.

B. Imaging Studies

Radiographs show infraction, fragmentation, and sometimes collapse of the metatarsal head. With a closed growth plate, the head might be enlarged and flattened.

Treatment

A. Nonoperative

Treatment consists of nonoperative measures, with or without casting. Different insets to relieve the pressure from under the second metatarsal head might be used. Metatarsal pad or custom-molded, pressure-relieving insets should diminish the pain and discomfort.

B. Operative

If a nonoperative approach fails to relieve the symptoms, a surgical approach should be considered. Exploration of the joint may be necessary, with cartilage shaving or resection of the head, and sometimes fusion of the second metatarsophalangeal joint. Arthroscopy of the joint, with articular cartilage reshaping and removal of possible loose bodies, has also been tried.

Return to Play

Return to sport should be guided by clinical symptoms.

PAINFUL OS TRIGONUM, FIBULARE, & SESSAMOID

The foot is well known for its accessory ossicles. Accessory navicular, os fibulare, os trigonum, and bipartite sesamoid are the most common. The accessory bones represent a failure of fusion of separate centers of secondary

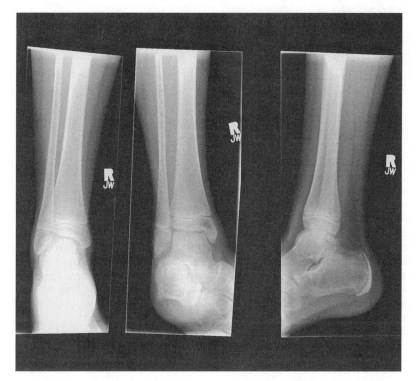

Figure 9–29. Symptomatic os fibulare.

ossification. They are very commonly discovered on radiographs taken for another reason. The bipartite or accessory bones may need treatment when causing pain or discomfort.

The accessory navicular was discussed previously. Painful os trigonum is caused by an acute injury to the bone, the unfused posterior process of the talus, or repetitive trauma. Pain at the posterior ankle with plantar flexion, especially in ballet dancers, should raise suspicion for possible os trigonum. The diagnosis might be confirmed by a bone scan or local injection of an anesthetic agent. The injection is also a therapeutic measure. Treatment includes a brief period of immobilization, modification of activity, avoiding excessive plantar flexion, ice, and NSAIDs. In resistant cases, os trigonum needs to be excised.

Os fibulare appears on a radiograph as a separate center of ossification just distal to the lateral malleolus. It becomes irritated after an inversion injury. Treatment is similar to the treatment of an ankle sprain, and frequently requires a short period of wearing a non-weight-bearing cast. Painful os fibulare may be treated surgically after prolonged nonoperative treatment has failed. Options include simple excision or ORIF with bone grafting (Figure 9–29).

Bipartite sesamoids occur in approximately 10% of the population, with 25% presenting bilaterally. The tibial sesamoid is more likely to be bipartited; it is also more prone to fracture or trauma of the bipartite form.

Symptomatic bipartite or fractured sesamoid requires quite a prolonged period of protected weight bearing. Insets with a metatarsal bar, NSAIDs, modification of activity, and cast immobilization may increase the success rate of nonoperative treatment.

Surgical treatment of the resistant, painful bipartite sesamoid might include ORIF with bone grafting, partial excision of the sesamoid, or shaving. Excision of the entire sesamoid is the most radical and potentially problematic solution.

Letts M et al: Surgical management of chronic lateral ankle instability in adolescents. J Pediatr Orthop 2003;23(3):392.

■ OTHER LOWER EXTREMITY PROBLEMS

CHRONIC EXERTIONAL COMPARTMENT SYNDROME

General Considerations

Chronic exertional compartment syndrome (CECS) is an overuse syndrome characterized by pain and sometimes dysesthesia or weakness of muscles embedded in a certain compartment. Symptoms are related to activity and subside at rest. CECS of the lower leg is well known; however, it frequently occurs in the forearm and thigh. Theoretically CECS can involve any muscle contained within a compartment. CECS of rare locations such as the gluteus muscles or muscles around the shoulder has been reported.

Pathogenesis

Muscles receive all necessary nutrients in the flow of blood, which occurs only during the relaxation phase of muscle contracture. During exercises, the muscles swell up, the arterial and venous blood flow slows down, and the intracompartmental pressure increases. Because the muscles are encased within very rigid compartments, there is no reserve space within them. As a result, blood flow is restricted, delivering an insufficient amount of oxygen and other vital elements. In addition, removal of potentially harmful products of metabolism is slower because of venous congestion. The organism reacts with pain.

The probable pathophysiology of the CECS is explainable based on present knowledge of physiology, anatomy, and physics. Why just limited numbers of athletes develop the symptoms is, however, unknown.

Clinical Findings

A. SYMPTOMS AND SIGNS

- Muscle pain during or after exercise.
- Hypoesthesia or dysesthesia.
- Tinnel sign.
- Pedowitz criteria: resting pressure is >15 mm Hg, 1 minute after exercise it is >30 mm Hg, and 5 minutes after exercise it is >20 mm Hg.

B. IMAGING STUDIES

Different imaging techniques have been employed to aid in diagnosing CECS. The different diagnostic tests are commonly more helpful in ruling out other causes of an extremity pain than in confirming the diagnosis of CECS. Radiographs help to diagnose fracture, tumor, or stress fracture. An MRI study facilitates the diagnosis of stress reaction versus stress fracture and may uncover other causes of pain. An MRI of the muscles involved in CECS may show a nonspecific, slightly increased signal on T2 images. T1 remains unchanged.

Near-infrared spectroscopy has been reported to be a valuable tool; however, its predictive value needs to be confirmed. A single-photon emission computed tomography (SPECT) bone scan with thallium-201 sometimes shows areas of ischemia, a rather late sign of CECS. A clinical history and measurement of intracompartmental pressure are still the gold standard of diagnosis.

Differential Diagnosis

- Stress fracture.
- Stress reaction.
- Fracture.
- Complex regional pain syndrome.
- Tumor (osteoid osteoma).
- Deep venous thrombosis.
- Peripheral vascular disease.
- Gastrocnemius strain.
- Medial tibial stress syndrome (Figure 9–30).

Treatment

Treatment of CECS relies on stretching, icing, and rest. Nonoperative treatment, however, has had limited success. Surgical release of the involved compartments is usually necessary to relieve symptoms of an established and confirmed CECS. Prior to surgery, other possible causes of pain of the extremity must be excluded.

In the case of confirmed, lower leg CECS, the standard of care is an open, four compartment fasciotomy. The release of the "fifth compartment," the tibialis posterior muscle compartment, may also be necessary. An endoscopically guided compartment release offers the advantage of a small incision and good visualization. Compartment release done through a very small incision (percutaneously), without endoscopic enhancement, seems to be the worst option, carrying the highest risk for nerve injury.

Return to Play

After successful surgery, return to sport depends exclusively on healing of the incisions, typically 6 weeks after the indexed surgery. On many occasions, the adolescent or pediatric patient resumes full activities much earlier, against official recommendations. This seems to have no detrimental effect on the final outcome of the treatment. With proper diagnosis and uncomplicated surgery, full recovery of function, return to sport, and relief of pain should be the expected outcome.

Aoki Y et al: Magnetic resonance imaging in stress fractures and shin splints. Clin Orthop 2004;(421):260.

Fraipont MJ, Adamson GJ: Chronic exertional compartment syndrome. J Am Acad Orthop Surg 2003;11(4):268.

Hutchinson MR et al: Anatomic structures at risk during minimal-incision endoscopically assisted fascial compartment releases in the leg. Am J Sports Med 2003;31(5):764.

Ota Y et al: Chronic compartment syndrome of the lower leg: a new diagnostic method using near-infrared spectroscopy and a new technique of endoscopic fasciotomy. Arthroscopy 1999;15(4):439.

Shah SN et al: Chronic exertional compartment syndrome. Am J Orthop 2004;33(7):335.

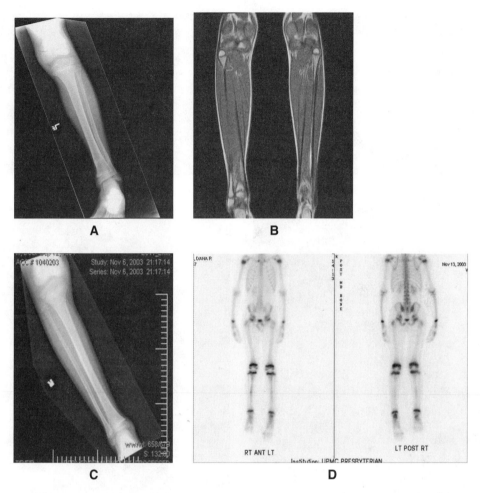

Figure 9–30. Stress fractures. Healed fracture of the distal tibia that happened 7 months ago. There is now pain over the proximal fibula of the ipsilateral leg. X-Ray shows periosteal reaction of the proximal fibula (*A*). MRI of the lower leg consistent with a stress fracture (*B*). Stress fracture of the right tibia in an 8-year-old baseball player (*C*). Bone scan shows increased uptake at the midshaft of the tibia (*D*).

INCREASED FEMORAL ANTEVERSION WITH INCREASED EXTERNAL TIBIAL TORSION: MISERABLE MALROTATION SYNDROME

In clinical practice, a small subset of patients will manifest with so called miserable (malignant) malrotation syndrome (MMS). This syndrome, which can be diagnosed after the age of 9–10 years, consists of increased internal rotation of the hip with coincidental increased external tibial torsion. MMS is more commonly observed among girls, and is associated with patellar maltracking problems and knee pain. A patient with MMS walks with an internally rotated patellae, with a neutral foot progression angle. A patient who tries to correct the position of the patella routinely rotates the feet outward as a result of increased external tibial torsion.

Initial treatment consists of physical therapy and a patellofemoral program.

With persistent pain and with no sign of other intraarticular pathology surgical intervention might be warranted. It is wise to document the MMS by rotational CT assessment of the femoral anteversion and tibial torsion prior to surgical correction of MMS.

To correct the MMS it is necessary to address both levels of the deformity. Delgado et al perform the osteotomies as close to the knee joint as possible. The authors prefer a derotational femoral osteotomy over a

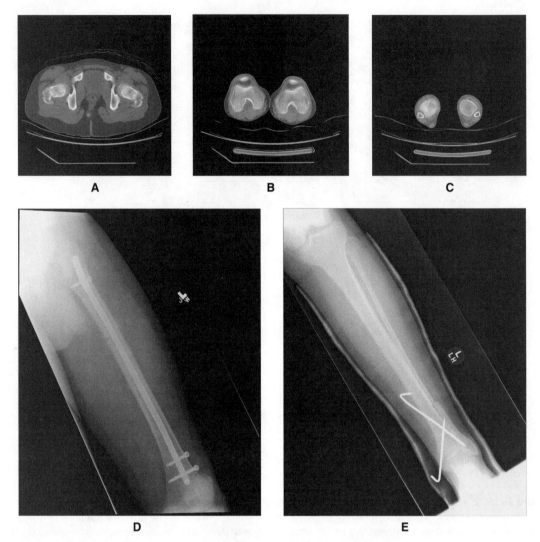

Figure 9–31. Three CT cuts necessary to evaluate the rotational profile: femoral neck orientation (**A**), position of the femoral condyles (**B**), and torsion of the tibia/lower leg (**C**). Miserable malalignment syndrome: derotational osteotomy using intramedulary fixation (**D**). Supramalleolar osteotomy of the tibia. Added osteotomy of the fibula allows for free derotation of the distal fragment. The osteotomy is stabilized by two smooth Steinman pins (**E**).

trochanteric nail for correction of the femur. Correction of the tibial torsion is usually addressed by a supramalleolar osteotomy with cross pin fixation (Figure 9–31).

The results of the surgical treatment are usually good. In a series of 14 patients with 27 affected limbs all patients were very satisfied with the results.

A bilevel osteotomy for documented cases of MMS should provide lasting relief of pain.

Bruce WD, Stevens PM: Surgical correction of miserable malalignment syndrome. J Pediatr Orthop 2004;24(4):392.

Delgado ED et al: Treatment of severe torsional malalignment syndrome. J Pediatr Orthop 1996;16(4):484.

Tonnis D, Heinecke A: Acetabular and femoral anteversion: relationship with osteoarthritis of the hip. J Bone Joint Surg Am 1999;81(12):1747.

CONTUSIONS

Pathogenesis

Contusions are probably the most common injuries that occur around the pelvis and lower extremities. They are caused by direct blows to the most prominent parts of the pelvic girdle or to a muscle.

Clinical Findings

A. SYMPTOMS AND SIGNS

Contusions are common in football (tackle), baseball (sliding), and soccer (direct kick). The contused part of the body hurts. Redness, swelling, and the formation of a subcutaneous hematoma follow. The hematoma is sometimes quite large. Contusion of the quadriceps manifests with subcutaneous hematoma and deep pain with palpation and stretching; swelling accompanies a more serious contusion. In severe cases, the hemorrhage may depose a large quantity of blood within a compartment, creating the possibility of compartment syndrome (Figure 9–32).

The hip pointer refers to a contusion of the iliac wing or greater trochanter. It presents with localized pain after direct injury. Pain sometimes is pronounced, accentuated by rotation of the trunk.

B. IMAGING STUDIES

A radiograph may be considered after more violent injuries to rule out fractures. An MRI should be obtained in cases of large, nonresolving swelling and hematoma.

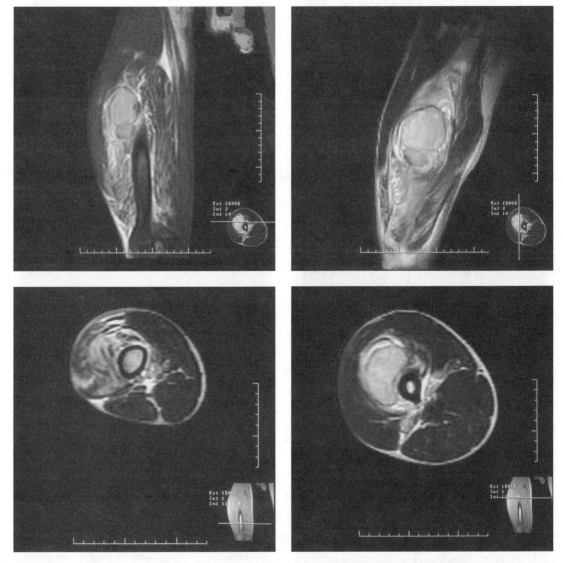

Figure 9–32. Large hematoma of a quadriceps muscle after a direct blow to the right thigh while playing football.

Differential Diagnosis

- Fracture.
- Avulsion fracture.
- Compartment syndrome.
- Apophysitis.

Treatment

A classic RICE approach is the standard treatment for contusions. A patient with the hip pointer should be allowed to rest, with return to sport guided by symptoms. ROM exercises and stretching will aid in providing a gradual return to full activity.

Very extensive quadriceps contusions, especially if accompanied by a large hemorrhage, should be approached cautiously. Initially, the RICE approach is sufficient. Immobilization of the lower extremity, with the knee flexed, prevents the quadriceps from developing a flexion contracture. Monitoring for possible compartment syndrome might be necessary. Classic compartment symptoms such as pain, numbness, tingling, and weakness might occur several hours after the initial injury or even the next day. A large hematoma with numbness and tingling, increasing pain impossible to control by oral pain medication, and pain with stretching of the flexors or extensors of the knee joint will be an indication to release all compartments of the thigh.

The need to address an evolving compartment syndrome is obvious; evacuation of a large hematoma is controversial. Based on the current literature there is no reason to evacuate a hematoma unless there are neurologic symptoms.

Rehabilitation & Return to Play

If a patient does not develop significant problems, return to sport is guided by subjective symptoms. A rehabilitation program designed to recover full strength and function of the quadriceps and hamstring muscles will aid in returning to sport within a relatively brief period of time.

Diaz JA et al: Severe quadriceps muscle contusions in athletes. A report of three cases. Am J Sports Med 2003;31(2):289.

■ UPPER EXTREMITY PROBLEMS

ANATOMY

1. Shoulder

A shoulder girdle is composed of a scapula, a clavicle, and the proximal humerus. The glenohumeral joint is a spheroid joint between the glenoid of the scapula and the proximal humerus. A shoulder is not mature until age 25 years, when the clavicle fully ossifies. Other important ossification centers and their age at fusion are the body of the scapula (appears at 8 weeks fetal), acromion and coracoid (both at 15 years), clavicle (at 5 weeks fetal), body of the humerus (at 8 weeks fetal), head of the humerus (at 1 year), greater tuberosity (at 3 years), and lesser tuberosity (at 5 years). The scapular as well as the humeral ossification centers fuse at age 20 years. Until completely fused, the physeal cartilage of an apophysis is inherently weaker than the muscles and ligaments that attach to it. Therefore, excessive forces may lead to avulsion fractures rather then ligament ruptures in an immature athlete (Figure 9–33).

The glenohumeral joint is the most commonly dislocated large joint in the body. Recurrent dislocation rates in children can reach 100%. Static restraints (articular

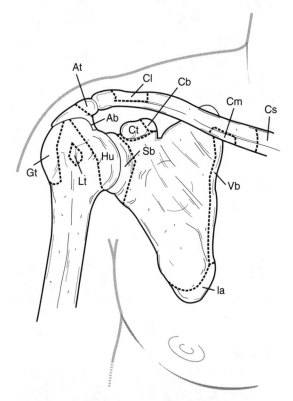

Figure 9–33. Schematic of the ossification centers of the clavicle (Cs, sternal border of the clavicle; Cm, medial clavicle; Cl, lateral clavicle), scapula (Sb, base of the scapula; Ia, inferior angle; Vb, vertical border; Cb, base of the coracoid; Ct, top of the coracoid; Ab, base of the acromion; At, top of the acromion), and proximal humerus (Hu, humerus head; Gt, greater tuberosity; Lt, lesser tuberosity).

anatomy, labrum, joint capsule and ligaments, negative pressure) and dynamic restraints (shoulder muscles and scapulothoracic motion) all work together to prevent dislocation. The acromioclavicular (AC) joint is a gliding joint with very limited ROM. It consists of a capsule, an AC ligament (primary restraint to AP displacement of the distal clavicle), and a coracoclavicular (CC) ligament (primary restraint to superior displacement of the distal clavicle). The CC ligament is further divided into a trapezoid ligament and a stronger conoid ligament.

Fifteen muscles move the shoulder. The rhomboideus major and minor, trapezius, latissimus, and levator scapulae connect the upper limb to the vertebral column. The pectoralis major and minor, subclavius, and serratus anterior connect the upper limb to the thoracic wall. The deltoid and teres major abduct and adduct the upper limb, respectively. Four muscles of the rotator cuff act to depress and stabilize the humeral head in the glenoid; supraspinatus, infraspinatus, and teres minor attach to the greater tuberosity of the humerus and externally rotate the upper limb; the subscapularis muscle attaches to the lesser tuberosity and internally rotates the upper limb. In contrast to degenerative muscle tears and tendinitis, which occur in the adult patient population, young athletes tend to develop avulsion fractures, since connection of a muscle to bone occurs usually via an apophysis.

The upper extremity muscles are innervated by the brachial plexus, formed by the ventral primary rami of C5–T1. The brachial plexus is protected underneath the clavicle and is organized into five levels: roots, trunks, divisions, cords, and branches. There are four preclavicular branches: the dorsal scapular nerve, long thoracic nerve, suprascapular nerve, and nerve to the subclavius. Preganglionic injuries to the brachial plexus can be differentiated from postganglionic injuries by the presence of scapular winging (injury to the long thoracic nerve) and Horner syndrome (injury to C8–T1, involving the stellate ganglion). Typical obstetric injuries to the brachial plexus result in Erb–Duchenne palsy at C5–C6, which involves the deltoid, rotator cuff, elbow flexors, as well as wrist and hand extensors, or Klumpke palsy at C8–T1, which involves Horner syndrome, wrist flexors, and hand intrinsics, and has a poorer prognosis.

LITTLE LEAGUE SHOULDER

General Considerations

Because Little League shoulder is a condition that affects mostly adolescent patients overusing their shoulder while pitching, preventive recommendations have been made by the USA Baseball Medical and Safety Advisory Committee. According to their guidelines a young pitcher should refrain from throwing more than 75 pitches per week (9–10 years old), 100 pitches per week (11–12 years old), or 125 pitches per week (13–14 years old). Athletes are at highest risk in their mid teens, when the growth spurt occurs and they develop more skillful and powerful pitching techniques (Figure 9–34).

Clinical Findings

A. SYMPTOMS AND SIGNS

A typical patient with a Little League shoulder is an adolescent baseball pitcher who presents with a gradual onset of pain localized to the proximal humerus and exacerbated by vigorous throwing. Pain is not restricted to a certain phase of throwing. Sudden onset of pain and residual pain after throwing are rare. The average duration of symptoms is between 6 and 9 months.

A tenderness to palpation over the lateral proximal humeral physis is the most common clinical finding. This was found to be reliable in 70% of patients. Pain with passive ROM and resistance to external and internal rotations can be seen. Weakness with external rotation occurs in up to 25% of patients. Swelling is uncommon.

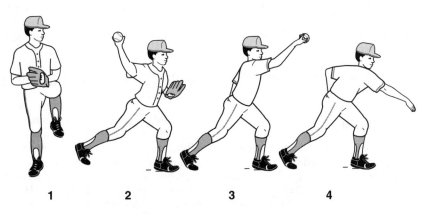

Figure 9–34. Schematic of the throwing phases: (***1***) wind up; (***2***) cocking; (***3***) acceleration; (***4***) deceleration.

B. Imaging Studies

Bilateral AP radiographs in internal and external rotation allow both proximal humeri to be compared. Radiographic widening of the involved proximal humeral physis is found in almost all cases. In 50% of the patients, lateral metaphyseal fragmentation or demineralization may be found, which is indicative of chronic changes. However, contrary to a displaced Salter–Harris type I fracture, reossification of the epiphysis takes between 8 weeks and 12 months. Plain radiographs can show the proximal humeral physis and are usually sufficient to diagnose a Little League shoulder.

An MRI may be necessary in the diagnosis of a Little League shoulder. It can be helpful in diagnosing associated conditions, such as epiphyseal fractures, infections, osteomyelitis, bone bruises, cysts, or tumors.

Differential Diagnosis

- Rotator cuff tendinitis.
- Biceps tendinitis.
- Multidirectional shoulder instability.
- Traumatic anterior dislocation.
- Traumatic posterior dislocation.
- Clavicular epiphyseal injury.
- SLAP lesion.

Treatment

Treatment of a patient with Little League shoulder starts with prevention and close supervision of young athletes, following the guidance of the USA Baseball Medical and Safety Advisory Committee. Treatment of Little League shoulder syndrome includes rest, ice, and NSAIDs.

Return to Play

An average recommended period of rest from throwing is about 3 months. A young athlete should be allowed to begin to throw again only after all symptoms have subsided. In the largest case series reported in the literature, 21 of 23 adolescent baseball players were able to return to asymptomatic pitching at the Little League level within 1–12 months (average 3 months) after being diagnosed with Little League shoulder symptoms.

ROTATOR CUFF TENDINITIS

Rotator cuff tendinitis is very common in the adult athlete engaged in activity involving overhead motion. In adolescents, it is relatively frequent in athletes with increased joint laxity and instability. With prolonged overhead activity, excessive motions of the humeral head in the glenoid cause inflammation of the rotator cuff muscles, with pain in the shoulder and decreased strength. Typically, pain starts during warm-ups and shows no improvement as practice or the game progresses. Late cocking, with the shoulder in maximum external rotation, and deceleration phases produce the most prominent symptoms. Tenderness over the rotator cuff muscles is the leading symptom, but there is no bony tenderness.

Treatment consists of nonoperative measures; patients generally respond well, depending on their cooperation with the therapy. Conservative treatment consists of rest, physical therapy, with special attention to strengthening the rotator cuff muscles, and NSAIDs. In severe cases involving acute tears, rotator cuff repair is recommended.

BICEPS TENDINITIS

The short head of the biceps muscle originates from the coracoid process with the long head attached to the glenoid labrum. Biceps tendinitis is an inflammation that causes pain at the insertion of the short head to the coracoid process. It results from overuse of the arm and shoulder, commonly related to overhead activities. Adolescent athletes complain of pain while moving the arm and shoulder, especially with extension and elevation. On clinical examination there is a tenderness to touch of the anterior shoulder over the coracoid process, along the biceps tendon and muscle. In growing athletes an apophysitis of the coracoid process may cause point tenderness at the origin of the short head.

Treatment is usually nonoperative, unless an acute tear of the biceps is involved. Conservative treatment consists of ice, in conjunction with physical therapy. A brief period of immobilization in combination with NSAIDs usually provides sufficient pain relief.

The goal of physical therapy is to ensure a safe return to sport. Adolescent patients may safely return to sports after an injured shoulder has regained a pain-free full ROM and normal strength, as compared to the contralateral shoulder. Tendinitis can best be prevented by following proper warm-ups and stretching exercises for the arm and shoulder, and by following guidelines of the athletic associations.

EPIPHYSEAL FRACTURE OF THE DISTAL CLAVICLE

AC injuries in the skeletally immature patient can be divided into five types. In contrast to AC injuries in the adult, the CC ligament never detaches from the periosteal sleeve of the distal clavicle. A type I injury is a contusion resulting from a direct force to the acromion, not violent enough to disrupt the AC or CC ligaments. In type II injuries the periosteal sleeve is partially torn with the CC ligament intact and AC ligaments disrupted.

Therefore the distal clavicle is not displaced. Type III and IV injuries present with completely torn AC ligaments and a tear of the periosteal tube, leading to unstable superior displacement. In type III injuries the clavicle is displaced only in a superior direction, whereas in type IV injuries the clavicle is also displaced posteriorly. In type V injuries the AC ligament is not in continuity with CC ligaments attached to the periosteal sleeve, and the distal end of the clavicle is buried within the trapezius or deltoid muscle. Type III–V injuries involve displacement of the distal clavicle and display the typical "piano key sign." A pseudodislocation of the distal clavicle due to unrecognized fractures has been described (Figure 9–35).

Type I, II, and III injuries can generally be treated nonoperatively with a shoulder sling or a figure-of-eight brace. Small bony prominences are generally accepted, as the risks of elective surgical repair outweigh the benefits of anatomic reconstruction. Interestingly, a new clavicle will remodel from the periosteal sleeve, and the displaced part of the broken clavicle will be reabsorbed over time. Open reduction and internal fixation may be considered for markedly displaced type IV and V injuries and for injuries involving neurovascular compromise during surgery. It is important to disengage the dislocated distal clavicle from underneath the trapezius and deltoid muscles, place it in the periosteal tube, and repair the periosteum. The deltoid–trapezius fascia imbrication over the clavicle will additionally stabilize the clavicle.

TRAUMATIC SHOULDER DISLOCATION

General Considerations

Most acute, first-time shoulder dislocations are related to sports injuries, whereas recurrent dislocations usually are not. Episodes of recurrent dislocation are reported at 75–100% in adolescent athletes. Anterior dislocations are far more common than posterior dislocations, which are usually the result of epileptic seizures or electricity-related injuries. Because the glenohumeral joint has the largest ROM of any joint in the human body, it is relatively easy to dislocate.

Pathogenesis

Young athletes with glenohumeral joint dislocation usually report one of the following mechanisms of injury: an aggressive jerk during contact sports (football, wrestling) or a minor trauma (swimming, pitching). Glenohumeral joint dislocation need not involve trauma; it can occur when reaching overhead or putting a jacket on. Anterior instability commonly presents with pain or apprehension with abduction, external rotation, and extension. Posterior instability is suggested by pain or

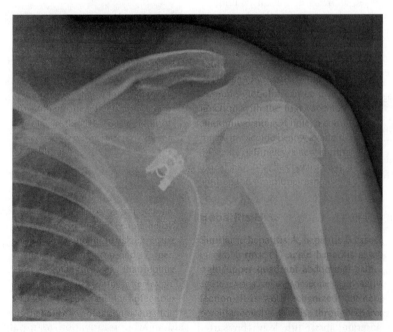

Figure 9–35. An anteroposterior radiograph of a 14-year-old soccer player showing a type III clavicular epiphyseal fracture.

apprehension during a flexed, adducted, and internally rotated position. An initial traumatic dislocation is usually difficult to reduce without the assistance of a physician. A patient with recurrent dislocation and associated joint laxity can easily self-reduce the dislocation.

Clinical Findings

A. Symptoms and Signs

Both shoulders should be examined to assess the difference between a noninvolved and an injured shoulder and to look for bilateral shoulder instability. Palpation of the shoulder reveals anterior tenderness in patients with anterior glenohumeral instability. ROM is full and the apprehension test with terminal external rotation, with the arm in the abducted position, is positive. Anterior and posterior drawer tests reveal laxity of the glenohumeral joint in the sagittal plane. The tests are performed at 0, 30, and 60° of abduction and at 0, 30, and 60° of external rotation. Laxity occurs in three grades. In grade I, the examiner can sublux the humeral head within the glenoid cavity. In grade II the humeral head can be subluxed onto the glenoid rim and in grade III it can be dislocated over the glenoid rim. During the anterior apprehension test, an anterior force is applied to the humeral head, with the arm held at 90° abduction and progressively externally rotated. A patient resists increasing external rotation secondary to discomfort and apprehension. With a relocation test, a patient feels more stable and experiences less apprehension as an examiner applies posteriorly directed pressure with a similar maneuver. A sulcus test is usually positive after traumatic dislocation of a shoulder, indicating inferior instability. For this test the arm is in neutral rotation, and a downward force is applied as the shoulder is relaxed.

B. Imaging Studies

Standard shoulder radiographs include an AP and a lateral view of the shoulder, a scapula-Y view, and an axillary lateral view (Figure 9–36). An AP view in internal rotation can reveal a posterolateral impression fracture on the humeral head, a Hill–Sachs lesion. The axillary lateral view is more specific for glenoid fractures, deformity, or glenoid hypoplasia. Abnormalities of the glenoid, seen on plain radiographs, may be evaluated by a CT scan. A CT arthrogram provides valuable information about the labrum, capsule volume, and bony geometry of the humerus and the glenoid. For a CT and MRI arthrogram, radiopaque contrast dye is injected into the glenohumeral joint space under fluoroscopic guidance, prior to the imaging. A defect of the capsule can be detected by the presence of extravasation of the dye. An MRI can identify anterior labral pathology (Bankart lesion). MRI arthrograms show more detailed images of the labrum, insertion of the biceps into the labrum,

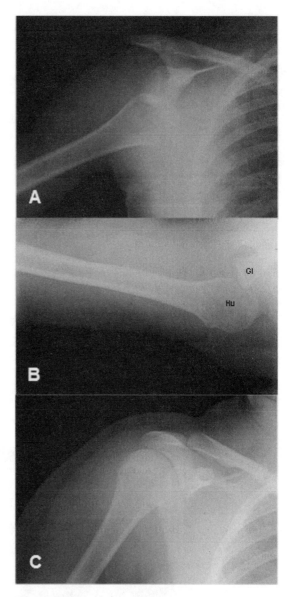

Figure 9–36. Radiographs of a 17-year-old female field hockey player; a first time, acute, traumatic, anterior shoulder dislocation. ***A:*** An anteroposterior radiograph showing an inferior dislocation. ***B:*** An axial lateral radiograph showing anterior dislocation and posterolateral impingement of the humeral head (Hu) under the glenoid (Gl). ***C:*** An AP radiograph showing relocation of the shoulder.

rotator cuff, and capsular anatomy. Invasive tests can add valuable information to the diagnostic work-up, however, indications for these tests should be very specific (Figure 9–37).

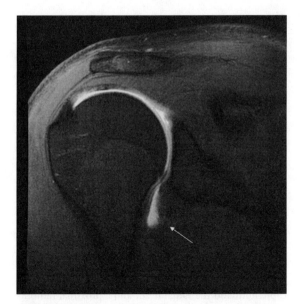

Figure 9–37. Coronal MR arthrogram of a right shoulder in a 17-year-old male soccer player showing an anterior labrum tear with extravasation of contrast inferiorly (**arrow**).

Sometimes examination under anesthesia (EUA) may be necessary for patients with guarding, pain, and discomfort during examination in the office, or who are extremely muscular. EUA will help in detecting the true magnitude and direction of instability, which may change the treatment plan. Diagnostic arthroscopy has been a wonderful tool, providing further information about the internal glenohumeral anatomy.

Treatment

A. NONOPERATIVE

Nonoperative treatment of traumatic anterior shoulder dislocation involves a closed reduction, preferably under conscious sedation, to prevent further damage during the reduction maneuver. The period of immobilization usually lasts 3–4 weeks. Restriction from sports activities for 6 weeks after the initial anterior shoulder dislocation may lower the recurrence rate. A physical therapy program designed to strengthen the rotator cuff and scapular muscles follows immobilization.

B. OPERATIVE

Operative treatment involves surgical repair of torn structures, performed either arthroscopically or using open techniques. Techniques for repair of a skeletally immature shoulder injury are similar to those for the adult population.

Deitch J et al: Traumatic anterior shoulder dislocation in adolescents. Am J Sports Med 2003;31(5):758.

Postacchini F et al: Anterior shoulder dislocation in adolescents. J Shoulder Elbow Surg 2000;9(6):470.

SUPERIOR LABRUM, ANTERIOR, & POSTERIOR LESIONS

General Considerations

Injuries to the superior labrum in overhead-throwing athletes have been divided into superior labrum, anterior, and posterior (SLAP) lesions, and classified into four subtypes. The incidence of SLAP lesions, however, remains unclear, although reports in the literature indicate involvement of between 6 and 26% of patients complaining of shoulder pain. Recently more and more young patients are being diagnosed with SLAP. Type I, which occurs in 10% of all SLAPs, is characterized by fraying of the superior labrum. It is usually degenerative, and is associated with rotator cuff disease. In type II lesions (40%), the biceps anchor is detached from the superior labrum with simultaneous fraying of the SLAP complex. A type II lesion occurring in younger patients is more frequently associated with traumatic instability compared to types III and IV. Type III (35%), a bucket handle tear of the labrum with an intact biceps tendon, progresses to a more extensive type IV (15%), which is a bucket handle tear and extension of the tear into the biceps tendon. Types II, III, and IV are more common in younger patients.

Clinical Findings

A. SYMPTOMS AND SIGNS

Traction and compression injuries may cause a SLAP lesion. Traction injuries are typical in baseball throwing. They also happen with attempts to brace during falls or after sudden pulls. Compression injuries may result from a fall onto an outstretched hand.

Patients usually complain of vague shoulder pain, exacerbated by overhead activity with popping, locking, or snapping. Sometimes torn and unstable fragments (type II–IV) block ROM of an injured shoulder, as they may be trapped between the humeral head and glenoid. Instability is usually not a part of a SLAP, but may be present with simultaneous Bankart lesions (Figure 9–38).

B. IMAGING STUDIES

Radiographic examination includes standard views of the shoulder: AP, an axillary, and an outlet view. An MRI and MRI arthrograms help detect labral pathology, especially with an intraarticular injection of gadolinium, which increases the sensitivity and specificity of detecting labral lesions up to 90%.

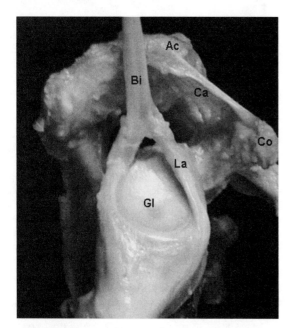

Figure 9–38. Anatomical preparation of a shoulder showing a type III superior labrum, anterior, and posterior (SLAP) lesion. Gl, glenoid; La, labrum; Bi, biceps tendon; Ac, acromion; Ca, coracoacromial ligament; Co, coracoid process.

C. PHYSICAL EXAMINATION

Clinical testing is still relatively subjective and not extremely predictable. The Speed biceps tension test is reported to be the most reliable, and is performed with the patient resisting downward pressure in 90° of forward elevation with the elbow extended and the forearm supinated. Pain as a result of inflammation, or damage of the superior labrum, is considered a positive test. In the O'Brien test, the patient's shoulder is held in 90° of forward flexion, 30° of horizontal adduction, and maximal internal rotation. Patients with a SLAP lesion report pain in response to resisted horizontal adduction and forward flexion of the shoulder. In a compression–rotation test, the patient is positioned supine. The glenohumeral joint is compressed with the shoulder at 90° of abduction and the elbow flexed at 90°. This test can trap the injured labrum between the glenoid and humeral head, which results in an audible clunk.

Treatment

Treatment for SLAP lesions is surgical. Type I lesions require debridement of the torn labrum. Type II lesions can usually be repaired with sutures, tacks, or suture anchors. Type III and IV injuries require resection of the unstable displaced bucket handle labrum fragment, followed by reattachment of the biceps anchor. Physical therapy is done after immobilization. The average return to sport for the young athletes is 6–9 months after surgery.

Bencardino JT et al: Superior labrum anterior-posterior lesions: diagnosis with MR arthrography of the shoulder. Radiology 2000;214(1):267.

Kim TK et al: Clinical features of the different types of SLAP lesions: an analysis of one hundred and thirty-nine cases. Superior labrum anterior posterior. J Bone Joint Surg Am 2003;85-A(1)66.

ANATOMY

2. Elbow

An elbow consists of a humerus, an ulna, and a radius. A humeroulnar joint between the trochlea and the trochlear notch, a humeroradial joint between the capitellum and the radial head, and a proximal radioulnar joint between the radial notch and the radial head connect these three bones. In a young athlete, a radiograph of the elbow shows unique, age-specific bony anatomy of the joint. It is therefore crucial to understand patterns of ossification of an elbow. An ossification center of the capitellum appears at 2 years, the radial head at 5 years, the medial epicondyle at 7 years, the trochlea at 9 years, the olecranon at 10 years, and the lateral epicondyle at 11 years. Distal humerus ossification centers fuse with the body of the humerus at age 16–18 years. The proximal radius fuses at 15–18 years and the olecranon fuses with the body of the ulna at 16 years (Figure 9–39).

The essential stabilizer on the lateral side is the lateral ulnar collateral ligament (LUCL). It inserts at the lateral epicondyle and the supinator crest of the ulna. Deficiency of the LUCL results in posterolateral rotatory instability of the elbow. The MCL consists of the anterior band, which is the strongest of the elbow ligaments and is tight in extension, the posterior band, tight in flexion, and the transverse band.

MEDIAL EPICONDYLITIS (LITTLE LEAGUE ELBOW)

General Considerations

Young athletes involved in throwing activities, such as pitching in baseball, commonly complain of medial elbow pain. During the acceleration phase of the throwing motion, an elbow is subjected to substantial valgus stresses, which increase tensile loads on the medial side and compression loads on the lateral side. Repetitive tensile loads onto the medial elbow may cause injury to

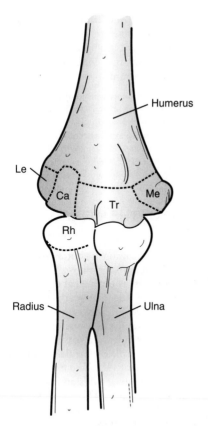

Figure 9–39. Schematic of the ossification centers of the elbow. Ca, capitellum; Rh, radial head; Me, medial epicondyle; Tr, trochlea; Le, lateral epicondyle.

a physis of the medial epicondyle. A medial epicondylitis in children and adolescents refers to a true apophysitis, also termed Little League elbow, whereas in adults a medial epicondylitis consists of tendinitis of the flexor—pronator tendons. Athletes with this condition are usually between 8 and 12 years old, commonly pitchers in baseball, with a history of heavy throwing.

Clinical Findings

A. SYMPTOMS AND SIGNS

Symptoms include medial elbow pain with insidious onset, in combination with a normal ROM of the affected joint, without locking or catching.

B. IMAGING STUDIES

Positive radiographic findings are not necessary to establish the diagnosis. Three views of the injured elbow, with comparison views, are usually sufficient. Until age 15 years, ossification centers of an elbow are at different stages of fusion, and multiple physeal lines make judgment of elbow pathology in an immature athlete difficult. The medial epicondyle and physis of a little league athlete's elbow may appear normal or may show widening of the physeal line.

C. PHYSICAL EXAMINATION

The diagnosis is usually made based on a clinical examination. Inspection of the elbow may reveal mild soft tissues swelling over the medial epicondyle. Palpation exposes tenderness over a medial epicondyle. A valgus stress applied to an elbow may reproduce the pain. A Tinnel test can be positive, with paresthesias in the ulnar nerve distribution, secondary to soft tissue swelling around the medial epicondyle, and its ulnar groove.

Differential Diagnosis

- Osteochondritis dissecans of the capitellum.
- Panner disease.
- Olecranon avulsion fracture.
- Supracondylar humerus fracture.
- Medial epicondyle fracture.
- Elbow dislocations.

Treatment

Prevention of Little League elbow is a multidisciplinary task, with parents, trainers, and coaches working together to protect young athletes. The USA Baseball Medical and Safety Advisory Committee recommends that pitching should be limited to six innings per week, and should include mandatory rest between sessions. Assessment of throwing technique is necessary to initiate appropriate, and gradually advancing, throwing programs.

Management of Little League elbow is usually nonoperative, with rest from throwing activities being crucial for the results of treatment. Application of ice to the elbow as well as antiinflammatory medications can help in the process. Research has shown that the number of pitches thrown during a certain time period is the strongest determinant of elbow pain. Therefore, patients with moderate to severe symptoms should refrain from throwing and pitching until symptoms have completely subsided; the athletes can then enter specific practice programs with progressive throwing. The number and velocity of pitching may slowly advance, not exceeding the recommended intensity.

Lyman S et al: Effect of pitch type, pitch count, and pitching mechanics on risk of elbow and shoulder pain in youth baseball pitchers. Am J Sports Med 2002;30(4):463.

PANNER DISEASE

The combination of repetitive trauma, caused by throwing activities in adolescent patients, together with the limited blood supply to the distal humerus in immature patients causes the typical symptoms of Panner disease, an avascular necrosis of the capitellum. During cocking and acceleration phases of throwing, the lateral elbow is subjected to compression loads.

The clinical presentation of Panner disease is very similar to an OCD, except for locking and catching, which usually are not present. The onset is insidious, with pain aggravated by activity, and there is usually a history of mild trauma or overuse. On physical examination, the extension of the involved elbow is limited to 20°. The primary difference between OCD of the capitellum and Panner disease is the age of presentation. Generally, patients 10 years and younger suffer from Panner disease. Intraarticular loose bodies are more commonly seen in older adolescents.

Radiographs reveal a flattened capitellum with areas of sclerosis, and a rough, or fragmented articular margin.

Management is similar to treatment for an OCD and requires complete rest from throwing, until revascularization of the capitellum is radiographically confirmed.

OSTEOCHONDRITIS DISSECANS OF THE CAPITELLUM

The etiology of OCD is not entirely understood, however, this injury is usually seen in elbows subjected to repetitive microtrauma. OCD is a pathologic condition of the capitellum, with abnormal subchondral bone in the body of the capitellum, and overlying cartilage. An osteochondral fragment may separate, and become a loose body, causing decreased ROM, or locking. Athletes are usually 12–16 years old and present with lateral elbow pain with associated locking, catching, and loss of full extension of the joint. Patients with acute OCD usually present with joint effusion. Tenderness to palpation over the radiocapitellar joint is common, but not pathognomonic.

Plain radiographs help to establish the diagnosis of OCD and to assess the severity of the disease. The capitellum usually reveals an area of radiolucency, or a radiolucent line demarcating an osteochondral fragment. Loose bodies can also be seen, and the articular contour of the capitellum may be irregular. In cases of suspected damage to the intraarticular cartilage, an MRI may further delineate the pathology.

Treatment of OCD of the capitellum depends on the severity of the disease and the integrity of the articular cartilage. With no clinical or radiographic evidence indicating cartilage pathology or absence of loose bodies, treatment may be nonoperative, with rest, immobilization, and NSAIDs. Rest is continued until full radiographic resolution of the defect is appreciated. In more advanced stages, surgical treatment may be indicated for removal of loose bodies, or to restore continuity of the cartilage. Cartilage damage represents a difficult problem that may lead to permanent loss of function and premature arthritis.

Kiyoshige Y et al: Closed-wedge osteotomy for osteochondritis dissecans of the capitellum. A 7- to 12-year follow-up. Am J Sports Med 2000;28(4):534.

Takeda H et al: A surgical treatment for unstable osteochondritis dissecans lesions of the humeral capitellum in adolescent baseball players. Am J Sports Med 2002;30(5):713.

Yadao MA et al: Osteochondritis dissecans of the elbow. Instr Course Lect 2004;53:599.

FRACTURE OF THE MEDIAL EPICONDYLE

Medial epicondyle avulsion fractures result from acute, excessive valgus forces to the elbow. They usually occur in adolescent athletes, as the medial epicondyle ossification center begins to fuse. Young athletes usually report a sudden "pop," or even "giving way" of the elbow during cocking or during the acceleration phase of throwing. The physical examination correlates well with the history, and reveals isolated medial elbow pain with swelling and decreased ROM. The most specific clinical test for medial epicondylar avulsion fractures is a valgus stress test at 30° of flexion. The test is positive when it elicits medial elbow pain. An injury to the MCL may present with similar findings.

Nonoperative treatment is the treatment of choice if there is no associated MCL injury and for fractures with less than 5 mm displacement. The elbow will be immobilized in a posterior splint, or cast at 90° of flexion, for 4–6 weeks. Protected active and passive ROM exercises will help regain full ROM.

Surgical treatment is warranted for displaced fractures and MCL-deficient joints. Surgery consists of an anatomic reduction of the displaced fragment. The MCL can be either repaired end to end or reconstructed. If indicated, an autologous palmaris longus tendon graft can be used, however, a high incidence of damage to the ulnar nerve is reported with reconstruction of an MCL.

Gradual return to athletic activity may be considered after several months of rehabilitation, with ROM exercises and progressive muscle strengthening. Moderate throwing will be allowed after 6 months with progressively advancing physical therapy programs.

SUPRACONDYLAR HUMERUS FRACTURE

Supracondylar humerus fractures are the most common fracture of the elbow. At our institution more than 200 supracondylar fractures, types II and III, are treated every year. Children are usually 5–8 years old and break their elbow after a fall onto an outstretched upper extremity. More then 90% of these fractures present as an extension type.

Garland classified supracondylar humerus fractures into types I, II, and III. Nondisplaced fractures are type I, angulated fractures with an intact posterior cortex are type II, and displaced fractures are type III. Children with these fractures should be evaluated carefully for associated neurovascular injuries, which occur in 5–20% of fractures. An inability to pinch (median nerve, anterior interosseous branch), to extend the wrist and thumb (radial nerve, posterior interosseous branch), or metacarpophalangeal (MCP) flexion and crossing fingers (ulnar nerve) indicate an injury to respective motor nerves (Figure 9–40).

Type I requires cast immobilization. Type II and III fractures usually need closed, or rarely open, reduction, and percutaneous pin fixation. The reduction maneuver consists of longitudinal traction, correction of medial or lateral displacement, hyperflexion, and pronation with

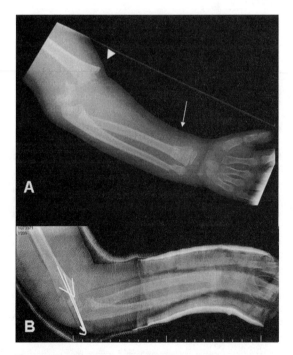

Figure 9–40. A: Lateral radiograph of a 4-year-old toddler who was run over playing football showing a type III supracondylar humerus fracture (*arrowhead*) and ipsilateral distal radius and ulna fractures; a "floating elbow" injury. ***B:*** Lateral radiograph of the patient in a long arm cast after closed reduction and percutaneous pinning of the distal humerus and closed reduction of both bone forearm fractures.

pressure on the olecranon. Crossed pins have classically been used, but similar clinical outcomes have been reported using lateral pins only, decreasing the risk of iatrogenic injury to the ulnar nerve.

Postoperative management consists of cast immobilization for 3–4 weeks. ROM is then encouraged. Patients return to full activity 4–6 weeks later. Complications include cubitus varus deformity in 5% and transient nerve palsies in 5–15% of patients. Compartment syndrome (Volkmann ischemic contracture) is a rare but devastating complication.

OLECRANON AVULSION FRACTURE

Young athletes with avulsion of the olecranon complain of acute pain, swelling, and decreased ROM. The predominant physical findings are tenderness over the olecranon and pain with extension. Radiographs reveal widening, or fragmentation of the olecranon physis, compared to the uninvolved contralateral side. Minimally (less than 2 mm) displaced fractures require a well-padded, posterior splint or cast for approximately 6–8 weeks. Displaced fractures, with significant step off, need to be treated using open reduction and internal fixation. Using either tension band wiring or cannulated screws stabilizes the fracture, however, patients need a cast to further protect the repair. They may return to sports roughly 3 months after an injury.

ELBOW DISLOCATION

Pathogenesis

Falls on an outstretched hand or forceful supination of a forearm may result in dislocation of an elbow. Dislocations usually affect humeroulnar and humeroradial joints. Typically, the ulna is displaced posteriorly in respect to the trochlea. Rupture of the ulnar collateral ligament and rupture of the anterior capsule are frequent, as are fractures of the medial epicondyle, coronoid process, and radial head. Associated fractures with elbow dislocations take place in 75% of patients. A Monteggia fracture is a fracture of the ulnar shaft, with dislocation of the proximal radioulnar joint (Figure 9–41).

Clinical Findings

A. SYMPTOMS AND SIGNS

Inspection of a dislocated elbow usually demonstrates medial and posterior displacement of the proximal forearm. Injuries to the ulnar, radial, and median nerves are common, with a rate of occurrence of 6%, 3%, and 3%, respectively. Vascular injuries occur in 3% of elbow dislocations.

B. IMAGING STUDIES

Compromised blood supply, following reduction, may require an angiogram.

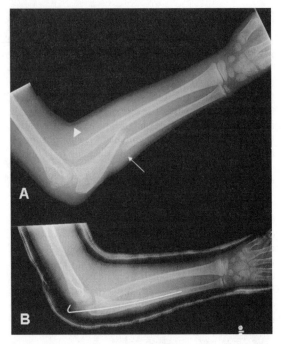

Figure 9–41. A: Lateral radiograph of a 7-year-old soccer player showing a displaced fracture of the proximal to middle one-third of the ulnar shaft (*arrowhead*) and dislocation of the proximal radioulnar joint (*arrow*); "Monteggia fracture." ***B:*** Lateral radiograph in a long arm cast status post closed reduction and percutaneous pinning of the ulna and closed reduction of the radial head.

Treatment

Reduction of the dislocated elbow on the field is controversial. From a practical standpoint, an athletic trainer or coach may try to reduce the joint on the field, using gentle traction. The elbow can be relatively easy to reduce, because swelling and muscle spasm develop later. It is advisable to explain to the parents that neurovascular injury can happen secondary to the reduction maneuver. Ideally, reduction of any dislocated joint should be done in a controlled environment, with conscious sedation and analgesia, and with the ability to manage possible airway problems. The reduction maneuver consists of supination of the forearm, a posteriorly directed pressure to the proximal forearm, with axial traction. The elbow is then gently flexed as axial traction is continued, until the elbow is reduced. An elbow will be immobilized in a 90° posterior splint. Nerve function is usually improved after reduction; however, in some instances nerve injuries can be inflicted by

a reduction. The likelihood of ischemic injury to the extremity is directly proportional to the time the elbow was left unreduced.

Loss of extension occurs in up to 30% of dislocations. Early active motion is therefore the key factor in rehabilitation of patients treated for elbow dislocations. Other symptoms include prolonged posttraumatic pain and increased valgus laxity of the joint.

Garland JJ: Management of supracondylar fractures of the humerus in children. Surg Gynecol Obstet 1959;109(2):145.

Kumar A, Ahmed M: Closed reduction of posterior dislocation of the elbow: a simple technique. J Orthop Trauma 1999;13(1):58.

Rasool MN: Dislocations of the elbow in children. J Bone Joint Surg Br 2004;86(7):1050.

Skaggs DL et al: Lateral-entry pin fixation in the management of supracondylar fractures in children. J Bone Joint Surg Am 2004;86-A(4):702.

GYMNAST WRIST

3. Wrist

General Considerations

Gymnastics continuously gains popularity in the United States. With increasing numbers of competitors, the rate of gymnastics-related injuries is on the rise as well. A gymnast with wrist pain sometimes presents a true diagnostic and therapeutic challenge.

Clinical Findings

A. Symptoms and Signs

Wrist pain affects about 75% of male and 50% of female gymnasts. The intensity and duration may vary, but most young gymnasts complain of wrist pain for 4 months or longer before seeking medical treatment. Axial loading combined with hyperextension, commonly seen in activities such as pommel horse, horizontal bar, vault, and floor exercises, place significant stress on the wrist. Most female athletes complain of an ulnar-sided wrist pain, whereas male athletes complain equally frequently of radial and ulnar-sided pain. Physical examination findings are usually unspecific; mild swelling and tenderness at the wrist may be present.

B. Imaging Studies

In children and adolescents, three views of a painful wrist, with comparison views, should be obtained. Until age 18 years, 29 ossification centers at the wrist are at different stages of fusion, making a precise diagnosis difficult. Stress-related changes can be seen as widening of the distal radial physis, epiphyseal cystic changes, beaking of the distal radial epiphysis, or metaphyseal irregularities. Premature closure of the distal radial epiphysis happens, with resultant positive ulnar variance in severe cases. An MRI helps to differentiate the pathology of cortical and trabecular bone, the articular surface, wrist ligaments, and the triangular fibrocartilage complex.

Treatment

Prevention of acute and chronic injuries is an important issue. The use of protective gear is as important as the setup of the training room and backups by spotters. As with any sports activity, proper warm-ups need to be emphasized, and rapid increases in intensity of exercises should be avoided. Treatment for patients with gymnast wrist is generally nonoperative. Ligamentous injuries, which are unusual in children and adolescent athletes, can be treated with immobilization or with surgical repair if they continue to result in instability and pain. Bony injuries require immobilization in a volar splint or cast. Cartilage injuries with disruption of the articular surface can be treated with debridement or repair, using open or arthroscopic techniques.

DISTAL FOREARM FRACTURES

General Considerations

The incidence of distal radius fractures, reported to be about 370 per 100,000 a year (2001), has been continuously increasing. The peak incidence corresponds to the peak velocity of growth, between 11.5 and 12.5 years of age in girls and between 13.5 and 14.5 years of age in boys. The mechanism of injury usually includes a fall on an extended hand.

Clinical Findings

A. SYMPTOMS AND SIGNS

The physical examination shows tenderness to palpation of the distal forearm, swelling, ecchymosis, and the presence of deformity.

B. IMAGING STUDIES

Standard AP and lateral radiographs are usually sufficient to make the diagnosis. Additional oblique views help detect subtle, nondisplaced, buckle fractures. Displacement, the presence and amount of comminution, distal radius articular surface tilt, radial length, radial inclination, and intraarticular extension dictate treatment for these fractures. Nondisplaced, Salter 1 fractures can be difficult to diagnose, as they may present with no changes on a radiograph, or with a mild widening of the distal radial physis. A history of trauma, with the presence of local tenderness over the distal radius growth plate, is sufficient to establish the diagnosis of a Salter 1 fracture (Figure 9–42).

Treatment

Treatment of displaced fractures requires a closed or open reduction and cast immobilization. Hematoma blocks, conscious sedation, or general anesthesia will diminish pain and discomfort during reduction. Acceptable limits of displacement and angulation vary depending on an athlete's age, location of the fracture, direction of deformities, and proximity to a growth plate. A well-molded cast will secure proper healing of the fracture and prevent fracture displacement. Immobilization time depends on the location of the

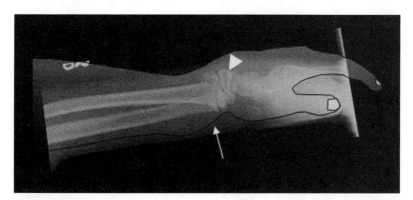

Figure 9–42. Schematic drawing superimposed on a lateral radiograph of a distal radius fracture (*arrowhead*) showing the silver fork deformity (*arrow*).

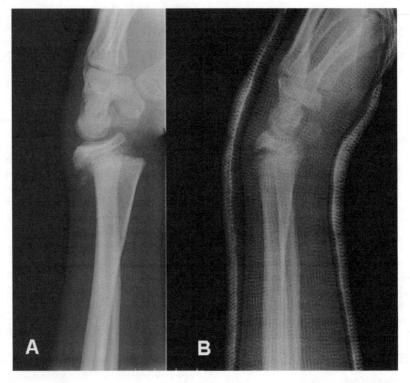

Figure 9–43. A: Lateral radiograph of a 14-year-old football player showing a Salter 2 distal radius fracture. ***B:*** Lateral radiograph in a short arm cast after closed reduction.

fracture. Distal radius fractures, with close proximity to the growth plate, usually require 4–6 weeks of immobilization, whereas mid-shaft fractures usually need a cast for a longer time (Figure 9–43). Progressive ROM exercises can follow immobilization with gradual return to sports. Open reduction and internal fixation, using pins, plates, or intramedullary flexible nails, may be required for severely displaced or unstable fractures. The probability that a patient will require surgery increases with age.

Khosla S et al: Incidence of childhood distal forearm fractures over 30 years: a population-based study. JAMA 2003;290(11): 1479.

The authors would like to thank Joanna Grudziak, BA, MA, for her help in preparing this manuscript.

Injuries Specific to the Female Athlete

10

Shane Seroyer, MD, & Robin West, MD

Since the initiation of Title IX of the Educational Assistant Act of 1972, requiring institutions receiving federal funds to provide equal access and funding to males and females in extracurricular activities, there has been an increase in the number of female participants in organized sports. The National Collegiate Athletic Association (NCAA) participation rate increased 69% for females versus 13% for males in a 15-year period after Title IX was passed. This increase in female participation in sports occurred at all levels of competition, from youth through the professional. Female participation in high school sports has increased 10-fold from the 1971–1972 to the 1998–1999 school years. This has been associated with more sports-related injuries in females and heightened awareness of the significance of proper physical training and conditioning in preventing injuries.

As the female athlete has flourished, a variety of gender-specific problems have emerged. The female athlete must contend with some issues unfamiliar to her male counterpart including several disturbing medical and musculoskeletal conditions. In 1993, the American College of Sports Medicine released the results of a consensus conference and coined the term the "female athlete triad," referring to the troubling syndrome of amenorrhea, disordered eating, and osteoporosis. Compared to males, female Naval Academy cadets were found to have a higher risk for injury from competition in intercollegiate athletics as well as from their military training. And compared to her male counterpart, the female athlete is more commonly affected by patellofemoral disorders, stress fractures of the pelvis and hip, spondylolysis, and noncontact anterior cruciate ligament (ACL) injuries (Table 10–1). The reasons for this predilection to injury remain uncertain. Once known, changes may be possible to improve safety for the female athlete.

Anderson J: The female athlete triad: disordered eating, amenorrhea, and osteoporosis. Connecticut Med 1999;60(11):647.

Arendt E: Anterior cruciate ligament injuries. Curr Women's Health Rep 2001;1:211.

Gwinn DE et al: The relative incidence of anterior cruciate ligament injury in men and women at the United States Naval Academy. Am J Sports Med 2000;28:98.

THE FEMALE ATHLETE TRIAD

The female athlete triad has received heightened consideration in the past 10 years. The three tenets of this condition—amenorrhea, disordered eating, and osteoporosis—are interrelated. Disordered eating in the athlete can vary from caloric restriction in excess of metabolic requirements to frank anorexia or bulimia nervosa. The latter may consist of self-induced vomiting, diuretic or laxative abuse, or fasting. Current societal pressures, especially the emphasis on appearance, impel many of the athletes to believe that they must sustain a thin, elegant body appearance to succeed or to be accepted. The form-fitting uniforms worn in certain sports such as swimming, gymnastics, and track may compound the issues. Sports in which the contestants are judged may also place an added pressure on the athlete to maintain a certain physical appearance.

There has been a long-noted association between weight loss and amenorrhea. The diagnostic criterion of anorexia nervosa is a weight loss resulting in a total body weight that is below 85% of ideal body weight. Primary amenorrhea, the absence of menstruation in females 16 years of age or older, must be differentiated from secondary amenorrhea, which is defined as the absence of three or more consecutive menstrual cycles after menarche. Athletic amenorrhea is thought to occur as a result of hypothalamic dysfunction. The loss in the normal pulsatile release of the gonadotropins, leutinizing hormone and follicle-stimulating hormone, may be induced by a negative caloric balance. This loss of the pulsatile release of leutinizing hormone and follicle-stimulating hormone acts at the ovaries to suppress the release of estradiol, resulting in the loss or absence of menses.

Table 10–1. Conditions affecting female more commonly than male athletes.[1]

Condition	Cause	Diagnosis	Treatment
Female athlete triad	Amenorrhea, osteoporosis, disordered eating	Combination of menstrual dysfunction, disordered eating, recurrent stress fractures	Multidisciplinary with early intervention, nutrition and psychological consult, oral estrogen replacement
ACL injury	Unknown: increased Q angle, narrow notch, hormonal influence, neuromuscular activation patterns	Large effusion after twisting injury, "pop," increased Lachman's, pivot shift	Neuromuscular training to prevent injury. ACL reconstruction to treat injury
Multiple direction shoulder instability	Increased laxity, hormonal influence	Complaints of shoulder pain, weakness, early fatigue, occasional instability	Therapy to strengthen rotator cuff, scapular stabilizers; capsular shift (open versus arthroscopic) to treat recurrent instability
Stress fractures	Hormonal influence, menstrual irregularities, anatomic variances	Localized pain, limp, limited motion, pain with weight-bearing, insidious onset	To prevent injury: normalize menstrual cycle, maintain well-balanced diet. To treat injury: limited WB, bone stimulator, ORIF "dangerous fxs" (lateral femoral neck) or nonunions

[1] ACL, anterior cruciate ligament; WB, weight-bearing; ORIF, open reduction with internal fixation.

Specific fat deposits rather than overall body weight may greatly influence the menstrual status of athletes. Weight regulation practices can reduce fat stores in regions around the hips, buttocks, and thigh, which may be essential for menstruating purposes. Eumenorrheic (ie, normal menstruating) college gymnasts have significantly greater fat stores in the lateral thigh than amenorrheic gymnasts. Menstrual irregularities occur with increasing frequency as exercise loads increase during competitive seasons, and are more prevalent in female athletes who experienced weight loss when compared to those who have maintained their weight during competition.

Much is known about the deleterious health affects of postmenopausal osteoporosis and its associated morbidities. The long-term effects of amenorrhea on the bones of young female athletes are unknown, but may be similar to postmenopausal effects. Amenorrhea is surprisingly common in strenuously exercising females, with a prevalence of nearly 20%. Amenorrheic athletes have significantly lower whole-body bone mineral density than control subjects, placing them at higher risk for injury. Decreases in bone mineral density in athletes who have been amenorrheic for more than 6 months resemble losses seen after menopause. These losses may be irreversible and lead to long-term sequela. Stress fractures have been shown to be significantly more prevalent in amenorrheic runners when compared to eumenorrheic runners, over the same time period with the same training mileage. A recent, large prospective study involving elite endurance athletes found that the rate of femoral bone loss in amenorrheic athletes was twice that found in the first year after menopause in nonathletic women.

Although their risk for stress fracture of the tibia may be equal to their male counterparts, female athletes are at increased risk for stress fractures of the pelvis and hip and for spondylolysis. Although controversial, support exists for the use of oral contraceptives to combat amenorrhea in female athletes in hopes of protecting them from stress fractures. Intervention through changes in life-style, training habits, and caloric intake, or through pharmacologic treatments such as calcium supplementation or hormone replacement, should be undertaken in the amenorrheic athlete to diminish further bone loss and reestablish a normal menstrual cycle.

The criteria for initiating estrogen replacement and the optimal dosing schedule have not been determined. However, the American Academy of Pediatrics recommends estrogen supplementation for amenorrheic adolescents if they are 3 years postmenarche and older than 16 years of age. Estrogen replacement should be considered in amenorrheic athletes who are unwilling to make life-style changes, who have been unsuccessful in reestablishing menses with life-style changes, who have been amenorrheic for 6 months or longer, and who have a history of a stress fracture.

Education concerning the dangers of the female athlete triad, as well as preventative strategies to combat its associated disorders, should be provided to all female athletes by their coaches and trainers. Attempts should be made to deemphasize physical appearance related to athletic performance and body fat measurements. A nutritionist should be available to educate athletes as to proper dietary habits and the dangers of inadequate nutrition. Peers should also be made aware of certain physical and behavioral clues that may indicate that a particular athlete is having a problem and may need help. Common warning signs include excessive criticism of body weight or shape, sudden noticeable weight loss, mood swings, depression, compulsive exercise or preoccupation with caloric intake, bathroom visits after meals, use of laxatives, chronic fatigue, anemia, abdominal bloating or upset, delayed wound healing, and frequent musculoskeletal injuries. Websites offered by the NCAA, American College of Sports Medicine, National Eating Disorder Organization, and National Association of Anorexia Nervosa and Associated Disorders provide helpful information on these issues.

Beals KA et al: Understanding the female athlete triad. J School Health 1999;69(8):337.

Braam L et al: Factors affecting bone loss in female endurance athletes. Am J Sports Med 2003;31(6):889.

ANTERIOR CRUCIATE LIGAMENT INJURIES

Anterior cruciate ligament (ACL) injuries occur two to eight times more frequently in female than in male athletes. A study of male and female midshipmen at the United States Naval Academy, all engaged in similar activities, has confirmed this. Although extensively studied, the reasons for this increased risk of ACL injuries in females remain unknown. Possible reasons include hormonal changes during the menstrual cycle, increased joint laxity, a knee structure that includes a narrow femoral intercondylar notch width, improper training and conditioning, and muscle activation patterns, all of which make females more prone to injury.

The role hormones play in ACL injuries is not known. Human ACL cells have estrogen receptors and fluctuations in the circulating concentration of estradiol may contribute to knee stability through the regulation of fibroblasts and collagen synthesis. Female athletes who sustained noncontact ACL injuries and had urine assays taken within 24 hours of injury to confirm the phase of the menstrual cycle had a much higher than expected rate of ACL injury during the ovulatory phase of the menstrual cycle. This phase coincides with a surge in estradiol that could relate to the effect of estrogen on the suppression of fibroblast function and collagen synthesis. But these findings are contradicted by the lack of association between ACL injury and the phase of the menstrual cycle in women taking oral contraceptives. In addition, ACL injuries are more common during the follicular phase of the menstrual cycle and knee laxity does not vary throughout the menstrual cycle.

Factors related to the structure of the knee, including notch width, the Q angle, and knee laxity, may contribute to ACL injury. The mean femoral intracondylar notch width is narrower in females, probably because they are, on average, smaller than males. Patients who sustained ACL tears may have had significantly narrower femoral intracondylar notch widths than uninjured controls. But a consensus conference in 1999 that addressed current available studies regarding notch width and its relation to gender found that the available data were inconclusive with regard to its relationship to ACL injury. It may be that the ratio of ACL size to femoral intracondylar notch width, rather than just the absolute width, is the relevant factor as cross-sectional area of the ACL in female athletes is significantly smaller than in male athletes. Or the femoral intracondylar notch may simply be proportional to the size of the athlete and not be important in causing ACL injury. Further study is needed. The Q angle is the angle created by the line connecting the anterior superior iliac spine and the midpoint of the patella and the line connecting the tibial tubercle and the midpoint of the patella. This angle may be larger in females, possibly due to a wider pelvic base. An increase in this angle may lead to increased medial stress on the knee. No definitive evidence has linked the Q angle to the increased incidence of ACL injuries in females. Joint laxity may also be greater in female athletes, but no causative relationship to ACL injuries has been established.

Many noncontact ACL injuries occur when an athlete lands from a jump, is decelerating, or is executing a cutting maneuver, all of which are performed, on average, in a more erect position in females than in males. These movements are associated with eccentric contraction of the quadriceps muscle. And high velocity, eccentric activation of the quadriceps muscle has long been thought to result in high ACL loads, especially with the knee in extension. Muscle activation patterns during proprioceptive activities and jump training have been studied to determine if there is a correlation with injury. The muscle activation theory contends that there are two main muscular activation or response patterns to anterior tibial translation or stress. In the first, which is quadriceps dominant and seemingly more prevalent in female athletes, preferential activation of the quadriceps occurs in response to anterior tibial translation. This action may accentuate the anterior translation and increase the ACL load. In the second, involving muscular activation or response patterns that may be more common in male athletes, hamstring dominant activation or simultaneous hamstring and quadriceps activation occurs. This muscular activation would decrease the anterior translation of the tibia and decrease the ACL load.

If improper training and conditioning as well as muscle activation patterns make females prone to ACL injury, then prevention programs with muscle training with special attention to the hamstrings as well as with proprioceptive training and plyometrics can be instituted. One study involving female high school soccer players showed that formal training of athletes with cardiovascular conditioning, plyometrics, speed drills, strength training, and agility decreased ACL injuries in the trained group compared to an untrained control group. A jump training program was tested to determine its effects on landing mechanics and muscular forces in female athletes. Plyometric training decreases the landing forces and increases the hamstring muscle power in these athletes. These programs may significantly affect knee stabilization and prevent knee injuries in female athletes.

Anderson AF et al: Correlation of anthropometric measurements, strength, anterior cruciate ligament size, and intercondylar notch characteristics to sex differences in anterior cruciate ligament tear rates. Am J Sports Med 2001;29:58.

Arendt E: Anterior cruciate ligament. Curr Women's Health Rep 2001;1:211.

Belanger MJ et al: Knee laxity does not vary with the menstrual cycle, before or after exercise. Am J Sports Med 2004;32(5): 1150.

Griffin LY et al: Noncontact anterior cruciate ligament injuries: risk factors and prevention strategies. J Am Acad Orthop Surg 2000;8:141.

Heidt RS et al: Avoidance of soccer injuries with preseason conditioning. Am J Sports Med 2000;28(5):659.

Huston LJ et al: Anterior cruciate ligament injuries in the female athlete. Clin Orthop Rel Res 2000;372:50.

Myklebust G et al: Prevention of anterior cruciate ligament injuries in female team handball players: a prospective intervention study over three seasons. Clin J Sport Med 2003;13:71.

Wojtys EM et al: The effect of the menstrual cycle on anterior cruciate ligament injuries in women as determined by hormone levels. Am J Sports Med 2002;30(2):182.

PATELLOFEMORAL DISORDERS

Patellofemoral disorders, described in more detail in Chapter 3, are more common in female than male athletes and are multifactorial in origin. This may be related to an increased Q angle, femoral anteversion, ligamentous laxity, external tibial rotation, forefoot pronation, and vastus medialis obliquus (VMO) dysplasia. Patellar disorders including lateral patellar compression syndrome and patellar instability are more common in females than males. These disorders are diagnosed by clinical examination, radiographs, and sometimes additional tests such as computed tomography (CT), magnetic resonance imaging, and bone scans.

Acute patellar dislocations can be treated with rehabilitation if there is no evidence of osteochondral injury and the patella is well centered after closed reduction. Recurrent instability often requires surgical intervention, including a proximal (eg, release of the lateral parapatellar retinaaculum and occasionally an imbrication of the medial parapatellar retinaaculum) and a distal (eg, tibial tubercle) realignment. Isolated lateral patellar compression syndrome can usually be treated with VMO strengthening, orthotics, patellar taping, and mobility. If after 3 months of rehabilitation the symptoms of lateral patellar compression do not improve, syndrome, a release of the lateral parapatellar retinaaculum can be performed. Hamstring stretching is also important in the treatment of patellofemoral disorder as it may decrease joint contact forces.

MULTIDIRECTIONAL SHOULDER INSTABILITY

Multidirectional shoulder instability (MDI), described in more detail in Chapter 5, is another problem more common in female than male athletes. It is a complex entity characterized by glenohumeral instability in two or more directions: anterior, inferior, or posterior. It may be more common in gymnasts and swimmers than in other athletes. A thorough physical examination reveals the sulcus sign and evidence of anterior and/or posterior instability. Imaging may reveal a patulous capsule that allows an increase in capsular volume. An incompetent rotator interval may also contribute. Rehabilitation aimed at improving muscle tone and coordination may result in a nearly 90% success rate. Failure after 6 months of such therapy in a compliant patient may be an indication that a surgical procedure, done with either an open or arthroscopic technique, should be performed. A goal is to tighten the patulous capsule.

Beasley L et al: The athletic woman: multidirection instability of the shoulder in the female athlete. Clinics Sports Med 2000;19(2):331.

STRESS FRACTURES

Another problem more common in female than male athletes is stress fractures. Stress fractures of the spine are discussed in more detail in Chapter 7. Spondylolysis, a stress fracture of the pars interarticularis of the vertebra, is more common in persons who participate in hyperextension activities such as dance, gymnastics, and diving. Progression to spondylolisthesis (ie, slippage of the vertebra) is also more prevalent in females. Athletes with this problem present with intermittent back pain that is usually associated with a specific activity. It may be diagnosed with plain radiographs and is most common at L5. Low-grade spondylolisthesis may be responsive to nonoperative treatment including rest, bracing, and physical therapy in up to 80% of athletes. The athlete may return to play when she is pain and symptom free. Higher grade slips (25–50%) may preclude an athlete from participating in hyperextension-type activities. Spondylolisthesis, with slips greater than 50%, and persistent pain with spondylolysis are conditions that may require surgical intervention, such as a spinal fusion. Athletes with spondylolisthesis may need to have their condition evaluated by a spine specialist before being allowed to return to play.

Stress fractures of the pelvis and hip are also more common in female than in male athletes. Pubic rami and femoral neck fractures are of particular concern in female athletes. The athlete with either of these conditions may present with pain in the groin, pain with activity, and limited ability to participate in particular activities. They can be easily mistaken for muscle strains or soft tissue injuries. Athletes affected by the "female athlete triad" are predisposed to stress fractures as decreased bone mineral density puts them at risk for these fractures. The etiology of the vertical stress fracture in the pubic rami is thought to be multifactorial and related to tight adductor musculature, crossover running style, and overstriding with running. Athletes with femoral neck stress fractures may, in addition, complain of anterior thigh pain in the distribution of the obturator nerve. Clinically they may have an adductor lurch with gait and experience pain with passive range of motion. They should remain nonweightbearing pending orthopedic evaluation. A stress fracture on the laterally based tension side (as opposed to the medial compression side) of the femoral neck has an increased risk of progression into complete fracture and warrants surgical intervention. Rest, physical therapy, and temporary withdrawal from participation in sport are the mainstays of treatment. The patient should not be allowed to return to play until she is pain free and has clinical and radiologic evidence of healing. This may take up to 3–4 months.

PREGNANCY & EXERCISE

In the past there had been concern that the physiologic responses to exercise during pregnancy could lead to fetal malformation, poor fetal growth, and premature labor. There were also concerns that poor fetal and maternal outcomes could result from the combined effects of exercise and the pregnancy-induced changes in hemodynamics, body temperature, circulating stress hormones, and caloric expenditure. However, these concerns have not been validated.

The physiologic effects of combining exercise and pregnancy are different than anticipated. The combination of pregnancy and exercise produces a maternal physiologic change in response to conditions of metabolic, thermal, cardiovascular, and mechanical stress. This change produces an extended margin of safety for both the mother and baby. Exercise and pregnancy have a synergistic effect by increasing maternal blood volume, heart chamber volumes, maximum cardiac output, the ability to dissipate heat, and the delivery of oxygen and nutrients to the tissue. Not only are cardiovascular, thermal, and oxygenation improvements made by both exercise and pregnancy, glucose and oxygen supplies for the baby are improved under most circumstances if the mother eats adequately and regularly. The musculoskeletal and ligamentous effects of regular exercise also protect the mother from injury and symptoms.

The maternal benefits of regular exercise during pregnancy are numerous. Fit women who continue to perform weight-bearing exercise throughout pregnancy and lactation at or above 50% of their prepregnancy levels have less weight gain, deposit and retain less fat, feel better, have shorter and less complicated labors, and recover more quickly postpartum.

The fetal benefits of regular maternal exercise are also plentiful. Infants of mothers who exercised during pregnancy have been shown to have fewer signs of distress, a decreased incidence of meconium-stained amniotic fluid, and a decreased risk in abnormal fetal heart rate patterns. APGAR scores of infants born to mothers who exercise are similar or higher than scores of infants born to sedentary mothers. Infants born to mothers who exercise when compared to infants born to sedentary mothers are more alert and more able to quiet themselves after exposure to stimuli. At 1 year of age, children of mothers who exercise had slightly better motor skills. At age 5, they were leaner and performed better on standardized tests of intelligence than the controls.

Healthy women with an uncomplicated pregnancy may safely continue or begin a regular exercise program during pregnancy. Maternal symptoms should dictate the intensity of exercise. The supine position should be avoided since it may lead to decreased cardiac output. Activities such as martial arts, which may cause abdominal trauma, should be avoided. Relative contraindications to exercise during pregnancy include bleeding in early pregnancy, anemia, arrhythmias, and an extremely overweight or underweight mother. Absolute contraindications include preterm labor, ruptured membranes, pregnancy-induced hypertension, persistent

Table 10–2. Absolute contraindications to exercise in pregnancy.[1]

Hemodynamically significant heart disease
Restrictive lung disease
Incompetent cervix
Multiple gestation at risk for preterm labor
Persistent second/third trimester bleeding
Placenta previa after 26 weeks gestation
Premature labor during current pregnancy
Ruptured membranes
Preeclampsia/pregnancy-induced hypertension

[1] Adapted from ACOG Committee Opinion, January 2002.

bleeding after 12 weeks, incompetent cervix, poor fetal growth, or multiple-birth pregnancy (Table 10–2).

ACOG Committee Opinion No. 267: Exercise during pregnancy and the postpartum period. Obstet Gynecol 2002;99:171.

Clapp JF: Exercise during pregnancy: a clinical update. Clinics Sports Med 2000;19:273.

Clapp JF et al: Neonatal behavioral profile of the offspring of women who continued to exercise regularly throughout pregnancy. Am J Obstet Gynecol 1999;180:91.

CONCLUSION

The Title IX Education Assistant Act of 1972 has had a profound impact on female athletes. Marketing of their sports has resulted in female athletes who are sports icons and role models. Female youth now share the same professional athletic dreams and ambitions as their male counterparts. Increased opportunities for these young women have also contributed to a healthier, more fit society. But this is not without consequence. Several musculoskeletal and medical conditions that frequently occur in females have resulted. Most alarming of these trends is the "female athlete triad." This condition, with devastating medical, physical, and emotional consequences, can be life-threatening. Fortunately, it is preventable through education, close monitoring, and deemphasizing certain societal pressures. The female athlete also has a predilection for ACL injuries as well as an increased incidence of stress fractures and patellofemoral disorders.

As the population of female athletes has increased, more research has been done to study their medical and musculoskeletal disorders. Our understanding of these conditions has already increased dramatically. For example, the healthy pregnant female with an uncomplicated pregnancy is now encouraged to exercise. Significant maternal and fetal benefits from exercise have been identified. In the future, a better understanding of injuries that have a predilection for female athletes will aid in preventing and treating these injuries in athletes of both genders.

Rehabilitation Principles

Tara M. Ridge, MD, Jennifer Swanson, DPT, & James J. Irrgang, MD

The ultimate goal of rehabilitation following an athletic injury is to restore symptom-free movement and function, allowing individuals to return to their prior level of activity in the shortest possible time. Rehabilitation includes the application of therapeutic exercise and physical agents. Physical agents include various forms of heat, cold, electricity, and massage that are used to relieve pain and swelling and to aid in the healing process. Therapeutic exercise includes a variety of movements designed to restore function to the greatest possible degree in the shortest period of time and to attain high levels of physical conditioning.

Establishment of appropriate goals during rehabilitation is dependent upon the ability to assess the extent of injury and functional status of the injured athlete. Subsequently, athletic trainers and physical therapists must be able to relate the effects of the physical agents and therapeutic exercise to the rehabilitation goals of the athlete for effective outcomes. Although an understanding of the pathology and the healing process is necessary to ensure appropriate rehabilitation, sports medicine professionals must also consider anatomy, kinesiology, and biomechanics when developing the rehabilitation program.

Rehabilitation of the injured athlete is a problem-solving process that can be depicted as a feedback loop. It includes assessment of the athlete and leads to development of needs, goals, and a plan of care. As the athlete progresses, the plan of care needs to be modified to allow for continued progress. Living tissues respond and adapt to the stresses placed upon them. For example, Wolff's law states that bone adapts to stresses such as weight-bearing activities and muscular contractions that result in increased bone mass. Soft tissue structures respond in a similar manner based on the SAID (Specific Adaptations to Imposed Demands) principle. This principle implies that tissues adapt to altered patterns of use. In essence, increased use results in specific adaptations of structure and/or function that enable those tissues to withstand the stresses imposed upon them. This is an important concept in rehabilitation. It implies that the degree of functional capacity achieved is dependent upon the intensity, duration, and frequency of exercise. During rehabilitation, tissues within the body must be stressed in a positive, progressive, and appropriately planned manner with the ultimate goal being to prepare the athlete to meet the demands of his or her sport, to achieve the highest levels of structure and function. However, as the load and demands of the athlete are progressively increased, continuous reassessment is required to avoid reinjury.

Rehabilitation begins immediately after the injury and progresses through the acute and subacute phases of injury or surgery, culminating in return to sport. For an athlete, it must also include a period of reconditioning to ensure optimal levels of fitness, which are necessary to achieve maximum performance and to minimize the risk of reinjury. Specific goals of rehabilitation are dependent on the phase of injury and include, but are not limited to, reducing or limiting inflammation, decreasing pain and swelling, improving mobility and flexibility, improving muscle strength and endurance, improving cardiovascular function, and, finally, promoting coordination. The ability to accurately evaluate and identify rehabilitation goals is critical to this process.

PRINCIPLES OF THERAPEUTIC EXERCISE

Therapeutic exercise is defined as those movements performed to restore the greatest possible degree of function in the shortest period, to attain high levels of physical fitness. Before initiating a therapeutic exercise program, the sports medicine professional must consider any precautions or contraindications to exercise as well as the nature and severity of the injury, as the intensity, frequency, and duration of the exercise must be appropriate for the stage of inflammation, healing, and conditioning. Next, the purpose of the exercise and the sequencing and progression of the program should be considered.

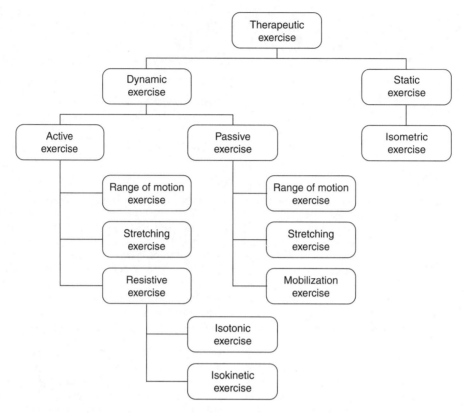

Figure 11–1. Categorization of the forms of therapeutic exercise.

Therapeutic exercise can be categorized into static or dynamic exercise (Figure 11–1). Static exercise includes isometric exercises in which no observable movement occurs. Dynamic exercise may be either active or passive. Active exercise occurs when voluntary contraction of muscles produces movement without the application of additional external resistance. It includes range of motion and stretching exercises. Active range of motion exercises include those movements *within* the available range of motion. Active stretching exercises are exercises in which the athlete utilizes voluntary effort to move *beyond* the restricted range of motion.

Active exercise occurs when voluntary contraction of muscles produces movement without the application of additional external resistance. It includes range of motion and stretching exercises. Range of motion exercises are performed to maintain motion, whereas stretching exercises are designed to increase motion. These exercises will be discussed in greater detail later in the chapter.

Motions in accessory, passive exercises include distraction, compression, rolling, gliding, and/or spinning of the joint surfaces. Individuals are not capable of producing accessory motions with voluntary muscle activation

and therefore a physical therapist or athletic trainer typically performs this manual technique to increase joint play (Figure 11–2). Joint mobilization is an example of passive, accessory motion that is performed at

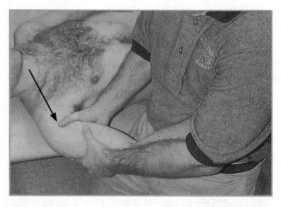

Figure 11–2. Joint mobilization can be used to reduce pain and increase range of motion. A distraction technique of the glenohumeral joint in the resting position is illustrated.

slow speeds and varying amplitudes; this will be described in further detail later in this chapter.

Kisner C, Colby LA: *Therapeutic Exercise: Foundations and Techniques*, 4th ed. F.A. Davis Company, 2002.

REHABILITATION GOALS

The ultimate goal of the rehabilitation program is to restore function as efficiently as possible, allowing the athlete to safely and quickly return to athletic competition. Although we are unable to "speed up" the normal healing process following an injury, we can optimize our plan of care to minimize delayed healing by designing an appropriate and functional rehabilitation program. Such programs must take into account the normal phases of healing and must address the sport-specific demands of the individual athlete. Failure to address normal healing parameters and sport-specific requirements will delay the return to competition, increase the risk for reinjury, and reduce the performance level of the athlete.

Although the inflammatory process is part of the normal healing process, prolonged or chronic inflammation may be deleterious to athletes who are trying to rehabilitate and return to athletic competition. By controlling the pain and swelling associated with the inflammatory process, athletes may be able to progress through the clinical rehabilitation goals and advance to functional activities more quickly. The cornerstone for managing the signs and symptoms of acute inflammation are rest, ice, compression, elevation, and nonsteroidal antiinflammatory drugs (NSAIDs). Whenever possible, they should be used concurrently for maximum benefits to facilitate a quick but safe progression through rehabilitation. Pain and effusion inhibit muscle activation and decrease strength and may result in additional injuries and reduced performance. Following an injury and the subsequent management of the acute signs and symptoms, rehabilitation should involve a variety of factors designed to prepare the athlete for return to sport. These factors include clinical goals for improving range of motion and flexibility, muscular and cardiovascular endurance, and, ultimately, strength. The program should culminate with functional goals for return to sport such as increasing power, speed, and agility.

Range of Motion

The range of motion available at a particular joint is termed "joint range" and is determined by the configuration of the joint surfaces and surrounding soft tissue structures such as the capsule, ligament, muscle, tendon, fascia, and skin. When discussing the available range of motion at a particular joint, we often consider the "muscle range," which is related to the functional excursion produced by muscles that cross the joint. It is important to note that the total joint range can be directly affected by the functional excursion and it is defined as the distance that the muscle is capable of lengthening and shortening. A one-joint muscle is expected to shorten and lengthen sufficiently to permit full active range of motion at the joint that it crosses. The functional excursion of multijoint muscles exceeds the joint range of any one of the joints that it crosses. Multijoint muscles, however, cannot lengthen or shorten sufficiently to simultaneously permit the extreme range of motion at all the joints that it crosses. For example, the hamstring muscle group cannot lengthen sufficiently to permit simultaneous full active knee flexion and hip extension. In this position, the hamstring muscle group is said to be actively insufficient. In the active insufficient position, the muscle fibers cannot shorten any further and are ineffective in generating additional tension.

A. NONCONTRACTILE AND CONTRACTILE TISSUES

To increase motion, the properties of both the noncontractile and contractile tissues that limit the motion must be considered. Noncontractile tissues include ligaments, tendons, capsule, fascia, and connective tissue components of muscle and skin. The contractile component is the muscle. The material strength of tissue is its ability to resist load or stress, and defined as tensile, compressive, and/or shearing forces. The mechanical properties of tissue are often plotted in a stress–strain curve that relates strain as a function of stress for a given tissue, whereas strain is defined as the deformation that occurs in response to stress and is typically expressed as a percentage of elongation (Figure 11–3). The toe region

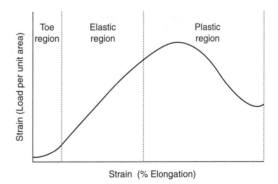

Figure 11–3. Stress–strain curve for connective tissue. The toe region is the area in which little stress is required to lengthen the tissue. The elastic region is the portion of the curve in which tissue returns to its original length when the stress is removed. The plastic region is that portion of the curve that results in permanent elongation when the stress is removed. (Modified from Kisner C, Colby LA: *Therapeutic Exercise: Foundations and Techniques,* 4th ed. F.A. Davis Company, 2002.)

occurs at the beginning of the curve and is the region in which very little force is required to elongate the tissue. This likely represents straightening of the wavy pattern of connective tissue fibers. The elastic range represents the area in which tissue returns to its original size and shape when the stress is removed. The elastic limit is the upper end of the elastic range and is the point beyond which the tissue will not return to its original size or shape when the stress is removed. The plastic range of the stress–strain curve represents the range beyond the elastic limit that results in permanent elongation when the stress is removed.

To increase range of motion there must be lengthening of connective tissue and this requires plastic deformation that results in gradual rearrangement of the connective tissue. Adequate time must be provided for remodeling to prevent fatigue and/or rupture of the tissue. Due to the viscoelastic nature of connective tissue, it exhibits properties of creep, relaxation, and stiffness. Creep is the elongation of tissue that results from constant loading, and can be increased by raising the tissue temperature. Relaxation is the progressive decrease in stress that occurs over time. Stiffness is the ability of the tissue to resist elongation and is determined by the slope of the stress–strain curve (Figure 11–4). Because connective tissue is viscoelastic, stiffness is dependent on the rate of loading. Therefore, an increased rate of loading is associated with greater stiffness. To maximize permanent lengthening, low- magnitude forces should be applied for prolonged periods of time. This process can be facilitated by the use of heating and cooling modalities in the lengthened position (Figure 11–5).

Another way of describing the noncontractile components of muscle is as series elastic and parallel elastic components. The series elastic component includes the tissue that connects the muscle fiber to bone, whereas the parallel elastic component consists of the tissue that

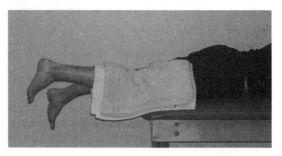

Figure 11–5. To maximize permanent lengthening, low-magnitude forces can be applied for prolonged periods of time. This process can be facilitated with heating and cooling modalities.

surrounds each muscle fiber. Lengthening of the musculotendinous unit lengthens both the series and parallel elastic components, producing a sharp rise in tension. Because muscle also consists of contractile components, as lengthening continues, mechanical disruption of the cross bridge begins as the actin and myosin filaments slide apart and an abrupt lengthening of the sarcomere occurs, known as "sarcomere give." Sarcomeres are elastic, therefore, when the short-term stretch is removed, they return to their original length. This implies that short-term stretching is not effective in increasing length of the contractile components of the muscle.

As mentioned earlier, plastic deformation, or permanent lengthening of contractile tissue, requires time for gradual rearrangement of connective tissue and can be achieved with prolonged immobilization. Prolonged immobilization is the lengthened position that results in the addition of sarcomeres and permanent lengthening of the contractile tissues and occurs to maintain the greatest functional overlap of the actin and myosin filaments. Conversely, prolonged immobilization in the shortened position results in a decreased number of sarcomeres and may result in contractures or a permanent loss of motion.

The neurophysiologic properties of contractile tissue must be considered when attempting to increase range of motion limited by musculotendinous structures. The muscle spindle is a sensory organ sensitive to muscle lengthening. Sudden stretching of the muscle results in lengthening of the muscle spindle and initiation of the monosynaptic stretch reflex. Consequently, sudden or ballistic stretching of the musculotendinous units may cause the muscle to contract as it is being lengthened, thus resulting in increased soreness or no appreciable change in length.

Another sensory organ, the Golgi tendon organ (GTO), is found in the musculotendinous junction and is sensitive to tension caused by passive stretching or active contraction of the musculotendinous unit.

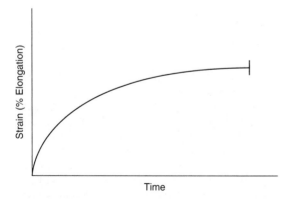

Figure 11–4. Tissue undergoes gradual elongation over time when subjected to constant stress.

Excessive musculotendinous tension causes the GTO to discharge, inhibiting the muscular contraction. Stretching techniques such as contract/relax utilize the GTO to inhibit the muscle contraction, allowing the muscle to lengthen. Similarly, reciprocal inhibition occurs when the antagonist muscle is inhibited as an agonist muscle contracts. This principle can also be incorporated into stretching techniques, such as contract/relax/contract and agonist contraction to facilitate muscle lengthening; this will be discussed in greater detail later in the chapter.

B. PASSIVE AND ACTIVE RANGE OF MOTION

Dynamic exercise can involve passive or active range of motion (Figure 11–1). Passive range of motion occurs without voluntary muscular effort on the part of the athlete and is the result of forces external to the body. Passive range of motion is indicated when the athlete is not able to move the body segment voluntarily or when voluntary muscle activity would be detrimental to the healing process. It limits the adverse effects of immobility and is used to maintain the available joint range of motion. However, passive range of motion will not prevent muscle atrophy or affect muscle strength or endurance, nor will it improve circulation to the same extent as voluntary, active exercise.

Active range of motion occurs when voluntary contraction of muscles produces movement without the application of additional external resistance. It includes range of motion and stretching exercises. Active range of motion exercises include those movements *within* the available range of motion. Active stretching exercises are exercises in which the athlete utilizes voluntary effort to move *beyond* the restricted range of motion. There is more information on active exercises later in this chapter in the section on strengthening.

Neither purely active nor purely passive range of motion, active assistive range of motion combines active voluntary contraction with an outside force to complete motion within the unrestricted range (Figure 11–6). Such exercises can be used when the athlete is able to actively contract muscles to move the segment and when there are no contraindications for active voluntary muscle contractions. Extremely useful during the early stages of rehabilitation, they can be used to limit the adverse effects of immobility and maintain contractility of muscles. In addition, these exercises provide sensory feedback and a stimulus for maintaining integrity of bone. Lastly, they can be used to improve coordination and motor skills necessary for functional activities.

C. TIMING OF RANGE OF MOTION EXERCISES

Range of motion exercise may be performed in anatomic planes, combined patterns, and sport-specific functional patterns incorporating movement in several planes simultaneously. Except when stretching is indicated,

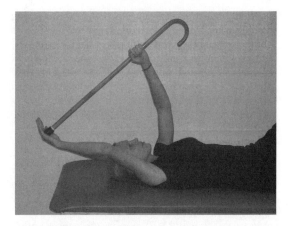

Figure 11–6. The athlete uses a cane to assist the voluntary contraction of the involved upper extremity within the unrestricted range of motion.

range of motion should be pain free and motion beyond the available range should not be forced. Generally 5–10 repetitions several times per day are adequate to limit the adverse effects of immobility. The athlete's response to range of motion exercises should be closely monitored and documented. Treatment must be modified as the athlete progresses and it is important to recognize signs of excessive exercise if range of motion exercises are performed acutely after injury. These signs include increased pain, swelling, warmth, redness, and loss of motion that persists for more than 1–2 hours after the exercise is completed.

Flexibility

Some definitions need to be clarified before continuing. Flexibility is the ability of a muscle to relax and yield to a stretching force. Tightness is a nonspecific term used to describe mild shortness of the musculotendinous unit that does not result in a significant loss of joint motion. Common in multijoint muscles such as the hamstring, rectus femoris, and gastrocnemius muscle groups, tightness can be improved by self-stretching or flexibility exercises. A joint contracture is a significant loss of motion from any cause. Contractures are described by identifying the involved joint and the direction of the contracture. For example, a lack of full knee extension would be termed a knee flexion contracture whereas a lack of full knee flexion would be termed a knee extension contracture.

Flexibility exercises are used to increase the length of the musculotendinous unit and the term flexibility exercise is often used synonymously with stretching exercise. Stretching exercises are designed to increase range of motion and lengthen pathologically shortened soft tissue structures. In active stretching, the stretching force is created by voluntary contraction of the athlete's muscles and allows for incorporation of the neurophysiological principles of stretching. Passive stretching movements are movements beyond the restricted range performed in an attempt to increase motion. External force may be applied by an athlete's own body, a machine, gravity, or another individual. The external force can be applied manually or mechanically. Manual passive stretching exercises are generally of short duration lasting 15–30 seconds per repetition. Passive mechanical stretching is performed by applying a low (5–10 lb) external load to the shortened tissues for a prolonged period of time (15–30 minutes). Passive mechanical stretching may be performed with the use of ankle weights (Figure 11–7) or other mechanical equipment. Prolonged mechanical stretch often results in greater permanent lengthening of contractile and noncontractile tissues, based on the TERT (Total End Range Time) Principle. This is the amount of time that the tissue is engaged into the restricted range. Increased time at end range facilitates remodeling of the connective tissue and plastic deformation occurs, permanently lengthening the tissue.

Neurophysiologic principles can be incorporated to relax muscles prior to elongation. This allows the contractile component to be lengthened more easily. These techniques can be used to stretch tight contractile structures more comfortably, such as those associated with muscle spasm; however, they do not generally result in a permanent increase in length. Examples of neurophysiologic stretching techniques include contract/relax and contract/relax/contract. Contract/relax stretching techniques involve isometric contraction of the tight muscle followed by lengthening of the muscle. The prestretch contraction of the short muscle results in stimulation of the GTO. A contract/relax stretching technique to address a tight hamstring muscle would incorporate contraction of the hamstring with simultaneous hip extension and knee flexion, followed by passive relaxation of the hamstring muscle and contraction of the quadriceps and hip flexor muscles as the hamstring is lengthened.

The athlete should be taught self-stretching techniques that incorporate the use of the athlete's body weight with active inhibition to stretch tight muscles. These should be performed following the passive stretching and active inhibition techniques described above. The athlete should also be instructed to perform self-stretching exercises several times daily to continue to make gains in motion.

Stretching exercises are indicated when the athlete demonstrates limited range of motion in the subacute or chronic phases of healing. Generally, stretches are held in the restricted range for approximately 15–30 seconds and should cause only mild discomfort. If stretching exercises cause a persistent increase in pain that lasts longer than 1–2 hours, the athlete should be instructed to decrease the intensity of the stretch by staying within less restricted ranges. In addition, aggressive stretching exercises during the acute stages of healing may jeopardize the healing tissue and aggravate inflammation and, therefore, should be avoided in the acute stage of soft tissue healing. Stretching exercises can also be used to correct muscle imbalances that result when an opposing muscle group is weak. Generally, the athlete should address the tight muscle group first with stretching exercises and then progress to a strengthening program of the opposite muscle. Stretching exercises may also be indicated before and after activity as a warm-up and after cool-down, respectively, to minimize the risk of musculotendinous injuries. Athletes should avoid stretching or forcing the joint beyond the normal range of motion. In essence, care should be taken to avoid creating a hypermobile joint.

Prior to stretching, local application of heat or active exercise is used to elevate body temperature and to increase soft tissue extensibility. In addition, massage may be employed to promote relaxation and decrease muscle spasm, making it easier to stretch tight muscles. Lastly, if mobility of a joint surface is limited, mobilization techniques should be utilized prior to stretching exercises to increase the accessory range of motion.

Joint Mobilization

Movement of the joint surfaces may include distraction, compression, rolling, gliding, and/or spinning. Rolling occurs when new points on one joint surface meet new points on an opposing joint surface, similar to a tire rolling along a road. Gliding of joint surfaces involves the same point on one surface, similar to a locked tire sliding over a road. Normal joint motion may combine both rolling and gliding of the joint surfaces to maintain congruency as the limb moves through the range of motion.

Joint mobilization techniques, designed to restore the normal gliding of joint surfaces necessary for physiologic

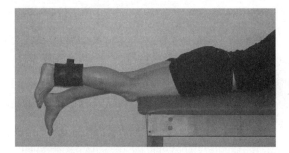

Figure 11–7. Passive mechanical stretching can be performed with the use of ankle weights or other similar equipment.

motion, are contraindicated during periods of active inflammation and hypermobility. In addition, the use of mobilization techniques following fractures should be delayed until there is radiographic evidence of union.

Joint mobilization can be performed using oscillatory or sustained movements. The Maitland or Australian system uses oscillatory techniques and are graded I through IV. Grade I and II oscillations are large-amplitude motions used to stimulate mechanoreceptors to decrease pain. Grade III and IV oscillatory movements are used to stretch tight structures in order to increase joint mobility and range of motion. The Kaltenborn or Norwegian system, which utilizes sustained mobilization techniques, has three grades of motion. Grade I, or piccolo motion, separates the joint surfaces just enough to equalize intraarticular and atmospheric pressure and is typically utilized to decrease pain. A grade II, or slack technique, removes the slack from the capsule and surrounding ligaments and can be utilized to increase range of motion. Grade III, or stretch techniques, utilize sufficient force to stretch joint structures to improve mobility. In general, the oscillatory motions of the Australian system are utilized for pain modulation whereas the sustained movements in the Kaltenborn system are utilized to improve joint mobility and range of motion.

Proper application of joint mobilization techniques requires a thorough examination of the involved joint to determine the tissues limiting motion as well as the stage of pathology. The mobilizing force should be correlated with the pain/restriction sequence. Pain occurring before resistance to motion is reached indicates an acute condition. Mobilization for acute conditions should consist of grade I and II oscillating techniques to decrease pain and maintain joint play. Pain synchronous with resistance to motion indicates a subacute condition. Grade III oscillatory or grade II (slack) mobilization techniques are appropriate for subacute conditions. A trial of gentle stretching should be utilized for subacute conditions. Pain engaged after the resistance to motion is indicative of a chronic condition and vigorous stretching is indicated. Joint mobilization techniques for chronic conditions include grade III and IV oscillatory or grade III (stretch) sustained techniques.

Joint mobilization techniques should be utilized only when mobility testing reveals decreased joint play. Hypermobile joints should not be mobilized. Generally, mobilization techniques are utilized when passive range of motion is limited from capsular contracture and joint play is limited in the direction of the restricted motion.

When performing joint mobilization techniques, the athlete should be positioned to promote relaxation and stabilization of the part to be mobilized. Initially, mobilization should be performed with the joint in the position at which the capsule has the greatest amount of laxity. This position generally occurs in the middle of the available range of motion and as range of motion

improves, joint mobilization techniques can be performed in the restricted position. Forces should be applied as close to the opposing joint surfaces as possible. The area of contact with the hand should be graded according to the stage of the condition and the intended goals of treatment as described above.

The direction of movement is dictated by the direction of the restricted motion and the shape of the joint surface. The treatment plane is a plane perpendicular to a line from the axis of rotation to the center of the concave articulating surface (Figure 11–8). When joint surfaces are distracted, the force should be applied perpendicular to the treatment plane. When gliding joint surfaces, force should be applied parallel to the treatment plane, utilizing the following convex/concave rule: Concave joint surfaces should be glided in the direction of the limited swing of the bone, whereas convex surfaces should be glided in the direction opposite to the limited swing of the bone. When performing joint mobilization techniques, angular motion of the bone should be minimized to reduce compression of the joint surfaces, which may damage the articular surface.

Oscillatory joint mobilization techniques should be performed at a rate of 1–2 cycles per second for 1–2 minutes. Sustained joint mobilization techniques should be performed for 5–15 seconds and repeated 10 times. Joint mobility and range of motion should be reassessed at the completion of joint mobilization and the athlete should perform range of motion and stretching exercises as a follow-up treatment to joint mobilization. The athlete may experience some increase in soreness; however, these symptoms typically subside within several hours.

Moore KL: *Clinically Oriented Anatomy,* 5th ed. Williams & Wilkins, 2002.

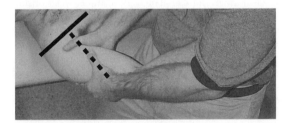

Figure 11–8. The solid line represents the treatment plane and is defined as the line perpendicular to the line drawn from the axis of rotation to the center of the concave joint surface. When joint surfaces are distracted, the force should be applied perpendicular to the treatment plane. When gliding joint surfaces the forces should be applied parallel to the treatment plane.

PRINCIPLES OF MUSCLE PERFORMANCE: STRENGTH & ENDURANCE

The development of strength and endurance is a key component related to overall muscle performance and must be addressed during the rehabilitation of athletes. Strength refers to the amount of force a muscle or muscle group is able to generate during a maximal contraction at a constant velocity. Force is defined as a linear measurement referring to an action that changes the state or motion of a body to which it is applied and is measured in newtons. Forces can be divided into two categories, internal and external, with the latter a result of gravity. Internal forces are generated by muscle, bone, and soft tissue deformation, and when applied to the musculoskeletal system, a muscle force produces a rotation of a joint about its axis. Torque is force applied at a distance from the axis of rotation. Muscle endurance is closely associated with muscle strength and refers to the ability to perform multiple contractions against a set resistance for an extended period of time. All of these variables play a key role in muscle performance and can be manipulated during rehabilitation to maximize improvement.

Strength

A. BASICS OF STRENGTHENING

Strength is defined as the maximum amount of force a muscle or muscle group can generate at a specified velocity. Muscle weakness or imbalance can result in abnormalities that can impair normal functional movement and must be addressed during rehabilitation from injury. Strength is mediated by a number of physiologic, biomechanical, and neuromuscular factors. Various forms of strength training are used to meet different goals and functional outcomes at each stage of tissue healing after injury or following surgical repair.

There are multiple factors that influence the strength of a normal muscle. There is a direct relationship between the physiologic cross-sectional area of the muscle fibers and the maximum amount of force that a muscle can generate, such that a larger muscle diameter correlates with greater strength. Force generation is also influenced by the length of the muscle at the time of contraction. According to the length–tension relationship, a muscle can generate maximal force at its resting length, defined as the position in which there is a maximum number of cross-bridges between the actin and myosin filaments. As the muscle shortens, the contractile force that a muscle can generate decreases due to the overlapping of myofilaments. Although the contractile force generated by a muscle decreases as the muscle lengthens, it is counterbalanced by an increase in noncontractile tension. Thus, the passive lengthening of the connective tissue results in a net increase in force. Therefore, the total force produced by the musculotendinous unit (including both contractile and noncontractile forces) increases as the muscle lengthens.

A number of contractile properties of muscle fibers contribute to production of force. Strength, endurance, power, speed, and resistance to fatigue vary based on the characteristics of different types of muscle fibers. Type I, slow twitch muscle fibers generate low levels of force and are resistant to fatigue. In contrast, type IIA and B, fast twitch muscle fibers have the ability to generate a large amount of tension but fatigue rapidly. Fiber-type distribution thus plays a large role in the ability of a muscle to generate force.

The order of muscle fiber recruitment is dependent upon the type of activity, the amount of force required, and the pattern of movement desired. Small motor neurons innervate type I, slow twitch muscle fibers and are initially recruited during low-intensity, long-duration endurance activities. As force requirements increase, large motor neurons innervating type II, fast-twitch muscle fibers are progressively recruited.

In addition to muscle fiber type, force generation is influenced by the speed and type of muscle contraction being performed. Greater torque is produced at lower speeds, and is related to the increased opportunity for recruitment of motor units. Eccentric contractions, in which the muscle is lengthened against resistance, produce the greatest force output. Tension increases as the speed of motion increases due in part to the facilitation of the stretch reflex and stretching of the series elastic component in muscle. In contrast, lower levels of force are generated during concentric muscle contractions. As the muscle shortens and the speed of contraction increases, there is an overall decrease in tension, as the muscle lacks adequate time to develop force. There is an inverse relationship between speed and force production during concentric muscle contractions. Adequate stores of energy and blood flow are also necessary to allow the muscle to contract efficiently, generate appropriate levels of tension, and resist fatigue. The amount of force generated by a muscle is also influenced by characteristics unique to the athlete, as the degree of motivation and willingness to put forth a maximal effort to generate maximum forces are dependent on the individual.

Neuromuscular changes that lead to increased strength include hypertrophy and hyperplasia. Hypertrophy refers to an increase in the size of the individual skeletal muscle fibers and is related to the increased contractile protein and the number of fibrils within the muscle fiber, as well as an increased density of the capillary bed surrounding individual muscle fibers. Increases in the connective tissue component of muscle may contribute to hypertrophy as well. Heavy resistance strength training has been shown to cause selective hypertrophy of type II fast-twitch muscle fibers. Rapid gains in strength during the early phases of resistance training are most likely attributed to recruitment rather than hypertrophy, largely due to motor learning that results in neural adaptations such as greater recruitment and synchronization of motor units. Hyperplasia refers to an increase in the number of muscle fibers resulting from the longitudinal splitting of muscle fibers. Although hyperplasia is controversial in humans, its presence has been demonstrated in laboratory animals exposed to heavy resistance training.

Strength is directly related to the amount of tension a contracting muscle can produce. To increase strength, the muscle must be progressively overloaded, such that it exceeds the metabolic capacity of the muscle. Overload is created by increasing either the resistance or the speed of the muscle action, or through a combination of both. Increasing levels of tension will develop in response to these loads, leading to hypertrophy and recruitment of motor units in the muscle.

B. ISOMETRIC, ISOTONIC, ISOKINETIC, AND VARIABLE RESISTANCE EXERCISES

The purpose of strengthening exercises is to increase the maximum force a muscle can generate. Strengthening is highly specific to the type of exercise and can be categorized into static or dynamic exercise (Figure 11–1). Static exercise includes isometric exercises in which no observable movement occurs. The length of the muscle appears constant, however, there is shortening at the sarcomere level. Isometric contractions occur when torque produced by muscle tension is equal to external resistance and no movement occurs about the joint. Isometric exercises may be initiated early in the rehabilitation program to help regain baseline strength lost to injury or disuse. These exercises can be used even when motion is contraindicated. One of the limiting factors involves the concept of joint angle specificity. Multiple-angle isometrics are necessary to develop strength throughout the entire range of motion whereas isometric exercises develop strength only at the position in which the exercise is performed.

Dynamic exercise can be passive, discussed above in the range of motion section of this chapter, or active. Active exercise can be resistive and includes exercises in which the individual utilizes voluntary muscle contraction to move against an applied resistance, such as isotonic and isokinetic exercises.

Isotonic exercises, by definition, should result in constant muscle tension through the range of shortening. However, this rarely occurs because motion against a fixed external resistance results in variable muscle tension due to the length–tension relationship of the muscle fiber and the changing mechanical advantage that the line of muscle action has on the skeletal system. Therefore, the term isotonic exercise has come to imply movement against a fixed resistance. Isotonic exercises are one of the most popular forms of strength training used in rehabilitative programs.

Isokinetic exercise involves movement at a constant speed. External resistance is variable and accommodating and is proportional to the effort put forth by the athlete. Isokinetic training encourages the muscle to generate maximum force throughout the full range of joint motion at different angular velocities. During the earlier phases of rehabilitation, isokinetic training should be performed at submaximal levels with maximal levels of training reserved for the final stages of rehabilitation as the individual is progressing back to sport or other functional activities. Resistance machines have been developed to provide variable resistance that matches the torque curves produced by a particular muscle or muscle group. In variable resistance exercises, the resistance is not accommodating and the speed is not controlled.

Resistance exercise programs can be designed to selectively recruit different muscle fiber types by controlling the intensity, duration, and speed of exercise. Specificity of training refers to the principle that the adaptive effects of training, including strength, power, and endurance, are highly specific to the type of training utilized and thus, whenever possible, exercises incorporated in the training program should mimic the desired function.

C. CONCENTRIC AND ECCENTRIC EXERCISE

Isotonic, isokinetic, and variable resistance exercises can be performed concentrically and eccentrically. Concentric contraction implies that the muscle shortens as it contracts, whereas an eccentric contraction implies lengthening as the muscle contracts. Concentric contractions are necessary to accelerate the body and eccentric contractions are necessary for deceleration. This information should be considered when choosing the most appropriate types of exercise and subsequent muscle contraction when attempting to match the demands of the sport. It is important to note that the force–velocity relationship is different for each type of contraction. During a concentric contraction, the force created by the muscle decreases as the speed of contraction increases. This type of contraction occurs when the internal force created by the muscle is greater than the external resistance. During an eccentric contraction, however, the force created by the muscle increases as the speed of lengthening increases. This type of contraction occurs when the external resistance overcomes the internal resistance created by the muscle and is often associated with increased muscle soreness and increased injury. The differing relationships related to force and velocity are believed to result partly from stretching of the connective tissue component within the musculotendinous unit and facilitation of the stretch reflex, both of which give rise to increased muscle tension with increased speed of lengthening.

D. MANUAL AND MECHANICAL RESISTIVE EXERCISES

The force in resistive exercise can be applied either manually or mechanically. Manual resistance is useful during the early stages of rehabilitation when the affected muscle is weak and can overcome only minimal to moderate resistance. It is also useful when working in a limited range of motion. In contrast, mechanical resistance is applied through the use of equipment or a motorized device. The amount of resistance can be quantitatively measured and progressed over time.

E. OPEN AND CLOSED KINETIC CHAIN EXERCISES

The type of exercise should be carefully chosen when developing the strengthening program. Open and closed kinetic chain exercises play an important role in both clinical and functional rehabilitations. Open-chain exercises occur when the distal segment moves freely in space. During closed-chain activities, the distal aspect of the extremity is fixed and thus motion occurs simultaneously at all joints that comprise the kinetic chain. The variables must match the requirements and demands placed upon the athlete during functional exercises in order for the exercises to be specific. Generally, muscle groups may be isolated during open-chain exercises, and more cocontraction of various muscle groups occurs during closed-chain exercises. Most activities incorporate some combination of both open and closed kinetic chain activities, with the latter particularly important during functional weight-bearing activities, and include exercises such as partial squats, step-ups, and lunges.

F. TIMING OF STRENGTH TRAINING

During the initial phases of recovery, rehabilitation focuses on pain modulation and restoration of joint range of motion and flexibility of the individual muscles. Next, strength training is introduced into the program. As the athlete progresses, the emphasis of the program shifts to functional training to develop balance, proprioception, and synergistic muscle activity required for sport-specific activities. Typically, strength exercises utilizing functional movement patterns that incorporate multiplane and multijoint movements are integrated into the program during the latter phase of the rehabilitation program.

It is essential to incorporate exercises performed at rapid speeds during later phases of rehabilitation and reconditioning, as it is reflective of the demands related to athletics. Thus, strengthening programs must progressively integrate individual muscle actions into functional muscle group actions, essentially transitioning from general exercises to sport-specific exercises designed to replicate movements common in given sports.

G. PRESCRIPTIONS FOR STRENGTHENING

Well-designed rehabilitative programs are structured with specific objectives and consider variables such as frequency, intensity, volume, progression, and recovery. According to the principle of specificity, training should include therapeutic exercises designed to target the desired muscle with the level of force production, velocity, and type of muscle contraction required by the sport. Strengthening should occur throughout the entire range of motion and reflect the pattern of movement (open versus closed chain) to match the desired activity.

The amount of resistance used generally reflects the intensity of the exercise and is based on a percentage of a one-repetition maximum (1 RM). This is the maximum amount of weight that can be lifted one time before fatigue prevents the completion of an additional repetition and is a function of the amount of resistance used.

Several specific exercise regimes have been proposed to improve strength. One technique of progressive resistive exercises (PREs) begins by establishing a repetition maximum. This is defined as the maximum amount of weight that can be lifted 10 times with proper technique. In this training program, three sets of 10 repetitions are performed, with the first set against one-half of the 10 RM weight. Resistance is increased during both the second and third sets, with three-quarters 10 RM and full 10 RM used in each set, respectively.

Another technique attempts to accommodate for the effects of fatigue such that the first set is performed against the full 10 RM weight and the third set is performed against one-half of the 10 RM.

Knight proposed a program consisting of daily adjustable progressive resistive exercises (DAPRE) in an attempt to utilize objective measurements to determine the amount and frequency for progressing the resistance. Initially a 6 RM weight was proposed, with the first set of 10 repetitions performed at 50% of this weight and the second set at 75% of this weight. The third set is performed for as many repetitions as possible at the full 6 RM weight. The number of repetitions performed during the third set is used to determine the resistance for the fourth set. If more than six repetitions are performed during the third set, the weight is increased. If less than six repetitions are performed then the weight is decreased. The number of repetitions during the fourth set determines the amount of weight to be used for the next session (Table 11–1).

Knight KL: Knee rehabilitation by the daily adjustable progressive resistive exercise technique. Am J Sports Med 1979;7:336.

Endurance

A. MUSCLE ENDURANCE

The term endurance refers to the ability of a muscle or muscle group to generate or sustain low-intensity repetitive forces until the onset of muscle fatigue or decline of proper technique. The effects of endurance training on muscle are different relative to those evoked when training for strength or power, as they result in a combination of central and peripheral adaptations, enhancing an individual's ability to sustain a given workload over an extended period of time.

Table 11–1. Knight's Daily Adjusted Progressive Resistive Exercise program.[1]

Number of Repetitions in Set 3	Set 4	Next Treatment
0–2	Decrease 5–10# Repeat set	Decrease 5–10#
3–4	Decrease 0–5#	Same weight
5–6	Keep weight the same	Increase 5–10#
7–10	Increase 5–10#	Increase 5–10#
11	Increase 10–15#	Increase 10–20#

[1] The program was developed to more objectively determine *when* to increase resistance and *how much* resistance to increase. The number of repetitions that the athlete is able to perform in set 3 dictates the amount of weight to be utilized in set 4 and the following treatment session.

Endurance training consists of high repetitions of moderate-resistance exercises. The development of muscle endurance is speed specific and, thus, rehabilitation activities must simulate the speed of athletic performance required for the return to competition.

Peripheral adaptations are localized to the muscle or muscle groups involved in the endurance training exercise, usually resulting in improvements in the oxidative capacity of muscle fibers. Physiologic responses to endurance training include adaptations to the respiratory, cardiovascular, and musculoskeletal systems. In terms of the respiratory system, adaptations include enhanced oxygen exchange and improved blood flow in the lungs and decreased submaximal respiratory and pulmonary ventilation rates. Adaptations to the cardiovascular system include increased cardiac output, blood volume, red blood cell numbers, and hemoglobin concentration, as well as enhanced blood flow to the skeletal muscle. Resting heart rate and heart rate at a given load both decrease in response to endurance training. A reduction in submaximal heart rate and improvements in thermoregulation also occur. In addition, the musculoskeletal system undergoes positive changes, reflected in increased mitochondrial size and density, increased oxidative enzyme and myoglobin concentrations, increased muscle bed capillarization, and increased atriovenous oxygen difference.

B. Cardiovascular Endurance

Many cardiovascular adaptations are associated with resistance training including a decrease in heart rate and in systolic and diastolic blood pressure, and a reduction in total cholesterol. A sufficient training stimulus is necessary for cardiovascular changes to occur in response to strength and endurance training. As the strength of a muscle increases, the cardiovascular response of the muscle improves, and results in an increase in endurance and power.

Table 11–2. Clinical example.

A 30-year-old female wants to increase her aerobic capacity and therefore needs to train at 70% of maximum heart rate. Her current resting heart rate is 80 beats per minute. At what intensity should she exercise?

$$HRmax = 220 - age$$

$$THR = (HRmax - RHR) \% \% \text{ of desired training intensity} + RHR$$

$$HRmax = 220 \times 30 = 190$$

$$THR = (190 - 80) \% \, 70\% + 80 = 165$$

The individual should exercise at an intensity great enough to reach and sustain 165 beats per minute.

Heart rate can be used to measure training over a broad range of intensities as well as set upper limits on training intensity to allow for recovery. Maximum heart rate (HRmax) can be estimated by using 220 minus the individual's age. To increase aerobic capacity for example, the training level or target heart rate (THR) can be established at 70% of HRmax. The equation used to determine target heart rate is THR = (HRmax–RHR) × % of desired training intensity + RHR (resting heart rate) (Table 11–2).

EXERCISE CONTRAINDICATIONS & PRECAUTIONS

The primary contraindications to exercise include active inflammation and pain. Use of resistive exercise in the presence of active inflammation can lead to further tissue trauma and aggravate pain and swelling. Resistive exercises should be modified or discontinued if they produce an increase in pain persisting more than several hours following exercise.

Given the potential intensity of resistance training, cardiovascular precautions should be noted and include avoidance of the valsalva maneuver, which may cause a transient, but marked increase in blood pressure, during resistive training. Careful attention must be given to ensuring that patients do not hold their breath during exercise, which may be facilitated by having patients count out loud or exhaling during exercise. In addition, athletes must be observed carefully when performing resistance exercises to detect substitute motions when the prime movers are weak or fatigued. Often, alternate muscles or compensatory motions are responsible for completion of the desired movement, thus further perpetuating muscle weakness or resulting in secondary tissue damage. Appropriate amounts of resistance, stabilization, and instruction regarding proper technique can reduce muscle spasm and prevent subsequent injury.

MUSCLE SORENESS

Resistance exercise can potentially result in the development of muscle soreness immediately after exercise or 24–72 hours following exercise. Immediate onset of muscle soreness develops during or directly following intense activity and generally subsides quickly with rest. It is thought to be related to muscle injury, ischemia, or the build-up of metabolites in the muscle itself, secondary to inadequate blood flow during exercise.

Delayed-onset muscle soreness develops 12–48 hours following vigorous exercise. Numerous theories have been proposed to explain this phenomenon, including lactic acid accumulation, Devries' pain–spasm theory, and microscopic tearing of muscle and/or connective tissue during strenuous activity, inducing an inflammatory response. Local muscular fatigue may also result from pain, discomfort, and inhibitory influences from the central nervous system. Decreased blood glucose or depletion of muscle and/or liver glycogen may be responsible for total body fatigue following prolonged resistance exercises.

According to the pain–spasm theory, a feedback cycle of a pain-induced reflex muscle spasm develops in response to ischemia and the build-up of waste products in the muscle. Prevention of exercise-induced muscle soreness includes a gradual increase in both the intensity and duration of exercise. In addition, adequate recovery time must be incorporated into the training program to avoid fatigue and promote the removal of lactic acid and the replenishment of energy and oxygen stores and is ultimately required to improve prolonged performance. Multiple studies have demonstrated the effectiveness of light exercise in the facilitation of recovery, justifying a gradual warm-up and cool-down following vigorous exercise.

FUNCTIONAL REHABILITATION GOALS

Power, speed, and agility are incorporated in the final phase of rehabilitation, with an emphasis on sport-specific skills. Prior to initiation of these activities, it is essential that the athlete have adequate strength, mobility, and endurance to safely and effectively execute speed and agility drills.

Power

Power is an important measure of muscle performance, requiring a combination of strength, speed, and skill. Power is defined as the rate of work performed per unit of time and is expressed in watts. Improvements in power occur by reducing the amount of time required to produce a given force, by increasing the distance over which the force is applied, or by increasing the amount of work a muscle is able to perform during a specified period of time. Although power is primarily a function of both strength and speed, it is the latter that is most often manipulated during training programs.

Maximum power occurs at intermediate velocities for concentric contractions. When training specifically for the development of power, exercises should be performed with lighter weights and at higher speeds relative to more traditional strength training programs.

Power is necessary to maximally accelerate the body and is an important component in a wide variety of sports skills. Effective use of power requires not only superior neuromuscular control and the ability to rapidly generate force, but also baseline strength at two speeds–slow and fast. Training for power must be performed at both the velocity and force specific to the demands of the desired activity.

Several different ways to improve power in the athlete are utilized in training programs. Plyometric exercises, one of the most effective interventions for developing power, facilitate the stretch-shortening cycle to (1) elicit a more forceful concentric muscle contraction and (2) increase the reactivity of the nervous system. Plyometric training consists of isotonic exercises that combine speed, strength, and functional activities. These exercises are incorporated during the final phase of rehabilitation, and should closely mimic both the movement pattern and the speed of execution of actual sports performance (Figure 11–9).

Speed

Speed, utilized to some degree in every sport or functional activity, must be addressed during the rehabilitation of athletes. The development of speed depends on the ability to rapidly generate force and optimize motor unit recruitment, and is often compromised after an injury. Activities emphasizing neural activation, motor unit synchronization, strength, and the development of a motor program for ballistic movements should be

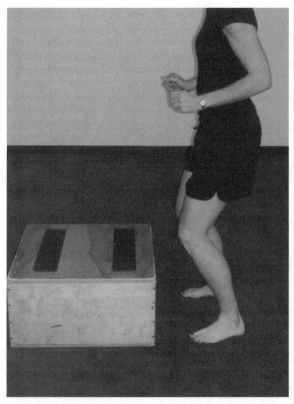 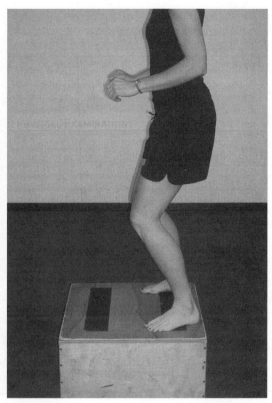

Figure 11–9. Plyometric exercises, such as box jumping, can be an effective way to increase power. These exercises combine speed, strength, and function.

incorporated into the training program to facilitate the return to sport. These interventions should match the speed of the functional movement or sport-specific activity as the speed of training is directly related to the speed at which strength gains occur.

Agility

Agility, which refers to the ability to abruptly change the direction of the body or to quickly shift the direction of movement in a controlled manner without losing balance, is imperative in most sports and is often more important than simply achieving or maintaining a maximum velocity. It is dependent on a combination of factors including strength, speed, dynamic balance, and coordination.

These skills require rapid force development and high power output, as well as the ability to efficiently couple concentric and eccentric actions into dynamic, explosive movements. Agility training emphasizes rapid decelerations, directional changes, and subsequent reaccelerations with the primary objective aimed at making these movements as automatic and efficient as possible.

Agility exercises should preferentially incorporate the movements and demands of the individual's sport. However, the ability to safely decelerate from a given velocity is a prerequisite before combining this skill with rapid changes in direction. Thus, it is essential to establish each athlete's ability to decelerate from varying speeds before changing directions and progressively advance accordingly.

Agility can be developed in many ways, initially incorporating activities such as shuttle runs, side-stepping, crossovers, and change in direction drills. At first, these exercises should be performed at submaximal speeds to allow the athlete to learn the appropriate body mechanics and ensure proper technique. The speed is progressively increased as these techniques are mastered to simulate game situations.

Once athletes have successfully completed a functional rehabilitation program, they must meet a series of clinical guidelines before returning to unrestricted sport. These criteria may vary slightly, depending on the athlete, the sport, and the recommendation of the sports medicine team. However, the premature return to sport places the athlete at risk for reinjury and will likely reduce the athlete's performance (Table 11–3).

Table 11–3. Criteria for full return to sports activities.

- The athlete should have complete resolution of acute signs and symptoms related to the injury.
- The athlete should have full range of motion and adequate strength and proprioception to perform sport-specific skills.
- The athlete should be able to perform sport-specific skills with normal mechanics and no observable upper or lower extremity deviations.
- The athlete should be able to perform sport-specific skills at prior level of function.

Rehabilitation of an injured athlete requires the restoration of function in the shortest time possible, allowing the athlete to safely and quickly return to competition. Although the normal healing process cannot be facilitated, the sports medicine team, when designing a therapeutic exercise program, can optimize the conditions for injury repair by taking into account the pathology of the injury and the normal phases of healing. A successful and efficient rehabilitation program should incorporate basic principles related to anatomy, kinesiology, and biomechanics to address the underlying impairments, while utilizing therapeutic modalities and exercise to ultimately promote functional speed, power, agility, and sport-specific activities.

Index

Note: Page numbers followed by "f" denote figures; those followed by "t" denote tables